August 14, 1997

MULTIPLE AIDS-RELATED LOSS

Kurt:

You are the foundation
which allows me to soar.

Love

MULTIPLE AIDS-RELATED LOSS:
A Handbook for Understanding and Surviving a Perpetual Fall

David Nord

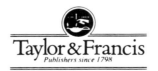

Taylor & Francis
Publishers since 1798

USA	Publishing Office:	Taylor & Francis 1101 Vermont Avenue, NW, Suite 200 Washington, DC 20005-3521 Tel: (202) 289-2174 Fax: (202) 289-3665
	Distribution Center:	Taylor & Francis 1900 Frost Road, Suite 101 Bristol, PA 19007-1598 Tel: (215) 785-5800 Fax: (215) 785-5515
UK		Taylor & Francis Ltd. 1 Gunpowder Square London EC4A 3DE Tel: 171 583 0490 Fax: 171 583 0581

MULTIPLE AIDS-RELATED LOSS: A Handbook for Understanding and Surviving a Perpetual Fall

1 2 3 4 5 6 7 8 9 0   B R B R   9 8 7

This book was set in Times Roman. The editors were Christine Williams and Kathleen Baker. Cover design by Michelle Fleitz.

A CIP catalog record for this book is available from the British Library.

(∞)The paper in this publication meets the requirements of the ANSI Standard Z39.48-1984 (Permanence of Paper)

Library of Congress Cataloging-in-Publication Data

Nord, David.
    Multiple AIDS-related loss: a handbook for understanding and surviving a perpetual fall/David Nord.
        p.   cm.—(Series in death, dying and bereavement, ISSN 1091-5427)
    Includes bibliographical references.

    1. AIDS (Disease)—Social aspects.   2. AIDS (Disease)—Psychological aspects.   3. AIDS (Disease)—Patients—Death.
I. Title.   II. Series.
RC607.A26N66   1997
362.1'969792—dc21   96-53419
                                                                                  CIP

ISBN 1-56032-581-X (case)
ISBN 1-56032-582-8 (paper)
ISSN 1091-5427

Contents

**PART TWO: THEORETICAL PERSPECTIVES
ON MULTIPLE AIDS-RELATED LOSS**

PART THREE: HEALING AND SURVIVING MULTIPLE AIDS-RELATED LOSS

Preface

> But even harder was trying to deal with the anxiety-provoking and otherwise deeply upsetting memories which constantly intruded, making it arduous to think objectively about the camps. Trying to be objective became my intellectual defense against becoming overwhelmed by these perturbing feelings. Consciously, I felt a great urge to write about the concentration camps, and in a manner which would make others think about them, make it possible for them to grasp what went on in them. It was a need which, many years later in the literature on survivors, we called their compulsion to "bear witness."—Bruno Bettelheim (1952/1980b, p. 16)

Persons living with and dying from AIDS have justifiably received most of the attention and compassion arising in response to the pandemic. Yet it is now time to acknowledge the impact on those who have survived AIDS-related loss. This was brought home to me as I sat with a client during a series of psychotherapy sessions. Although I had lost a large number of friends to AIDS, I never realized the impact of multiple loss until Brad started talking about his experience of constant grief, misdirected anger, and lack of interest or pleasure in anything and his emerging tendency to drown his feelings in alcohol. Unexpectedly, I was seeing myself through part of my client's experience. As I listened to him gradually connect the cumulative impact of multiple loss to his symptoms, I was amazed that I had not realized it sooner: Multiple AIDS-related loss had broadly and significantly disrupted my life and the lives of many friends and coworkers. I soon discovered that hardly anyone else had realized it either.

Thomas Mann said, "A man's dying is more the survivor's affair than his own" (Staudacher, 1994, p. 94). This book discusses the survivor's affair, specifically, the experience of surviving multiple AIDS-related loss, an experience that is made more difficult by the lack of attention it has received. Lack of understanding of survivors' experiences results in few resources and little support for survivors. This book offers specific suggestions for coping with multiple AIDS-related loss.

As the years of AIDS-related suffering and death mount with no end in sight, it is increasingly clear that survivors of multiple AIDS-related loss face a disaster similar to some of the world's worst disasters, but a disaster that also has historically unique traits. Namely, surviving multiple AIDS-related loss has cumulative and continuous effects, while stigmatization and the absence of traditionally available support systems handicap recovery.

Survivors will discover through this book that they are not alone. I am continually struck by the consistent response I hear from survivors who have read or heard my message about multiple AIDS-related loss. Nearly always, survivors proclaim, "I did not think that anyone understood!" This book is meant to legitimize the profound pain experienced by many survivors of multiple AIDS-related loss. Normalizing the abnormal experience of survivors is an important coping strategy that is discussed throughout this book. This task parallels the often-stated goal of Holocaust survivors to bear witness to the horrors they endured. This book is intended to be useful as a testament to the survivor's experience, but it also offers hope through suggestions that have proven helpful to many survivors.

Professionals who work with survivors of multiple AIDS-related loss need a resource for understanding and treating victims of this disaster. Among those who may benefit are counselors, psychotherapists, caregivers, volunteers, case managers, social workers, thanatologists (those who study death and grieving), and traumatologists. Academic interest may bring others to this book. The extremes of human experience are frequently instructive about more general truths. Lifton (1979), who has devoted his life to understanding the effect of traumatization, observed that extreme environments "can epitomize and illuminate more ordinary ones" (p. 148). Scientific inquiry has regularly pushed limits to determine something about the common. Unlike nearly all historic disasters, which are studied after they have ended, multiple AIDS-related loss gives us the opportunity to look within the experience of individual and communal disasters as they occur. This book will provide a resource for historians and libraries to inform the citizens of future generations about the tragedy survivors are now enduring.

Thanatologists interested in death anxiety and the variety of grieving responses will find this book valuable. Thanatologists have defined death attitudes almost exclusively in terms of affect while "leaving crucial cognitive and especially behavioral features of these attitudes virtually ignored" (Neimeyer and Van Brent, 1995, p. 129). This book includes emotional, cognitive, and behavioral responses to multiple AIDS-related loss.

Multiple AIDS-related loss informs us about a number of human traits and responses. These include the capacity of humans to cope with ongoing loss that devastates an existing community and preexisting social systems. We learn the value of families of choice and origin by observing the family's importance and function in response to crisis. Continuous bereavement teaches us about grief. The effects of ongoing traumatization are illuminated. The impact of stigmatization is multiplied by its effect on a prestigmatized group.

This book begins where it should, with the real-life stories of survivors of multiple AIDS-related loss. Chapter 1 presents the experiences of two survivors in their own words. Steve is a gay man who tests negative for HIV and has seen his world significantly disrupted by AIDS. Debra is the mother of hemophiliac sons with HIV whose loss includes the deaths of nephews and many hemophiliac friends. It may feel easier and safer to look at the survivor's experience strictly through the limited lens of theory, analysis, and intervention strategies, but these survivors' stories are informative and compelling because they are heartbreaking. They give a flesh-and-bones, heart-and-soul, here-and-now focus to the remainder of this book by exposing the pain and hope of actual survivors.

Chapter 2, "An Awakening Awareness," outlines the historical context of AIDS. A number of factors contribute to the psychological devastation of AIDS. The term *AIDS epoch* is used throughout this book to acknowledge the distinctive social, cultural, political, and personal effects compelled by the realities of AIDS. The AIDS epoch began in 1981 with the earliest recognition that a terrible scourge was emerging and continues to the present day. Chapter 2 outlines a model for a four-stage process through which survivors move in their experience of multiple loss.

Chapter 3, "Understanding Multiple AIDS-Related Loss," explores unique characteristics of this disaster. Losses from AIDS are more than death events. Various levels of loss, both quantitative and qualitative, affect survivors. Among these distinguishing factors are characteristics of AIDS, its focus of impact on discrete communities, its cumulative and ongoing nature, and stigmatization.

Chapter 4 presents the stories of two more survivors. Keith is a gay man who has HIV and lost his life partner and countless friends to AIDS. Terry is a heterosexual woman who has, through her volunteer and professional work as an AIDS caregiver, had many losses.

Chapter 5 explores grieving multiple loss. Traditional theories of grief provide a background to this experience but are inadequate to fully explain its unique consequences. Grieving focuses on two levels of loss: individual and global. Individual loss needs to be grieved systematically. An overshadowing death may exist and stymie other grief work until it is resolved. Global losses include a host of community-wide and individual loss. Fresh losses are best addressed as they arise, although this approach means that other grief work waits. Anniversary reactions are discussed. Unresolved grief and complicated bereavement may be the norm, given a number of factors considered in this chapter.

Chapter 6 outlines the problems faced by survivors as they grieve and adjust to multiple loss. Intrapsychic difficulties include withdrawal and isolation, contrary attitudes, and diffuse anger. Survivor's guilt arises in most survivors and often presents itself subtly though pervasively.

Chapter 7 discusses traumatization as a component of the survivor's experience. Multiple AIDS-related loss is a traumatic experience as formally defined in psychology. Survivors suffer traditional symptoms of traumatization, including emotional numbing and withdrawal as well as intrusive thoughts and recollections. One's assumptive world is severely disrupted. Secondary stress reactions are common in survivors, especially caregivers. Many survivors suffer from learned helplessness.

Chapter 8 looks at the impact of multiple AIDS-related loss on families of origin and families of choice. Traditionally recognized families of origin are sometimes hard hit by AIDS, especially the families of persons with hemophilia. Families of choice fulfill the same functions and roles as families of origin. They often include nonmarried couples and close friends. The interface of these two family systems is often fraught with difficulties, but it also offers potential for healing.

Chapter 9 explores issues of self-identity and existential anxiety. One's sense of self is forever altered by this experience. It has become commonplace for populations most affected by AIDS to describe themselves as *being* HIV positive or negative, in contrast to how people describe having almost any other disease (e.g., one does not say "I *am* cancer"). Developmental stages are often jumbled by surviving multiple, ongoing loss. Survivors may themselves be engaged in tasks and following priorities traditionally associated with elderly persons, including regular attendance at memorial services, reading obituary pages, and living on after friends have died.

Existential anxiety is provoked by direct contact with suffering and death, yet this anxiety offers opportunities to make purposeful choices. A striking similarity among survivors is their insistence on questioning the meaning of life and determining their own personal meaning in light of multiple AIDS-related loss. This chapter is transitional. It begins to shift focus from an exploration of the problems and characteristics of surviving to a focus on healing approaches. The ancient Chinese had a word for *crisis* that is made up of two ideograms, one for danger and one for opportunity (Kliman, 1981). This perspective summarizes the combination of despair and choice survivors face. Recovery from multiple AIDS-related loss necessitates a look at existential and spiritual issues.

Chapter 10 is about the recovery process. The importance of seeking help is stressed, and giving help as a volunteer is encouraged. Suggestions are offered for dealing with problems such as diffuse rage, stigmatization, anxiety, and self-destructive behaviors and attitudes. Problems outlined in the chapters on grief and trauma are addressed here.

Specific suggestions to help survivors of multiple loss are presented in chapter 11. It begins by addressing the outlook and attitudes of those who fare better. A shift of perspective from victim to survivor is central. The task of bearing witness is explored. This chapter also offers a model for support groups for survivors of multiple loss. Several rituals for healing are presented.

Chapter 12 is addressed to the professional caregiver, psychotherapist, social worker, or counselor working with survivors of multiple AIDS-related loss. Survivors are likely to seek professional help. Professionals must be aware of the special issues presented by the survivors. Assessment requires attention to factors unique to this event. This chapter discusses issues such as counter-transference that have direct relevance to the helping professional but also in-cludes information that is useful to survivors.

Chapter 13 offers some conclusions that arise out of the extreme nature of multiple AIDS-related loss. Some of the lessons learned from this experience may apply to other crises. The inadequacy of existing diagnostic categories is made plain by this experience. Predictions are made about the future.

The Epilogue presents my experience with multiple AIDS-related loss. It is a personal perspective on this disaster, exploring my journey of suffering and healing.

The Appendix offers an opportunity for readers, alone or in a group, to experience a guided imagery exercise that takes them through the experience of surviving multiple AIDS-related loss. It is a powerful and enlightening ex-perience.

The impact of multiple AIDS-related loss has focused on certain communi-ties, namely those of homosexuals, hemophiliacs, and intravenous drug users (IVDUs). This reality contrasts with most historic tragedy where survivors are dispersed, able to return to communities that remain intact and capable of pro-viding support. In comparison, many survivors of multiple AIDS-related loss rely on support from the same community whose devastation creates the need for support. When support is most needed it is least available. Certainly, the gay community staggers under this load. The impact of multiple AIDS-related loss on gay and bisexual men is not uniform. Living in an urban gay setting greatly increases one's risk for suffering multiple loss, especially for socially and politi-cally active individuals. In addition, those who test HIV positive have a distinct experience with multiple AIDS-related loss. Gay men who test negative for HIV face uniquely challenging issues as well.

Less attention has been given to those with hemophilia, many of whose families have suffered merciless loss. Many hemophiliac persons formed com-munities to cope with the blood disorder and then suffered compounding loss from their mutual association during the AIDS epoch. Unfortunately, the hemo-philiac experience with AIDS has been largely ignored. Throughout this book, there is a concerted effort to include their experiences.

Caregivers are another group that have been hard hit by multiple AIDS-related loss yet have received little attention. These special persons responded to AIDS by deciding to be involved. They have volunteered their physical and emotional energy to lessen the suffering of those affected by AIDS. This far into the pandemic, hardly anyone is involved by chance. So, when I refer to caregivers or volunteers I mean everyone who chooses to be involved and in-clude health care workers, psychotherapists, hospice volunteers, chore service workers, case managers, emotional support buddies, or "just" friends. These caregivers deserve recognition because they all volunteer themselves for chal-lenging and painful work. In whatever capacity they choose to be involved, caregivers face unique challenges: how to balance overwhelming need with the risk of burnout, how to assess for secondary stress response in one's self and colleagues, and how to maintain strength for the future.

Surviving multiple AIDS-related loss is a challenge for which there is no exact historic precedent. We cannot look to an event that happened before and say, "It is just like. . . ." However, to make sense of this particular experience this book looks to previous disasters that have similarities in terms of either the characteristics of the event or the survivor response. Throughout this book, reference is made to historic disasters to provide a point of comparison. The Holocaust, for example, is used because its survivors have been well studied and analyzed regarding the long-term impact on their lives. In addition, a number of similar survivor responses are observed.

Survivors pioneer a wilderness of grief, trauma, identity, spirituality, and meaning. Survivors confront these issues and are forced to respond. One response is to ignore, deny, withdraw, and hide. Although one must respect the pain and fear that prompt these responses, this book proceeds down a different path when it offers suggestions for optimal coping.

Personal perspective influences the way this book explains multiple AIDS-related loss. The reader deserves to know that my perspective of this tragedy is one of a participant: I am a survivor of multiple AIDS-related loss. I intend a voice of objectivity but acknowledge a passion for this topic that undoubtedly sways my way of looking at it. The reader should benefit from this tension between my desire for objectivity and the reality of personal experience.

Survivors regularly say that no one who has not lived through this experience could understand it. They often report that people outside the immediate world of multiple AIDS-related loss "don't get it." Mainly, I believe this assertion is true. An example may help. In a group I facilitate for survivors of multiple loss, the 1995 bombing of the federal building in Oklahoma City was intensely discussed following the event and at the 1-year anniversary. Group members were enraged that so much attention was devoted to the deaths of fewer than 170 people while their tragedy was ignored. Passion was as strong as it has ever been in the group. Jealous, frustrated anger was vented against the media and the public for paying so much attention to Oklahoma City. These group experiences demonstrate the depth of alienation felt by survivors of multiple AIDS-related loss and the perception that their experience is ignored and belittled. As a rule, no one truly understands another's experience, and this rule is even more valid at the extremes of human experience. Although we cannot always walk in another's shoes, we can learn from the experiences of others. That is one purpose of this book.

Psychology provides the primary framework and vocabulary used in this attempt to understand the many issues raised by multiple AIDS-related loss. Sociological and existential perspectives are also included. This book is meant to be helpful to both professionals and nonprofessionals, although it will not thoroughly explain subjects that are covered elsewhere. Although there are lots of books on AIDS, grief, trauma, psychotherapy, gay relationships, and so forth, there are none on multiple AIDS-related loss.

AIDS has focused its impact on gay men in the Americas and Europe. Even so, study, analysis, and information on AIDS has disproportionately focused on the impact of AIDS on gay men. This is unfortunate because a dearth of information is available about AIDS and IVDUs, hemophiliacs, bisexuals, heterosexuals, and minorities. IVDUs, for example, face uniquely challenging issues that may be very different than those of gay men and that affect their caregivers and friends.

> In addition to their illness, these folks may be dealing with addiction, homelessness, and hunger. For some of them, a diagnosis of AIDS is secondary to where their next fix or their baby's next meal will come from. . . . These clients are frequently African-American and Hispanic people whose needs are quite different from the middle class gay white men who brought AIDS to the attention of the nation. For the caregiver, it may be a whole new world with a whole new set of rules and priorities. (Garfield, 1995, p. 6)

The fact that most available information stems from the gay experience unavoidably influences the material presented in this book. I have diligently sought out and incorporated information about the true variety of survivors of multiple AIDS-related loss, especially those with hemophilia. The nongay reader should be able to identify with the information about gay survivors of multiple AIDS-related loss and, where necessary, to extrapolate from the gay experience useful information. The similarities far outweigh the differences.

The title of this book came from listening to a survivor naming his experience "a perpetual fall." It is an appropriate title for a few reasons. First, the reality of a continual, ceaseless, recurring perpetual loss marks the survivor's experience. As this book demonstrates, this persistent reality affects both the survivor's experience with and efforts to adjust to multiple loss. Survivors of multiple AIDS-related loss face a perpetual fall.

D. W. Wincott observed that traumatization relates to a fear of annihilation. "Falling forever" is among the "primitive agonies" that compose this fear (Davis & Wallbridge, 1990, p. 44). Traumatization is part of survivors' experiences, in part because their identity risks annihilation as their interpersonal foundation crumbles beneath them. Survivors lose the grounded foundation of normal expectations, normal developmental stages, and normal connections that provide stability and security from the risk of a perpetual fall. Not surprisingly, therefore, one hears survivors regularly speak of feeling helpless, despairing, and victimized. They flail about, out of control, in a fall where there is no bottom.

The title also carries a metaphorical meaning pertaining to seasons. Speaking of mourning, Oda (1992) wrote,

> In the dark winter of grief, the promise that time will heal rings hollow. We are unable to contemplate a day when the great cloud of sorrow will be lifted. But

healing will come, or more accurately, we will come to healing, if we accept mourning as a process that must run its course until it is fully spent and we emerge, strengthened and renewed by the experience. (p. 5)

Grieving normally occurs as a response to an event that has happened. We grieve someone or something that *was* lost. The event of loss is past tense, permitting survivors to view their "winter" as something that will run its course. In most grief experiences, the belief that things will get no worse provides solace and hope that grief work will bear the fruit consistent with the image of spring. The survivors of multiple AIDS-related loss may not yet live in the midst of their metaphorical winter. Rather, they may exist in a season of perpetual fall, where the future offers a dark winter of grief.

In the region in which I live, fall is a time of leaves falling and salmon spawning. Both cycles seem to end in death, decay, and rot. Yet rotting leaves provide nutrients to living plants, and salmon lay the eggs of future life. Those survivors who develop positive coping responses to multiple AIDS-related loss consistently report personal, collective, and spiritual growth arising from the ashes of this tragedy. One is struck by survivors' insistence that meaning be found amid the suffering. Despair is transformed by choice.

If AIDS has helped "us open our eyes, to raise our consciousness, to open our hearts and minds, and to finally see the light," as Elizabeth Kubler-Ross (1987, p. 12) asserted, then something good is accomplished. In the world of AIDS, nothing is taken for granted. As a result, this experience has brought many, many persons to a place of deeper spirituality, closer connection with others, and a more fulfilling life.

Although AIDS has exposed some of the worst in human nature, it has certainly exposed the very best. In the early years, when fear dominated, love was sometimes stronger and the dying were held and comforted. When social, medical, and political efforts seemed forever insufficient, persons with vision and persistence demonstrated what was possible. When caregivers grew tired, utterly worn out by a crisis without end, self- and mutual care became a priority.

Although a part of me finds value in this horrific experience, a part of me will never accept that this value was worth the cost of anguish it required. I must hope that one day, AIDS will be no more. Michael Callen (1988), a long-term survivor of AIDS and multiple loss, summed it up best:

We the survivors must bear witness to the horrors we have endured. But even as we grieve, even as we honor the memory of those who have fallen, we must at the same time fix our hearts and minds on a clear image of the day when AIDS is no more. (p. 35)

Let it be.

Acknowledgments

I wish with all my heart that this book was never written, that this book was never needed. It is a terrible thing to feel compelled to acknowledge that massive suffering has made this book possible. Each teardrop of multiple loss survivors ought to be individually acknowledged, but the buckets of anguished tears overwhelm my ability to properly salute the suffering that serves as the imperative for this book.

Personally, I could not have endured the crisis of these recent years without my family. Foremost in my family foundation is my partner, Kurt Kirstein. No one should have to put up with the moodiness that marked the months of this book's writing. No one should be expected to put up with the roller coaster ride of emotional and physical ups and downs that sometimes mark our life. No one should be expected to endure the uncertainty and risks that our love entails. But Kurt has done all these things and more. He is my best friend, my confidant, my lover, my companion in life's travels.

Gerald Greenblatt, perhaps the dearest friend I will ever know, has done more to sustain me than he will ever know. He has been my buttress and ally. Terry Johnson encouraged me through my darkest days and championed the potential within me before I could see it. Kathi Zemke has gently cradled me while encouraging me to my highest hopes. Phyllis Perry, my mother, has never wavered in loving me, and a mother's love is irreplaceable.

The content of the book was improved by the careful proofreading of Billy Brennan, Ned Farley, Kurt Kirstein, Kathi Zemke, and the helpful editors at Taylor & Francis: Elaine Pirrone and Bernadette Capelle. Dr. Robert Neimeyer not only provided a careful eye to the manuscript, he emboldened me with encouragement through the early days of this project. I am completely indebted to those survivors of multiple AIDS-related loss who have touched my life, especially members of the 1995–1996 support group at the Seattle AIDS Support Group.

Finally, but most importantly, I dedicate this book to the too many loved ones, friends, and heroes I have lost to AIDS.

Part One

The Experience of Surviving Multiple AIDS-Related Loss

Surviving multiple AIDS-related loss is a world of heart-shattering experience. Chapter 1 presents the stories of two survivors of multiple loss: a gay man without HIV and a hemophiliac mother. The second chapter explains the historical perspective that frames the survivor's experience. Two more survivor stories are offered in chapter 3: a gay man with HIV and a heterosexual caregiver to persons with AIDS. These survivors all come from different backgrounds, but they all face similar impacts from multiple, ongoing loss. The fourth chapter explains exactly why the phenomenon of multiple AIDS-related loss is historically unique and what specific factors contribute to the survivor's experience.

Chapter 1

Survivors' Experiences: I

We read to know that we are not alone.—C. S. Lewis

A true understanding of the ordeal faced by survivors of multiple AIDS-related loss is inaccessible without hearing the intimate, real-life experiences of these survivors. Theory alone is inadequate to the task. This book focuses heavily on theory and analysis. Thus, it is important early on to present the real-life experiences of survivors of multiple AIDS-related loss.

Two survivors tell their stories in this chapter. After the following two chapters, which orient the reader to the characteristics of multiple AIDS-related loss, two more stories are offered in chapter 4. These stories may help the reader empathize with and better appreciate the survivor's experience. Steve is a gay man who has recently tested HIV negative and has survived multiple loss. Debra is a hemophiliac whose family of origin is suffering multiple AIDS-related loss. All except Debra asked that their real names be used.

A guided imagery exercise is offered at the back of this book as an appendix. It explores the experience of surviving multiple AIDS-related loss and is meant to provide a personal glimpse into the experience and world of survivors.

STEVE PARSONS: A GAY MAN WITHOUT HIV

Steve: *In 1981, we were sitting around talking over Thanksgiving dinner. There were a few of us there including a doctor and his partner at the time, my lover at the time, and a friend. There was about six or seven of us. We were sitting at a table, and I remember the doctor mentioned GRID* [gay-related immune disorder]. *It was this disease that was horrible. It was like everyone was just terrified; everyone was like "Oh, my god!" What is it? What's causing it? Everyone just thought it was poppers. After the dinner everyone was shaken by it.*

They called it GRID, the gay plague. Then everyone started talking about ramifications, what it all means. They don't know how it's being transmitted. It was a terrifying day. You started hearing about it, a little bit, in small articles in the papers, the gay news, whatever.

David: *What was your first personal contact with AIDS?*

S: *In 1983, Tom Davies came into the flower shop. He was the first person I knew. He died in 1984. Then it was just like someone had pulled their finger out of the dike. And it all collapsed.*

That's how it all started happening: rapidly. Out of that table, three people are dead, one or two more are positive. I guess that out of those six people only a couple of us are. . . .

D: *You have lost a lot of people.*

S: *Yeah, Tracy—he was one of my lovers who died, and then there was Tony. He was another partner who died. They were both former partners. Actually, they died within 2 weeks of each other. And then* [Steve takes a long, deep breath] *I've had boyfriends, several boyfriends who have died. And then I try to think of how many people I've been with sexually that have died. I don't know. . . .*

Because of my flower business, I got to know a lot of people who would come to the shop, and I'd see them. I didn't know them, but I recognized them by face. They were familiar, a lot of people in the community.

D: *Have you ever tried to quantify how many?*

S: *Hundreds.*

D: *A person who was straight or somehow oblivious to this problem might hear you say that and say, "Oh, he's exaggerating."*

S: *Which happens, at work. I go to work, and 8 years ago I was gun shy about it, but then, it was like, these people don't have a clue about what is going on. So I decided to make it a quest to let these people know of my personal losses. I'd go in and say, "Hey, I lost two people last week," and they would be just horrified. And I would continue doing this and pretty soon you would look at their face or eyes and they were like "oh," like in disbelief or they thought I just wanted attention. Whatever, they just didn't want to hear it. So, pretty soon, I just stopped, like in the last year or so I just stopped telling people. Their reaction was not sympathetic or empathetic. It was more like denial or "I just can't deal with you." It was them shutting down.*

It was an empty feeling, like being out there in the battlefield by yourself, struggling, looking around and yelling "help." There were times I felt helpless.

And then at the same time the government was doing nothing. Sometimes I was so angry.

D: *Do you see that anger changing over the years?*

S: *Well, this year was really hard for me.* [Steve lists off people who have just "died in 2 months," including his psychotherapist, two long-term friends, and a respected Washington state senator, Cal Anderson.]

I don't know. I've just resigned myself. It's like the numbing is there. It's like, after 14, almost 15 years now, I can't get on the roller coaster ride anymore. I am burnt out about getting emotionally involved anymore. So I guess there is some kind of resolution. You can't get too attached.

D: *You used the word* resignation; *is that the way you would describe your attitude now?*

S: *Only because I am trying to preserve myself.*

D: *When you said that I heard a little bit of guilt.*

S: *Yeah, because I don't want to turn my back on my friends, but how much. . . . How many. . . . In what other period of history have survivors had to endure 15 years on an emotional roller coaster ride? How long can you handle that? So, you kind of pull back emotionally. You have to continue your life, right? You just can't stop.*

I use the analogy of a conveyor belt of all your friends coming and they're dying and they're going by and it's like you can't reach the switch to turn the conveyor belt off so you're just there watching this, grieving, and trying to stop it but you can't, you don't have enough time to grieve the last one who died before the next one is coming.

[Wondering about the tone of guilt in his words, David asks if there is any survivor's guilt, especially with him testing HIV negative.]

S: *Yeah, I think there is a division in the community. I don't feel like I have a right, even in my loss and grief group, to talk about my losses when there are people in the group who are HIV positive.*

D: *What losses, other than deaths, have you experienced?*

S: *In the early 80's, when I was coming out, there was like a party atmosphere. I feel like the celebration is over. Gay liberation has hit a wall, a big wall. We can't have the same political aspirations we had. Sexual freedom, being able to express yourself sexually is dead.*

There's been some loss of spirituality. The anger about why has God done this to us? So it's been a shift, a reevaluation of what my spiritual values are. [Observes that spirituality has become a lot more important.] *I've looked at my values, what's really important. It isn't possessions, new cars, looking good. My life priorities are changed. I went back to school. I try to find a purpose in life and live by my values.*

D: *What other changes have you noticed?*

S: *My real estate business has changed, not that it's a big priority, but clients I would have sold to, and my network, are dead. In other ways*

*my business has increased. I don't know how many houses I have sold
"for the estate of."*

*My core group is almost all gone. How can you replace friends?
You want to get old with people. When I was younger we used to talk
about having the first gay nursing home. That's kind of funny, but I'll
never be there with my friends from when I was 20 years old.*

*New friends are different, losing history; I don't have a history. I
can't say to someone, "You remember in 1980. . . ."*

*And the community spirit, like when Cal Anderson died. He was
an icon. Now, who do we have? He had a history in politics. We don't
have that history, the leaders, the leadership anymore.*

*The arts, all the designers. It's kind of funny; who will design for
us?*

D: *What are your memories of hospital visits and memorial services?*
S: [Smiles, telling a funny story that happened in the hospital room of
a friend, Larry, who knew that his time was short. (He died 2 days
later.) Larry had a bottle of Marinol (a synthetic form of marijuana
used to stimulate appetite) that he knew he would never finish.] *Larry
and his friends had a party* [laughing], *I guess they were really gone,
singing and dancing in the hospital room. He knew he was dying and
he was stoned and they were stoned.*

[wistfully] *You know, a man of 38 or 40 should not be having to
spend so much time in hospitals. He shouldn't have to spend half
his time volunteering to care for terminally ill friends. He shouldn't be
so familiar with hospice care. Does he need to know how to be an
executor of a will? He shouldn't have attended 40 or 50 memorial
services.*

D: *So, how do you cope?*
S: *Personal, individual psychotherapy. I don't know what I'd do without it. But, last summer my therapist died from AIDS.*

*Support groups help too. Last summer, when there were all those
losses in a couple months, the [multiple loss] group was really helpful.
Knowing that I am not alone is really helpful. I get that from our
support group.*

D: *What rituals or ways of commemorating your losses do you use?*
S: *The AIDS walk this year was really emotional. I found myself with
tears. The Memorial Vigil is important, especially the scrapbook. Attending the Friday Feast is important.* [Steve notes that the feast, a
weekly dinner at the Seattle AIDS Support Group house, reminds him
of a Jewish Sabbath tradition, and therefore, is especially meaningful to
him. His many volunteer efforts are a direct response to his experience
with multiple AIDS-related loss.]
S: *If I didn't do that, I wouldn't feel good about myself. I look at it as
a battle. How could I not help in the battle when all my friends are
dying?*

Steve does not avoid memorial services, though he understands why some
persons do. These are important events that help him work through his grief.

> **D:** *Do you ever think that you will feel resolved or be able to reach a state of acceptance about these losses?*
>
> **S:** *No, how could you be? I don't know how anyone could be. It's like a scar, a big burn. The wound may heal, but a scar always remains, and every time a burn, even though it is healed, gets close to heat, it hurts again. It's the same with this. Every time I have another loss, I feel all the others.*
>
> **D:** *What does the future hold?*
>
> **S:** *As long as the disease continues, I will be in the front. That's my choice.*
>
> **D:** *Is there anything else you would like to add?*
>
> **S:** [Offers a topic hardly ever mentioned, wondering how much energy it will take to adapt to a time when AIDS is no more.] *It will be like having your sunglasses ripped off your eyes.*

Steve believes that if such a day ever comes, it will require a tremendous amount of readjustment for the gay community because "we have had to do so much adjusting to living with AIDS. . . . There is a sense of connectedness that exists now. It has glued us together to make us more connected instead of divided." Steve notices this especially in the bonding between lesbians and gay men. He gives lesbians a lot of praise for their work and believes that "they have not been acknowledged for all their efforts."

DEBRA GALLAGHER: A MOTHER WITH HEMOPHILIAC CHILDREN

> **David:** *How has AIDS changed your life?*
>
> **Debra:** *My life is AIDS. It has totally changed, on every conceivable level. Every decision I make somehow reflects that experience.*
>
> *My kids want a new pair of jeans but they cost $65.00 and I don't have any money left, so I charge it because I have this weird thing in the back of my head that says, "You know, if you spend the rest of your life paying off credit cards because you were giving your children quality, and they only have a certain amount of time, it's worth it." I want them to have things! It's like every day is a "Make a Wish" kind of day, but this is not the way I would have been if AIDS wasn't in their future.*
>
> *When Matthew dropped out of school, some would say it was just a teenage phase. But I have to look at his perspective, seeing his cousins die and knowing that his brother has HIV and he has HIV. You know? How do you deal with that? How do you live with that?*
>
> *Everything is affected. My life is totally AIDS infiltrated. It's like living in a totally different world from everyone else.*
>
> *This year was a real tough phase for me. I feel like I'm moving into this new phase, this transition: healthy asymptomatic to things aren't right. We have to worry. All these things that are just not normal. We don't know what they are and we have to investigate them. There are no clear-cut answers about what to do, and that's totally*

frustrating. It's ambiguous, everything's all ambiguous. The treatment's ambiguous. This might work, maybe it won't. And there's always these risks. It's not like it's simple things that you can fix. So, I just feel like there's this shift.

I met this person who's wonderful and he happens to have HIV and hemophilia. I am planning on spending the rest of my life, uh, his life, with him. We are talking about getting married.

Evan and I have been able to get along really well. We haven't encountered AIDS-related issues that we haven't been able to get through. I knew going in and so did he, so we've been able to talk about things. We find a way to talk about these things. But, yesterday, he had a cut in his mouth. So he said that we couldn't kiss that day. It was the first time that I really thought AIDS was really everywhere. It's in my kids, it's in my lover, it's always interfering.

Sometimes just in casual conversation it comes up. He's not only dealing with it himself, but he has this whole circle of friends. This summer we met a fellow at a hemophilia conference who was really sick when we met him. He was a kid, like 19 years old, not much older than Nick [her son]. He was so close to Nick's age, but he was really, really sick. During the conference, he had to go to the emergency room for something that was going on. Suddenly I could see Nick in him. Well, he hasn't called, and we've sort of lost contact. We don't know whether or not he is alive. That happens. Is the family going to know who to call? That just came up in casual conversation, you know, how's this guy doing?

Right now, Evan has the attitude "I am not going to get sick!" When I've talked about my concern for the kids he says, "Well, they are going to be OK. We are all going to be OK." So, these issues come up in our house; you know, dead nephews! That is the reality. Not that I am being a pessimist, but death is a real issue and you can have all the optimism in the world but. . . .

I don't want to take away his hope or his coping mechanism, but I still need to be validated for my feelings that I am having at the moment, which are real. I don't want to get stuck there and start making funeral plans and fall into despair. Yet, there is a certain amount of reality you have to face, and pain that you have to feel in order to get to a place and make a decision and do something. You have to acknowledge that there is a problem there.

In a relationship, how can you talk about feeling afraid that my children are going to die without interfering with his healthy denial that is his way of coping?

I also worry about him. He's strong and healthy and promises to take care of the kids, but then the reality is. . . .

Then, I have flashes about what am I going to do if he gets sick. What will I do when *he gets sick. I don't think about it every day, but I find myself overwhelmed by loss of control. It's frightening; I can't even imagine what life will be like 6 months or a year from now.*
David: *Two of your nephews died?*

Debra: *Brian died a year and a half ago, and he was 13. Three years ago Bert died, and he was 12.*

They were both sick for 7 or 8 years. They got sick right from the beginning. It got so you could count the days when Bert didn't have to be on antibiotics. There was always an infection going on, almost from the beginning.

They were all given a worst case prognosis: 2½ years, that's all they have—2½ years. Regardless of what their T cells were or whether or not they have opportunistic infections. So, basically, you are dealing with the loss of a normal life. And a loss of a future. Not only for my nephews but for my sons. A loss of any sort of future planning or normal decision making.

The fact that they have a terminal illness. The living with the not knowing how long you have. We were told it wouldn't be longer than 2½ years.

David: *How many persons have you lost to AIDS?*

Debra: *Before Bert died, 7 adult men in our community who were active members of the board, regulars at adult camp. . . . Wait a minute, it's more than that. It's probably more like 14 now. People like the camp director. Some of them were people that I knew just as acquaintances, and others were* [draws a deep breath], *were guys who really taught me a lot about hemophilia, the people that, 18 years ago, helped me learn to deal with hemophilia. They were an important loss because they were the first example I saw of an adult with hemophilia. It was such a relief to realize that my children could actually become adults. So, then when they died it was also the loss of that dream.*

It doesn't follow the normal patterns of grief when you have one on top of another. Maybe, in your lifetime, or occasionally you hear about a family member or child who has lost one family member, and they spent their whole life having to deal with that on some level. It colored their whole experience because they experienced that. But what happens when you have lost two people that you were really close to? What happens to their psyche, what goes on in their head? How can you help them when they are also afflicted with the same illness that they saw their cousins die from? And how do they live day to day looking at their brother wondering who will die first, who will get sick first? When you throw all of those things in there, it's hard to even name them all, much less sort them out and tell them, "Here is how you can deal with it and live a good life."

David: *Was there ever a specific moment in time when you realized what was happening, when you realized, "Oh my God, look what's happening?"*

Debra: *Yeah! It was in 1987. My sister found out on her own, by calling an AIDS hot line, not through the hemophilia treatment centers, not from the infectious disease doctor they were seeing. They were saying that Brian's pneumonia has nothing to do with AIDS, his skin things have nothing to do with AIDS. They told her to flea bomb her house and she did it three times, but it was an AIDS dermatitis thing* *going on. She found out by calling an AIDS hot line that he had what was then classified as ARC. So, even when she went to all these specialists, she had to find out herself.*

That was happening at the same time I was doing a research paper for school on AIDS. I came across a Scientific American *article that said, "Everyone who is infected will eventually develop AIDS and die." I was blown away, sobbing and crying. I guess I still wanted to believe that some people won't get sick and die and that would be nice. For me, that was when. . . .*

It sent me into hell and despair that lasted for weeks. I felt like I spent a couple weeks in hell. Everything was dark and gloomy. It was like a big, dark cloud looming over me everywhere, and nothing made sense. Nothing looked right anymore. Everything was just gray.

It was like if you knew a plane was going to crash and everyone was going to die and you can't do anything about it and every person on that plane you know. That's what it felt like. I suddenly became aware because I knew all these people who were positive. I not only knew that my kids would die, but I also had this awareness of all those people who would die.

David: *How do you cope with your losses?*

Debra: *SASG* [Seattle AIDS Support Group] *is my main coping place now.*

Since so many people have died, and my kids are the only ones left, there isn't any other support group [in the hemophiliac community]. *For me, the group at SASG is a major coping mechanism, but it also has its down side because I get to know people who are sick and that hurts because it's another loss. You worry, and there is anger, because you just don't want one more person to get sick or die from it.*

A more painful aspect of being a part of the hemophilia community is that we were *a support group for each other. When we began, we had support group meetings about how to deal with our infants and our toddlers, when they start walking, what to do with injuries. There were eight people, and my sons are the only ones, of the children, still alive.*

Then, after the kids have died, you lose contact with all the rest of the family because they don't want to relive it. They don't want to look at your children. They don't want the pain. So, it's easy for them to drop out of the group. The spouses of the guys who died are no longer involved in the community. So, it's not only the death of that individual; you lose the whole family. I can't think of anybody, that once the person who is infected has died, stays active in the community.

Especially, with the guys, who as they got sick you saw less of them. A lot of the men, because I wasn't really close to them, there was a couple of years of no contact. So, the relationship sort of ended then, but it didn't really end until they died. Then, I found myself going back to the beginning of when I first met them and going through their whole life and how they affected me and grieving for that person.

David: *Do you think you will ever reach a point of resolution?*

Debra: *It is never totally done. I think of everybody, and it comes up again and again. Particularly when someone dies; I can never just grieve for one person. It always triggers something about someone else's death.*

Also, there is a counselor that I see, usually once a week. Sometimes I just go in there and cry. The grief builds up behind a dam because I try to function and carry on my life as normal as possible, but sometimes the dam breaks. Sometimes there is a reason for it and sometimes there is not. It's just grief consuming my consciousness and I have to quit and cry. At one point I used to run from it, but now I know that there is no escape from the grief. I've learned that just because I feel the despair, it doesn't mean that I have to stay there. So, I am not afraid of being in despair. Being stuck there used to be a fear.

David: *Besides counseling, what do you do to cope with multiple loss?*

Debra: *One of my coping mechanisms today is, "If I can find something to do, I do it." You take some kind of step, however small, whether it's a phone call, making an appointment, reading an article; I just have to do something. Being stuck in despair and being immobile is the worst thing. As long as there is something to do, some tiny step, like "try this new vitamin," I think we all feel better. When I told the kids, when we first talked about their status, I said, "We are going to do whatever we can to stay as healthy as we possibly can." That's the attitude that they have had.*

Whether or not it's a placebo effect, I think they benefit. When their cousins were sick and in the hospital time and time again, they needed to know they were doing something different than their cousins. So, I made sure there was always a treatment program for them. If, in their minds, they feel like they are doing something, it helps.

When I'm wanting to go there and deal with it, the sooner I do, the better. So, sometimes, especially if someone dies, I will play their favorite music or look at some photographs and bring on the grief, remember those good times.

Debra keeps a scrapbook of persons she has known who died of AIDS. Mainly the photos are of children. She has written tributes to their short but important lives. Included in it are her nephews.

David: *How are you doing, yourself?*

Debra: *I have a lot of physical problems with my back and neck that I know are stress related. Because your brain sort of functions and you keep going, but it has to come out somewhere. So I meditate and try to do relaxation, but nothing is ever enough because this is overload. There is never really enough recovery time.*

David: *Maybe you could say something about hemophilia and why it has been so directly connected to HIV infection.*

Debra: *With severe hemophilia, you can have spontaneous bleeding, with no known cause or trauma. My boys have severe hemophilia, so* *it's not possible to just tell my kids not to do this and you won't bleed because they will bleed anyhow.*

The blood factor that is used now is pooled from 20,000 units of plasma. They take out the clotting factor that is used for people with hemophilia. So, a person with hemophilia could be exposed to between 20,000 and 500,000 a year because of the way the product is made.

They [the blood companies] *didn't heat treat or screen the product correctly. They didn't take a lot of measures that could have minimized the risk from HIV, and hepatitis, and about 20 other things.*

There is a lot of anger because we keep finding out new information about how things were handled when the AIDS epidemic first began. It seems that decisions were made based on money. Even though they had ways to screen the blood product, and they also had ways of destroying the virus with heat-treating processes. In the early '80s, they choose not to do it because it wasn't cost effective.

So, we don't trust them. I don't think a trusting relationship will ever be restored because there is a dominating sense of betrayal. It keeps the anger going.

David: *Does stigmatization affect you?*

Debra: *For the most part, people with hemophilia choose to remain secretive about their disorder. They never have been real comfortable about admitting they had hemophilia, even before AIDS happened. From the beginning it was a closet disorder, following the Romanovs' tradition. When AIDS came into the picture, it just compounded that phobia and the tendency to be secretive. We, as people in the community who have tried to be involved in the larger community and other AIDS organizations, have constantly had to deal with people who didn't want to be labeled as gay or IV drug users. The people who felt the strongest about it were the parents who had small children, that it would have a negative effect on their children, that they would be discriminated against. So, they resisted the chapter's efforts to do anything, even walking in the AIDS Walk carrying a hemophilia banner. People didn't want that to be on the news because they thought someone would discriminate against their kids.*

[Debra is not the real name of the person interviewed here. She has conflicting thoughts about her current need to maintain her family's confidentiality.]

Debra: *My kids are not public, so I can't use any of the real names until. . . .*

I have to respect their decision on this. You need to change all the names. Don't identify me by my position, either. You can say I am a hemophiliac patient advocate, that's all.

David: *If it were not for your sons, would your decisions about confidentiality be different?*

Debra: *Oh, yeah! I definitely think so. I am constantly challenged by the decision. There are things happening in health care reform where I am functioning as* [her official occupational title], *and I know I could be so much more effective if I could give my story. There has been that* *challenge over the years. People say, "It would make such an impact if you could talk about it." I was even referred to the medical advisor of the president, during Bush's term, and I just had to say no, [not] unless I could protect my children. Someday I hope to tell Bert and Brian's story, to give voice to Bert and Brian. To tell their stories, to somehow make a difference, to give meaning to their lives. Not that their lives didn't have meaning, but so they didn't go through the suffering without any. . . .*

If some good could come from it, if someone else can benefit from the experience, I would like to be out there.

I know of a woman who has chosen not to tell anyone that her child has hemophilia. She has made the decision for him that no one will know that he has hemophilia.

David: *Has your family been available to support you?*

Debra: *Well, we think very differently about spirituality and life and death. During the time that my nephews were sick and dying, I really didn't get much support from them. Because they were in need of support themselves. It was like our family was drowning, and you could only save yourself. If you tried to save someone else, you would just pull each other down. That was true, especially for my sisters. Each one in my family was so overwhelmed with pain that we have not been the best person to be strong for each other because we had to take care of ourselves.*

That's why marriages break up so much when the child dies. Parents go through this pain. When they need each other the most, they don't have anything more to give. They are both hurting in a huge way. One of my sisters' marriages broke up, and the other one's is struggling. I won't be surprised if it breaks up. It's so sad because that's one more loss. The families in the community are totally decimated.

Some of the guys who died had spouses who became infected and also died. So, I have heard stories of people losing their mother, father, and a couple kids, then having a couple sets of those in the same family. There was one huge family with 12 kids; 6 of them had hemophilia and got HIV. Then, they passed it on to their wives and kids. It totally wiped out this family.

I know a woman who adopted three children with bleeding disorders because she thought this was an easy disease to manage, and she could take care of it. Well, all of those boys got HIV. I think two of them have already died.

Sometimes, the mother and one of the kids die. Then, a father is left trying to raise an infant. All these heart-wrenching stories. It is indescribable. It is hard to explain. Just a whole web of impact.

New parents of hemophiliacs, those with kids from 1 to 5 years old, still worry about getting HIV. They don't trust that the blood products are safe. Although they are not out there advocating for people with AIDS, they are advocating for a safer blood supply. They know that it is very real that history could repeat itself, maybe with some new virus that is not detected yet. I know parents that won't treat the way they are supposed to. They are very, very conservative because they are terrified that this is going to be the dose that infects their kids with AIDS. That is exactly what parents were doing in the early '80s. Then, the National Hemophilia Association and the blood companies were encouraging more use of blood products. Their slogan was "Treat Early, Treat Often." It's really hard to separate the monetary aspect of it because they make so much money off of Factor. So, how can the consumer ever be comfortable with someone who is making so much money off it?

David: *How has the hemophiliac community supported each other?*

Debra: *We tried to set up a support group for men in the community. HIV wasn't even going to be a focus. One individual assumed, I don't know how, but he assumed that we would be out there advocating for gay rights. He was nervous about being in the support group. I don't know. Where is the connection? It's almost laughable. He was very afraid of being put in a position that he didn't think was correct from his religious position.*

Then, there was another group that, after hearing my speech on hemophilia, the disease, had to have major clarification to make sure that their position against homosexuality would never be challenged.

In the beginning, people needed someone to blame. If you had a religious conviction that said homosexuality was wrong, then they were a perfect target. I think every single parent I know of was in that place. Maybe some still are, but they don't talk about it. A couple of the guys that were infected said they had to go through a time of being angry.

Mainly what changed a lot of people's feelings about gay people was being forced to go to the gay community for information and treatments. That was the saving grace. Two things happened. One, it was the only place you could get help, and also a lot of people had an opportunity to meet someone who was gay and see that he was a person too. That was how they would come to terms with it.

One of the issues that we have to deal with is how unprepared our community, and society as a whole, has been about all these issues, not only the medical aspects. There are not books out there about multiple loss that effectively address the needs of children who experience it. There may be something about cancer, but with HIV it's so complicated by the fact that you don't talk about it. You keep it a secret. You don't have the freedom, my children don't have the freedom, to talk about it and deal with all the emotional impact of the loss. Because of the stigma, because of the fears, it keeps them silent. There isn't much information out there about how to deal with it.

I have heard other people say that "You are a pioneer" because you are having to live through this experience without any markers or maps or another's experience to use as a guide. You sort of pick up fragments here and there, but [for] the most part you are all alone. There is no one else I know, personally, who has two teenage sons who have HIV who also lost two nephews, in a short span of time, and is also engaged to someone who has hemophilia and HIV.

David: *Is there anything more you want to add?*

Debra: *My life has taken on a much more intense appreciation for living in the moment and one day at a time: the concept of impermanence that you can't escape from. I find comfort in the Eastern tradition. I mean, I don't have anything to hold on to. I can't hold onto my children. I won't have grandchildren. I have no future. I didn't plan my life for my children to die before I did. Nothing prepared me for all this uncertainty. That is the theme of this life. That is the biggest way that AIDS has changed my life. There is so much that I cannot control. There is so much that I have to let go of and so much reality that is grief, despair, and pain. You have to witness so much suffering that the only way I can survive is to find the joy in each moment that I can. And that's a challenge in itself because life sucks a lot. I still have to work. I still have to do things that are really unimportant in the big picture. I have to balance and juggle a lot.*

CONCLUSION

Steve and Debra's experiences with multiple AIDS-related loss are informative. As a gay man, Steve experienced the fear of AIDS from its earliest days and has lost many of his dearest friends—members of his family of choice. Even though Debra's background is different than Steve's, she shares the perception that AIDS has changed everything in her life. She has also lost, and risks losing, many members of her family. Both Steve and Debra have been helped by seeking support from other survivors of multiple loss and both have re-evaluated their spiritual priorities as a result of this crisis.

Chapter 2

An Awakening Awareness

I most certainly never thought then about the survivors, but always about those who fell in the war. . . . I was as if delirious or crazy, surrounded by three or four people with mutilated bodies.—Hermann Hesse (1956), *The Journey to the East*

Much has changed from the time when AIDS first emerged. Gradually and recently, people became aware of multiple AIDS-related loss as an experience distinct from the individual losses that result from AIDS. The history of attitudes and values assigned to this pandemic are important to understanding multiple AIDS-related loss.

This chapter is not meant to be a linear or thorough history of AIDS. The history keeps changing because survivors live in an ongoing event. It is the future's charge to recapitulate, with perspective, this experience. The intent here is to contextualize the emergence of this phenomenon through the facts, attitudes, and experiences that affect survivors of multiple AIDS-related loss. This is offered, in part, through a four-stage model through which both individuals and communities move. Future challenges are considered in light of today's trends.

THE CONTEXT OF AIDS

AIDS emerged at a time in world history that uniquely imprinted the survivor's experience. A variety of social and political factors influence the survivor's experience with multiple AIDS-related loss, making it an entirely different experience than it would have been only 20 years before. Technological advances, social changes, political priorities, and cultural attitudes all combine to uniquely mold the survivor's experience.

A Century of Tragedy

The tragedy of AIDS caps off a century already overflowing in tragedy. Technological advances have simultaneously made humans more adroit at inflicting horrors on each other while permitting more and speedier awareness of human and natural disasters. Overshadowing the century was the risk of terrible war, beginning with the use of gas in World War I and taken to historically new heights of terror by the nuclear threat in World War II. Two hot world wars and one cold war kept citizens of the Earth continually aware of apocalyptic threat. "That even an apocalypse can be made to seem part of the ordinary horizon of expectation constitutes an unparalleled violence that is being done to our sense of reality, to our humanity" (Sontag, 1989, p. 93).

Shock arises from surprise and suddenness. In the 20th century, massive, methodical murder is mundane. Repeated, systematic slaughter of one human group by another barely shocks global consciousness and inspires little action. The century has contained an accelerating history of horrors: the Chinese atrocities against the Japanese early in the century, the Nazis' final solution, atomic warfare against Japan, the political terror of Stalin, the killing fields of Cambodia, the brutal slaughter of the Tutsis in Rwanda, and the ethnic cleansing of Bosnia.

Catastrophic reports and predictions regularly fail to stun a gorged public or incite action. The "end of the world" has come and gone too many times. A stoic attitude was expressed by Stephen Jay Gould (in Sontag, 1989) when he compared a nuclear war to AIDS. Even if it killed a quarter of the human race, he said, "there will be plenty of us left and we can start again" (p. 86). Sontag concluded that "perhaps it is only a little less monstrous to be invited to contemplate on this horrendous scale with equanimity" (Sontag, 1989, p.86).

Awareness of these, and other disasters, was expanded by communications system advances; however, awareness of the magnitude and constancy of suffering had a cost. There was too much to bear. How could anyone genuinely respond to the continual barrage of suffering? Solace was found in the comforting knowledge that these tragedies were mainly happening to someone else and far away. These tragedies were distant, unrelated to one's self, someone else's problem.

A Brief History of AIDS

The debate over where AIDS originated is largely irrelevant to the survivor of multiple AIDS-related loss. Not irrelevant to the survivor's experience is the controversy that still surrounds so much speculation about AIDS and its origin. A variety of theories have been promulgated about its origin, the most credible being a route from central Africa, the most far fetched being a plot by right-wing factions of the CIA intent on killing minorities. There are still some who downplay or deny the role of HIV as the cause of AIDS, notably Peter Duesberg (Burkett, 1995). Controversy that still exists about its genesis is minor compared with controversy about its social, cultural, and political implications.

This continuing controversy must be recognized in the context of multiple AIDS-related loss because AIDS, unlike most other diseases or disasters, is constantly associated with controversy, judgment, and politics. As Larry Kramer (1994) said, "There is nothing in the whole AIDS mess that is not political" (p. 110). This reality has significant implications for persons with AIDS, care-givers, and survivors. What follows is not a comprehensive history of AIDS and is not a balanced presentation of the political history of AIDS. Rather, it is meant to provide a perspective of events, attitudes, and milestones that shape the survivor's experience.

1981   On July 4, 1981, *Morbidity and Mortality Weekly Report* publishes a report titled "Kaposi's Sarcoma and Pneumocystis Pneumonia Among Homo-sexual Men—New York City and California."

1982   Most scientists at the Centers for Disease Control (CDC) are con-vinced that GRID is an intectious disease. *GRID* replaces *gay cancer* in the evolving lexicon of AIDS. A virus, HTLV-III, has been identified and linked to the syndrome.

Although media attention is sparse, Dan Rather of CBS News reports,

> Federal health officials consider it an epidemic. Yet you rarely hear a thing about it. At first, it seemed to strike only one segment of the population. Now . . . this is no longer the case. (as cited in Shilts, 1987, p. 172)

1983   The New York State Funeral Directors Association recommends that its members refuse to embalm anyone who appeared to have succumbed to AIDS.

Jerry Falwell speaks about AIDS: "You cannot shake your fist in God's face and get by with it. . . . I don't hate homosexuals," he says, just their "perverted life-styles" (as cited in Shilts, 1987, p. 347).

Bathhouse owners in San Francisco attack appeals to close bathhouses by saying that "only 1,279 of us" have AIDS (as cited in Shilts, 1987, p. 307).

President Ronald Reagan's Secretary of Health Margaret Heckler confi-dently proclaims, "I want to assure the American people that the blood supply is 100 percent safe" (as cited in Shilts, 1987, p. 345).

1984   Nearly 2,300 Americans are reported to have died of AIDS, with total cases topping 5,000, although the numbers of AIDS cases are consistently underreported. Especially in the early years, euphemistic causes of death (e.g., natural causes, liver cancer, long illness) are reported on death certificates and in obituaries.

Rock Hudson flies to Paris for treatment with the experimental drug HPA 23 (Hudson & Davidson, 1986).

The Reagan administration requests no increase in federal AIDS funding.

Blood industry spokesman Dr. Joseph Bove says that "more people are killed by bee stings" (Shilts, 1987, pp. 433–434) than by transfusions causing AIDS. Blood bankers argue that testing would add $12 to the cost of each unit of blood.

1985 A threefold increase in European AIDS cases is reported by the World Health Organization during the previous year (Shilts, 1987, p. 500).

The presidents of France and the United States agree to name Robert Gallo and Luc Montagnier "codiscoverers" of HIV and to share the royalties from HIV blood test royalties (Shilts, 1987).

Rock Hudson dies.

1986 Ninety-one percent of persons diagnosed with AIDS in the United States have died (CDC, 1987).

1987 President Ronald Reagan makes his first speech on AIDS. He focuses on the need to test heterosexual persons applying for marriage licenses, barely mentions education, and never mentions gay men.

The National Institutes of Health, allocated $47 million to test new AIDS drugs by a Democratic Congress, fails to spend it (Kramer, 1994).

The Nation of Islam suggests that Jewish doctors mixed HIV into the vaccines given African American children. The United Front Against Racism and Capitalism-Imperialism charges that AIDS was a product of "germ warfare by the U.S. Government against gays and blacks" (Burkett, 1995, p. 187).

AZT, a herring and salmon sperm extract developed in 1964 as a possible cancer treatment, is approved for use against HIV by the Food and Drug Administration (Burkett, 1995, p. 81).

The AIDS Coalition to Unleash Power (ACT-UP) is formed with a mass demonstration planned for March 24th on Wall Street against the Food and Drug Administration and for the release of experimental drugs.

1989 Fewer than 1% of hospital admissions have HIV, but 30% of admitted male African Americans between the ages of 25 and 44 have HIV (Burkett, 1995, p. 179).

Kimberly Bergalis grabs attention by bitterly claiming that her dentist infected her with HIV. She says she is a virgin although admits having had oral sex and recurring "near penetrations" by her boyfriend. A gynecological examination indicates genital warts and an irregular hymen. She comes to embody the "innocent victim" of AIDS (Burkett, 1995).

1990   "A Miracle Drug Against AIDS—At Last!" is trumpeted in the *Weekly Review* of Kenya. The drug, Kemron, is a minuscule dose of interferon. Bitter charges of racism ensue when the traditional medical community denies its efficacy.

Although women of color make up 19% of the female population, almost three quarters of women with AIDS are African American or Hispanic.

Magic Johnson announces that he has tested positive for HIV. Vice president of the United States Dan Quayle, touting the government's new-found prioritization of AIDS, says, "And wouldn't it be wonderful to have a cure for AIDS in the marketplace before Magic Johnson gets AIDS?" (Burkett, 1995, p. 269).

1992   Bill Clinton is elected president of the United States. Hope soars that a serious and dedicated government effort will make a difference.

Within 5 months of taking office, President Clinton is declared a failure by ACT-UP, which distributes bumper stickers that say "25,000 Dead Since Jan. 20, Thanks for Nothing Bill."

1993   More than half the AIDS cases in the United States are among minorities. The AIDS rate among African American men is five times that for White men. For African American women, it is 15 times higher than among White women.

1994   A glossy and trendy magazine, *POZ*, dedicated to the HIV community, begins publication.

The National AIDS Clearinghouse compiles a list of 18,402 AIDS service organizations in the United States.

The rate of new infection among 20-year-old gay men is the same as a decade earlier.

1995   More San Franciscans die of AIDS than have died in the four wars of the 20th century combined and quadrupled (Odets, 1995).

Over 450,000 cases of AIDS have been reported in the United States, over 125,000 in Europe. Worldwide HIV infection is 18.5 million (World Health Organization).

In December, the first protease inhibitor, saquinavir, is licensed by the FDA.

1996   Combination drug therapies result in dramatic improvements for the health of many PWAs. HIV is undetectable in the bodies of some of those taking these new "drug cocktails" and there is hope that, with time, the virus may be cleared from the body. AIDS cases in the United States top a half million (Hill, 1996), and there are 21 million worldwide (King, 1996).

THE LANGUAGE OF AIDS

Language changed to include the experience of AIDS; an extensive vocabulary developed. Before this new vocabulary was available, reliance was placed on the vocabulary of historical tragedies. An example of this use of historical vocabulary is the insistent comparison of AIDS to the Holocaust, which devalues both. AIDS may be a holocaust, but it is not the Holocaust (see Bettelheim, 1980a). Survivors of multiple AIDS-related loss have no need to rely on the tragedy of others to justify their own tragedy.

Choice of language says much about response to AIDS. Much of the AIDS vocabulary has a siege perspective that supposes a foreign threat (e.g., "the war on AIDS"). Susan Sontag (1989) provided a survey of this military vocabulary.

> It was when the invader was seen not as the illness but as the microorganism that causes the illness that medicine really began to be effective, and the military metaphors took on new credibility and precision. Since then, military metaphors have more and more come to infuse all aspects of the description of the medical situation. Disease is seen as an invasion of alien organisms, to which the body responds with its own military operations, such as the mobilizing of immunological "defenses," and medicine is "aggressive, as in the language of most chemotherapies." (p. 9)

Persons infected with HIV are "exposed" to a dangerous, external enemy, and those who are infected become a type of enemy because they are infectious.

The language of AIDS separates "high-risk groups" from the "general population." Because there are "innocent victims" there must be "guilty victims." Even well-meaning attempts to educate the public reinforce these divisions. A campaign by the American Foundation for AIDS Research said that "the AIDS virus is an equal-opportunity destroyer" (Sontag, 1989, p. 82), a phrase that subliminally affirms what it means to deny. The message implicit in every assertion that AIDS can affect anyone is that the opposite is true.

Dread and stigma imprint the language of AIDS. Horrible, mutilating, and painful symptoms evoke dread. The tendency to invest AIDS with morally judgmental meaning adds to the suffering of victims and survivors. The very reputation of this illness adds to the suffering of those who have it. This results in the common experience, among persons affected by AIDS, of feeling shame or disgust, which hinders their willingness to talk about their problem and receive support. In her classic work, *Illness As Metaphor*, written before AIDS, Sontag (1978) observed that "disease widely considered a synonym for death is experienced as something to hide" (p. 8). AIDS provokes secrecy unlike any other disease.

The reluctant, sometimes squeamish, avoidance of frank and open conversation about AIDS has done more than handicap support. It has significantly hampered prevention strategies. Other than injecting the blood of a person infected with HIV into the blood of someone uninfected, anal intercourse is the most likely way to contract HIV, but penetrative intercourse is not an easily discussed subject, much less anal penetrative intercourse. AIDS prevention efforts require frank discussion of sex and sexuality, topics about which many people in the United States have conflicted and contradictory attitudes.

Language affects the survivor's experience. It defines how survivors perceive their identity and how they interpret their world. Lack of adequate language inherently minimizes the experience of survivors of multiple AIDS-related loss by denying them an adequate way to express their experience. This lack of language impedes grief by handicapping efforts to express grief, a crucial task in grief resolution.

THE FOREIGNIZATION OF AIDS

AIDS is the quintessential disease of "otherness." The general public distances itself from those affected by AIDS by making the victims, and the source of infection, foreign. Xenophobic overtones provide a way to distance one's self and community from AIDS while providing a context of blame. The "unhealthy" are separate from the "healthy." Survivors of multiple AIDS-related loss are viewed as part of the others, culpable for their suffering.

The tendency to blame foreigners for the spread of plague has a long-standing history. The Egyptian plagues described in the Bible were the fault of those who suffered. As plague spread through Asia and Europe in the 1340s, it was regularly regarded as an invasion from outsiders (Ziegler, 1969). Cotton Mather, a theocratic leader in early America, called syphilis a punishment of God. Preachers in England in 1832 connected the cholera epidemic with drunkenness.

The foreignization of AIDS occurs on an explicit and implicit level. Explicitly, foreigners are blamed for AIDS. In 1985, *Literaturnaya Gazeta*, a Soviet Union weekly, published an article claiming that AIDS was engineered by the U.S. government at Fort Detrick, Maryland. This news story was reported on Moscow radio, featured in London's *Sunday Express,* and appeared in newspapers in Kenya, Mexico, Nigeria, Peru, Senegal, and the Sudan (Sontag, 1989). It is common practice in nearly all nations to bar visitors and immigrants who test positive for HIV. AIDS is thought to have started in the "Dark Continent," Africa, then to have spread to Haiti, to North America, and to Europe. Foreign culprits are blamed for AIDS throughout the world, consistently viewed as harbingers of the virus, although who exactly is considered foreign differs.

AIDS is also seen as a foreign threat from internal foes. In the West, AIDS is manifested mainly among three groups: inner city minorities, homosexuals, and IVDUs. Its prevalence among these groups is not seen as accidental. These groups are considered high risk because of promiscuity, irresponsibility, and immorality. A language of separation surrounds AIDS. This forced separation requires attributing to victims something more than weakness. "Unlike me," they are indulgent, sinful, delinquent, and deviant. Jerry Falwell proclaimed that "AIDS is God's judgment on a society that does not live by His rules" (cited in Sontag, 1989, p. 61), and Patrick Buchanan condemned AIDS by mocking "the poor homosexuals [who] have declared war on nature, and now nature is exacting an awful retribution" (cited in Shilts, 1987, p. 311).

Infection is equated with punishment. Blame and judgment surround sexuality and addiction in unparalleled ways. Getting a disease from sex or drug use is considered almost willful, thus worthy of explicit blame, and blame has a comforting appeal. Primitive and modern societies have consistently sought an explanation for tragedy. Disasters always evoke questions of meaning. Survivors strive to make sense out of their experience. Partly, this language of blame results from fundamental confusion and disagreement on the ultimate cause and meaning of suffering, but mainly it maintains AIDS as a disease of otherness.

Robert Crawford (1994) made a compelling case for an evolving separation of the healthy and unhealthy.

> For the expanding middle class of the commercial and industrial societies of Europe and America, the goal of health became an essential component of what it meant to be modern, progressive, rational, and distinctive. The language of health came to signify those middle class persons who were responsible from those who were not, those who were respectable from those [who] were disreputable, those who were safe from those who were dangerous. (p. 1349).

This division between healthy and unhealthy has widened "since the mid-1970's as the middle class embarked on projects of personal reconstruction and renewal" (p.1352). The healthy were responsible about their diet, did not smoke, and worked out. Health is a "metaphor for self-control, self-discipline, self-denial, and will power" (pp. 1352–1353). The unhealthy possess the opposite characteristics.

The survivors of multiple AIDS-related loss are affected by the foreignization of AIDS. Their suffering is attributed to their familiarity with the blamed others. It is guilt by association. Either they are one of the others or they have purposefully put themselves in contact with the other. They get what they deserve; they are culpable for their pain and therefore unworthy of sympathy.

COINCIDENCES OF HISTORY

Coincidences of history combine with characteristics of this virus to heighten its potential devastation.

Social Capitalism

Underlying the coincidences of history described below are two trends related to freedom. A particular notion of freedom dominates basic assumptions of the late 20th century, one that prioritizes the individual above the collective. Also, a mushrooming capacity for freedom is shaped by technological advances in communications, transportation, and health care.

A model of freedom, social capitalism, based on rugged individualism and personal fulfillment, now dominates the world. Success is defined by one's capacity to do as one wishes. "The ideology of capitalism makes us all into connoisseurs of liberty—of the indefinite expansion of possibility. Virtually every kind of advocacy claims to offer first of all or also some increment of freedom" (Sontag, 1989, p. 77). Indeed, the value of individual freedom is assumed, especially any freedom that can be practiced alone. Personal responsibility or obligation connote shame, standing as antonyms to freedom and choice.

These values foster consumption, growth, expansion, and possibility. The dominating economic system and sociopolitical philosophy encourage pushing the limits of possibility. Doing what one wants brings prestige and is prioritized. The catastrophe of AIDS demands constraint and limitation. This conflict between a culture of unlimited consumption and necessary limits was a distinguishing characteristic of early responses to AIDS, especially in the gay community and the boardrooms of blood suppliers. Sontag (1989) connected this broad trend of history with sexuality and, therefore, AIDS.

> Given the imperatives about consumption and virtually unquestioned value attached to the expression of self, how could sexuality not have come to be, for some, a consumer option: an exercise of liberty, of increased mobility, of the pushing back of limits. Hardly an invention of the male homosexual subculture, recreational, risk-free sexuality is an inevitable reinvention of the culture of capitalism, and was guaranteed by medicine as well. (p. 77)

The spread of the virus has been greatly assisted by the expanded possibility for, and reduced cost of, transportation. The number of annual airline passengers soared from 170 million in 1970 to 538 million in 1995 (Samuelson, 1996). Only in recent decades have trips all over the world been possible for so many. This reality permitted the burgeoning spread of HIV that could not have occurred previously. French AIDS researcher Jacques Leibowitch called AIDS "the charter disease" (cited in Shilts, 1987, p. 248). There is some opinion that HIV has existed in the world for decades but only began spreading recently because of the greatly reduced cost and greatly increased availability of travel.

Sexual Freedom

An unprecedented acceptance of sexuality combined with its easy access arose at the same moment in history that medical advances made sexually transmitted diseases nothing more than annoyances. These minor inconveniences were outweighed by a distinctive fashion of sexual voracity. A new sexual freedom emerged, especially in gay men who were expressing themselves in open, spontaneous sexuality that in the past had been severely restricted. Given the mode of transmission of this virus, ghettos of gay men and the institutions of urban gay life served to concentrate the risk of transmission. A more voluminous, efficient, and rapid system of infection could hardly have been invented.

One of the earliest persons with AIDS was a handsome, sexually active, gay flight attendant, believed to have been instrumental in spreading the virus throughout much of North America. Chilling accounts of Gaitan Dugas's indifference to the risk he inflicted on others abound. Health officials referred to him as "Patient X" and were well aware of the danger he embodied. Many of the earliest cases of AIDS, in New York, Los Angeles, San Francisco, Alberta, Edmonton, and Vancouver are traced to him. Shilts (1987) presented several incidents that document the fact that Dugas knew the harm he was causing. When advised by his doctor in 1982 to quit having sex, Dugas told him, "Somebody gave this thing to me. I'm not going to give up sex." Shilts reported that

> it was around this time that rumors began on Castro Street about a strange guy at the Eighth and Howard bathhouse, a blond with a French accent. He would have sex with you, turn up the lights in the cubicle, and point out his Kaposi's sarcoma lesions. "I've got gay cancer," he'd say. "I'm going to die and so are you." (p. 165)

Medical Factors

One aspect of medical history that significantly affected access to experimental treatments in the early years of the AIDS epoch and that contributed to intense anger among AIDS activists was the debacle with thalidomide. A sedative widely prescribed in England and Germany to relieve morning sickness, thalidomide left the medical community a legacy of caution. Especially in the Food and Drug Administration, ultracautiousness about any new drug treatments was preferred to risk taking. The lessons learned from thalidomide, and the rules governing drug approval that pertain to slower, less fatal illness, should not have been applied to a disease like AIDS, especially when so many of the infected were willing to serve as guinea pigs for experimental drugs and protocols (Kramer, 1994).

Despite some paranoid beliefs that have surrounded this virus, it is actually quite difficult to transmit. Direct contact between heavy concentrations of the virus and the blood system is the way HIV is transmitted. Some bodily fluids carry the HIV virus, but only in concentrations too low to result in HIV transmission. For example, it would take a few gallons of saliva to infect someone with HIV. It so happens that anal intercourse is a nearly ideal way for transmission to occur because of the propensity for semen to enter the bloodstream through tears and abrasions. Other populations who were exposed to direct blood-to-blood contact were at high risk. IVDUs, who were compelled to share needles, often shared blood and the virus.

The invention of Factor VIII (Factor), a substance that helps the blood of those with hemophilia clot normally, greatly extended the life expectancy of hemophiliacs who, before Factor, had a life expectancy of only 20 or 30 years. People with hemophilia lack one molecule in the genetic code that determines whether blood will clot to stop bleeding; therefore, bleeding is common and often profuse (thus the name of the disorder, hemophilia, or "love of blood"). It is passed genetically from mother to son. Before Factor, the lives of hemophiliacs were filled with frequent hospital visits and blood transfusions that accomplished nothing but replacing lost blood.

Factor is a condensed version of the blood of up to 100,000 different donors. Obviously, the risk of having an HIV-infected blood donor infect those with hemophilia was magnified by the number of donors required to produce one treatment of Factor. Hemophiliacs, who relied on blood factor to control bleeding, were exposed to HIV at astronomic rates. Before 1986, between 70% (CDC, 1987) and 94% (Jason, Stehr-Green, Holman, Evatt, & Hemophilia-AIDS Collaborative Study Group, 1988) of hemophiliacs were infected with HIV.

In 1982, a hemophiliac patient died of Pneumocystis carinii pneumonia, a disease that would later be widely identified in persons with AIDS. At the time, this particular form of pneumonia was so rare that it caught the attention of the hemophilia expert at the CDC, Bruce Evatt, who assured the patient's concerned doctor that the filtering process for Factor prevented transmission of bacteria and protozoa, and therefore PCP. He was technically correct; however, smaller microbes such as viruses could escape this process. HIV was one such virus that was not screened for while hemophiliacs were relying more heavily than ever on the blood supply.

HIV's long incubation period differentiates it from many other viruses. Persons with HIV often do not know that they have the virus until they are tested. Many are still confused about the HIV test. The most common test, the ELISA test, is actually a test for HIV antibodies that develop in persons exposed to the HIV. One important consequence of its being an antibody test rather than a virus test is that it sometimes takes 3 to 6 months before the body produces the antibodies detected by the test. Therefore, a person can be exposed to HIV and test negative for a period of time.

Many viruses quickly fade away simply because they kill off their host, and in doing so prevent their spread. Ebola, for example, although a particularly virulent and horrific virus, vanishes relatively quickly because it quickly kills most of its victims, eliminating the hosts of transmission. Because HIV can remain undetected so long, the opportunity for infection by people who do not even know they carry it is heightened.

Political Coincidences

In the early years of the AIDS epoch, political coincidences heightened the devastation of AIDS by severely handicapping prevention efforts among homosexuals and IVDUs while allowing neglect of the blood supply's safety (see Kramer, 1994; Shilts, 1987). Ronald Reagan's leadership is held responsible by many for the infection, suffering, and death of hundreds of thousands. A more indifferent, ill-disposed, and unfriendly leader could not have arisen at a worse time. Burkett (1995) offered a broader context to the political environment when she wrote,

> Ronald Reagan's refusal to confront the epidemic was not just a conspiracy of indifference to the fate of gay Americans. It simply did not fit America's emerging self-concept. The 1980's were the quintessential feel-good era. In that "morning in

America," wars were to be short and successful, with all but the victorious moments hidden from the press. AIDS was hopelessly out of synch with the times. (p. 303)

One's mind and heart shudder at the possibilities squandered in the earliest years. It is impossible to overstate the lost potential for reduction of harm. A national leader who had the compassion, intelligence, and foresight to forcefully promote prevention through safer sex education, clean needles, and maintaining a safe blood supply could have prevented untold infection.

Denial of Death

Our townsfolk were not more to blame than others; they forgot to be modest, that was all, and thought that everything still was possible for them; which presupposes that pestilences were impossible. . . . They fancied themselves free, and no one will ever be free so long as there are pestilences.—Camus, *The Plague*

HIV swept the world at a unique time in history. For the first time, disease seemed controllable, and the denial of death was at a zenith. Seligman (1994) commented that tragedy used to be a normal part of life, "the life condition." Until very recently, most people

thought that life was a vale of tears. Not so now. It is not unusual to go through an entire lifetime without tragedy. Bad things still happen to us all too frequently: Our stocks go down, our aged parents die, we don't get the job we had hoped for, people we love reject us, we age and die. . . . Once in a while, however, the ancient human condition intrudes, and something irredeemably awful, something beyond ordinary human loss, occurs. We are then reminded how fragile the upholstered cubicles we dwell in really are. (p. 136)

This is obviously written from a Western perspective. The denial of death is the dubious luxury of citizens in the industrialized, prosperous nations of the world. It is not one shared by citizens of developing nations (e.g., Kenya and Uganda, where AIDS is rampant), where sickness and death regularly occur at home among family and friends.

Medical advances had demonstrated stunning success at eliminating or treating the world's worst maladies. Massive infectious epidemics were confidently assumed to be a thing of the past. Advanced scientific understanding of disease made absurd any attempts to moralize about epidemics. In his book *Living while Dying*, Benita Martocchio (1982) explained the transformed attitude toward death in the latter part of the 20th century.

The physician rather than the dying person struggled with death and death reflected the physician's failure to win the battle with death. As in primitive societies, someone or something external to the individual could be blamed when death triumphed. . . . Deaths became clinically avoidable and thus premature. . . . This view of death as clinically unnecessary created problems for all, but especially for survivors. It evoked feelings of guilt or anger, as well as the need for self-punishment, retribution, reevaluation of prior decision, actions, or professional expertise, depending upon the individual's role in the situation. These problems and dilemmas were compounded when death was perceived as premature. The thought of someone being "struck down in the prime of life" has always aroused fear and consternation. What is unique to the twentieth century, however, is that regardless of a person's age or attendant circumstances, death is usually seen as premature. . . . There is thus a need to avoid death, deny its existence, or treat it as an abnormal event distinct from life. (p. 25)

Much of what Martocchio wrote applies directly to AIDS, a disease that evokes guilt and is perceived as resulting in premature death. If death was denied and distant, even more so was tragedy, an event that only happened to someone else.

The early years of this pandemic were marked by an optimism that proved false. More than erroneous, the unmet expectations for a cure or vaccine provoked a greater sense of tragedy. Although history is replete with examples such as plague or war killing the young, an assumption that such disaster was now inconceivable and impossible predominated. Thus, reactions of anger, despair, and depression were more pronounced than in a time when society was more aware of the threat of sickness, death, and life's tenuous nature. Rage and resentment surround the way the government, drug companies, blood companies, and the medical establishment responded to AIDS. The assumption that a cure should be found is implicit in much of the reaction to the diseases and deaths associated with AIDS.

Death seems unsanitary and obscene in the modern age, so modern humans separate themselves from it. Examples of this abound. Public displays of the deceased are now rare, whereas they were common in the past. Today, most people have never seen a dead body. Dying occurs in hospitals or hospices, rarely at home. It is supposed to happen to elderly people, not to young people. The messy details of disease and dying are assigned to professionals: doctors, nurses, and trained volunteers.

AIDS has changed all that, especially for survivors of multiple loss. The human body's frailty, its fluids and sores, have been exposed. Survivors regularly witness the withering of friends, whose skeletons stretch their skin. Excrement is made public as incontinent 30-year-olds are forced to wear diapers and condom catheters lead to plastic jugs that sit between friends. Bodily fluids became synonymous with the risk of infection, so survivors sometimes wear rubber gloves to touch their friends. Survivors have felt the weight of bone and ash and have literally let friends slip through their fingers.

Understanding the Survivor's World

Understanding the survivor's world requires appreciation for the epidemiology of AIDS, the psychosocial influences that framed responses to AIDS, and the historical context and social situation in the late 20th century. The world in which AIDS appeared is a world awash in suffering, overwhelmed by need, and increasingly more interested in self-protection. At first, AIDS was very "out there," arising only in others. A joke that circulated early in the epidemic has someone disclosing his AIDS diagnosis to someone who responds by saying, "I didn't know you were Haitian."

A regular scattering of celebrity deaths occasionally brings AIDS into public recognition. Red ribbons, movies, benefit concerts, and celebrity appearances help to counter faltering public attention, a task necessitated by the freshness required by today's private media news and the lingering perception that AIDS happens only to someone else.

STAGES OF SURVIVING MULTIPLE AIDS-RELATED LOSS

Individuals proceed through four stages of response to the experience of multiple AIDS-related loss. These stages are conceptually useful because they provide a way to organize the survivor's experience, a task necessitated by the nearly universal survivor response of feeling overwhelmed. Rather than suggesting a way to divide various responses to multiple loss, these stages are intended to provide a context, a framework for better understanding the survivor's experience. They will be useful to what follows later in the book.

Movement through these stages is not always linear. Boundaries between stages are not precise; rather, they are somewhat fluid. What follows is a concise summation of these stages. More detail about characteristics of these stages is provided throughout the remainder of the book. The stages are (a) shock and denial, (b) overload and confusion, (c) facing reality, and (d) reinvestment and recovery.

Unlike most tragedies, multiple AIDS-related loss has an impact on communities and individuals that not only is interrelated, but is circularly synergistic. *Synergism* normally refers to the simultaneous actions of separate agencies that together have greater total effect than the sum of their individual effects, an apt description for the experience of survivors of multiple loss. These stages assume an interrelationship between individuals and communities. The impact of multiple AIDS-related loss on the community exacerbates the impact on individuals, and the impact on individuals exacerbates community-wide impact. These stages may also be applied to communities when multiple loss affects a distinct community, namely a community of urban homosexuals.

Shock and Denial

Denial is anxiety management. Emily Dickinson said, "The truth must dazzle gradually, or else every man be blind" (as cited in Fulton, 1995). Shock is a normal response when people's formerly realistic expectations about their world and future are smashed. At first, survivors were left reeling by the sudden appearance of death among their young friends. A danger that could not be pinpointed was clearly present, but uncertainty about it predominated. Ovid said, "Where belief is painful, we are slow to believe" (cited in Staudacher, 1994, p. 14). For some survivors, shock and denial blended together for a long time. Attention was focused, at first, on loss and grief connected to singular, distinct losses, but a looming threat of danger predominated. A hunch that something tragic and unstoppable had begun took shape.

Rollo May (1981) wrote that "the mass of citizens react as a neurotic would react: we hasten to conceal the frightening facts with the handiest substitutes, which dull our anxiety and enable us temporarily to forget" (p. 15). There is no better description of the denial that many survivors still maintain long after the realities of multiple loss have been made clear. Even within communities that are hardest hit, blatant denial is common. In the gay community, especially among young people, multiple AIDS-related loss is frequently viewed as a reality only for older gay men. This delusion is supported by the long incubation period of HIV infection. In the hemophilia community, AIDS-related loss and grief are frequently urgent problems for families only until their familial loss has passed, then the subject of AIDS is avoided. An inexhaustible repertoire of methods are invented to divert the survivor's attention from the persistent fact of AIDS-related loss. Use of mood-altering chemicals, isolation, and withdrawal are some examples of denial.

A problem with denial is that it leaves survivors most vulnerable to the very perils against which they have tried to defend themselves. Although denial may commence as a conscious process, it soon becomes an unconscious one; otherwise it would never work so well, "and so completely" (Bettelheim, 1952/1980a, p. 84).

Overload and Confusion

Individual confusion is often marked by bereavement overload (Kastenbaum, 1969). The cumulative effect of multiple AIDS-related loss begins to take its toll on the survivor. This is the time between initial shock and later acceptance of reality. For many, it begins as a feeling of utter helplessness and hopelessness. Friends and family are dying. There is no way to be sure why some get sick and others do not, but there is plenty of guessing. A survivor may be frantic to exert control.

The fury of angry and confused AIDS-affected persons was embodied in ACT-UP, which was especially active during the Reagan and Bush years when there was a widespread perception that the highest levels of government were inattentive, or even hostile, toward persons with AIDS. ACT-UP's embodiment of community anger in the gay community frequently alienated potential supporters. Juxtaposed against this demonstration of rage were calls to quarantine all infected persons in locked camps. On the broadest community level, society was confused about its response to AIDS.

The controversy surrounding Larry Kramer typifies the confused response of the gay community. In Spring 1983, Kramer had written his famous (or infamous) article "1,112 and Counting." In that article Kramer wrote,

> If this article doesn't scare the shit out of you, we're in real trouble. If this article doesn't rouse you to anger, fury, rage, and action, gay men may have no future on this earth. Our continued existence depends on just how angry you can get. . . . Unless we fight for our lives, we shall die. In all the history of homosexuality we have never before been so close to death and extinction. Many of us are dying or already dead. . . . There are now 1,112 cases of serious Acquired Immune Deficiency Syndrome. (p. 1)

Kramer ended his perspicacious article by listing, one by one, the 20 persons he knew who had already died from AIDS.

Reactions to this article (and to others by Kramer) were vicious attacks. Robert Chesley, a New York writer, wrote several letters to the editor of the *New York Native*. He warned Kramer that

> being alarmist is dangerous. I think that the concealed meaning of Kramer's emotionalism is the triumph of guilt: that gay men *deserve* to die for their promiscuity. . . . Read anything by Kramer closely. I think you'll find the subtext is always: the wages of gay sin is death . . . something else is happening here, which is also serious: gay homophobia and anti-eroticism. (as cited in Shilts, 1987, pp. 108–109)

This confusion is still prevalent, though mainly unrecognized, in the gay community. A "completely uncontrolled epidemic—a psychological one" (Odets, 1995, p. 7) rages in survivors, especially those who still test HIV negative, but Walt Odets (1995) noted that his public recognition of it brought "criticism about the impropriety—or sheer effrontery—of my addressing the issues of HIV-negative men while men with AIDS were dying" (p. 7).

Understandably, survivors may seek any method of holding back, or at least curbing, devastation to their lives. A portion of survivors will remain at this stage. Some avoid contact with their feelings and shun persons associated with AIDS. Some react by attempting to flee the crisis by moving to another city.

Various, sometimes contradictory, emotions may emerge. Chronic depression, severe anhedonia, sleep disturbances, and self-destructive behavior arise in some. Anger, rage, cynicism, pessimism, and despair arise in others. Still others respond with anxiety, feelings of vulnerability, insecurity, or guilt. Hemophiliacs, for example, frequently experience particular types of guilt, anger (Goldman, Miller, & Lee, 1993), fear of stigmatization (Mason, Olson, Myers, Huszti, & Kenning, 1989), tendencies toward secrecy (Brown & DeMaio, 1992), and disruption of future expectations. Always remember that the survivor's experience is entangled in the same variety of reactions, fears, hopes, and cycles that are experienced by the family member, friend, or acquaintance with AIDS. Survivors experience vicarious reactions to the experiences of their loved ones. One survivor of multiple loss who is losing her son said "when he feels up, I feel up; when he feels down, I feel down."

In the early 1980s, there was no HIV test, no way to know who had it. All manner of "preventive" strategies were used. Some committed themselves to radically restrictive diets, others sought out the latest chemical treatments in Mexico and France. Others took on the cause of AIDS as their primary purpose in life, becoming politically active or directly helping those with AIDS. Other survivors responded by separating themselves from perceived risks. They become sexually celibate or emotionally cut off in order to insulate themselves.

An example of one trend that arose a few years into the AIDS epoch depicts the roller coaster ride of sky-high hopes to crushing despair experienced by many with AIDS and by the survivors of multiple loss. Fostering a positive, healing attitude through self-affirmations was popularized. One guru of this movement was Bernie Siegel, who in his video *Hope and a Prayer* said, "When a person changes, the new personality does not need the old disease." Louise Hay was immensely popular among persons with AIDS and their supporters in the mid- to late 1980s. Her appeal has waned significantly. Although her message may have improved the quality of life for many (especially gay men) by bolstering self-love, this proved to be no physical cure. In *The AIDS Book: Creating a Positive Approach* (Hay, 1988), she told people with AIDS,

> When we discover that we have been "tested positive," it is not the end of our world. It is merely a loving message from our bodies telling us that we have gotten off track and need to make some positive changes in our way of living. . . . "Testing positive" is a warning symptom of an underlying cause, an attempt of your consciousness to communicate. Our job can be to find and eliminate the underlying cause. If we heed the warning, then our condition may not need to expand further into ARC or AIDS. (p. 17)

Although these messages seem grossly oversimplistic and naive from the perspective of the second decade of AIDS, their popularity speaks volumes about the confused urgency for, and shortage of, hope. For all the naivete of this response, it also contains a core truth. For survivors, all refuge from the surrounding storm was being eliminated. Their last hope for control, for meaning, for surviving themselves, was in their own personal attitude. The survivor, although overloaded, starts to see beyond the confusion. This is the crucial transition point between confused overload and facing reality.

Facing Reality

Realization that the underlying occurrence of loss cannot and will not be stopped is the main task of the third stage. Apprehension, which some survivors describe in retrospect as a sense of impending dread, changes into a resigned or dreadful certainty that there is no end in sight. The future holds ongoing loss. In the preceding chapter, Debra described this moment: "It was like if you knew a plane was going to crash and everyone was going to die and you can't do anything about it and every person on that plane you know."

Some survivors note a specific instance in time when they realized the magnitude of what was happening. This threshold is sometimes crossed suddenly, in an "ah ha!" moment of clarity that corresponds to a personal crisis such as the diagnosis of one's self or significant other with HIV. In some cases, as it was in Steve's story, it may be a day when friends are gathered together and notice, together, the impending calamity. Many survivors report such a moment when they knew that everything changed. Uncertainty about the nearly inevitable course of HIV infection gives way to certainty that most everyone who is infected will die, and this realization is personalized: "My friends will die!" Others experience a gradual, evolving realization. Circumstances combine to force the survivor to face reality, such as the cumulative toll of many sick friends, hospital visits, deaths, and memorial services. These events make the reality concrete.

Chris Tollfree (personal communication, 1996), a psychotherapist who works with survivors of multiple loss, observed that early in the AIDS epoch there was "a lot of drama associated with AIDS." He described "drama queens" who almost enjoyed the excitement and emotion of confronting death and suffering. As AIDS continued, the titillating appeal was replaced by a realization that "we had to be in this for the long haul." A certain amount of detachment was necessary.

An individual's identity in connection to HIV itself fosters a perspective on reality. This is especially true in the gay community where everyone has an HIV status whether it is positive, negative, or undetermined. The HIV antibody test ushered in an era of division. The experience of surviving multiple AIDS-related loss is different for these groups.

Reinvestment and Recovery

Despite survivors' recurring and urgent prayer that losses cease, they will not. They must decide between victimized existence and making vital choices to live with their destiny. As Miguel de Unamuno (1921/1954) said, "The instinct of knowing and the instinct of living, or rather of surviving, come into conflict" (p. 115). "Whether he likes it or not, he must believe, because he must act, because he must preserve himself" (p. 117). The survivor's recovery necessarily includes action.

Adjustment to an environment where multiple AIDS-related loss is accepted as a past, present, and future reality is the main task of this stage, although there are as many ways to approach this task as there are persons who engage it. Chapters 8 and 9 discuss these choices in detail. Survivors are challenged to decide how they will cope. Survivors choose either to reinvest themselves in life or to merely survive. These decisions are always evident in behavior.

Reinvestment and recovery include acceptance of the reality of multiple AIDS-related loss. For some survivors this attitude is summarized in the Serenity Prayer: "God, grant me the serenity to accept the things I cannot change, courage to change the things I can, and the wisdom to know the difference." At this point of acceptance, survivors face the daunting task of deciding what to do given the irrevocable disruption wrought by multiple AIDS-related loss. Survivors face vital questions: How will I choose to live in this new world? With whom will I have a relationship? How intimate will I let myself become? What are my values? Where do I find meaning in the midst of so much apparent meaninglessness? Will I keep exposing myself to more potential pain? These are the fundamental existential questions of life, and they are inevitably faced by the survivor who chooses this course.

"We taught the world style and taste, now we teach it how to die." This assertion was the summary of one gay survivor of multiple AIDS-related loss. This assessment of the gay community's adaptation to, and of, the tragedy of AIDS is a testament to affirmative adjustment. Kayal (1994) analyzed the gay community's adjustment to AIDS, noting that the Reagan and Bush presidencies "put the responsibility of AIDS, in cause, prevention, and service delivery, into the hands of gay people" (p. 53). Gays responded with determination and magnanimity, especially after the realities of HIV infection became known and its virulence was experienced.

Cultural outpouring is an adjustment to the reality of AIDS that continues in a way unprecedented by any other disease. In contrast, cancer, which has killed more people, has engendered virtually no art (Kimmelman, 1989). Examples include, but are certainly not limited to, plays by Tony Kushner and Larry Kramer; John Coigliano's Symphony Number One; fiction by Paul Monette, David Feinberg, and many others; photographs by Nicholas Nixon; and paintings by Ross Bleckner and Keith Haring. This heritage of culture arising from the tragedy of multiple AIDS-related loss is primarily an achievement of the gay community. Exactly why AIDS has provoked so much cultural wealth is not altogether clear, but it is an area for future investigation. It is vastly interesting, however, that it does arise in this context. This cultural outpouring must, by its wealth and force, say something, either about the unique characteristics of AIDS or about the persons most affected. It is likely the combined impact of a uniquely tragic disaster on a uniquely creative and energetic community.

Two stark realties shaped the gay community's response to multiple AIDS-related loss: First, the crisis was going to continue, and second, little assistance was forthcoming from outside the gay community. Thus, the "responsibility of AIDS, in cause, prevention and service delivery" (Kayal, 1994, p. 53) was in the hands of gay people. The gay community responded impressively to the reality of AIDS with unprecedented cohesion (Stulberg & Smith, 1988) and the development of community-based AIDS service organizations (Lloyd, 1992). This response was so effective that most AIDS sufferers and survivors outside the gay community have relied on services established by the gay community.

In contrast to the stage of confusion, these responses are marked by purposeful intent. Choices are made in order to adjust to new realities. Although this process occurs at mental and spiritual levels, it is observable in specific, behavioral changes. Specific tasks are undertaken. These might include working as a volunteer, attending support groups, doing the work of grief, participating in psychotherapy, and actively seeking out and deepening relationships.

The survivor who chooses to survive in a shut-down state is not negatively judged. The pain and confusion that motivate these responses must be met with sympathy. The radical disruption to the survivor's world, identity, and personal view of meaning make it entirely comprehensible that responses of psychic and physical withdrawal ensue. Given the amount of loss endured, and the ensuing pain it provokes, it is natural that means to avoid future loss and pain through a stance of fundamental emotional and relational conservatism are sought.

One strategy to avoid the potential of pain inherent in personal relationships is to avoid them, especially relationships with persons who are likely to become sick with or die from AIDS. This decision exerts a heavy cost by means of the loss of support, friends, and relationships.

Avoidance of feelings is chosen by some survivors of multiple AIDS-related loss. Otherwise well-functioning survivors sometimes constrict their range of emotions to such an extreme that they are rarely sad about another death or happy about a positive event in their life. This goal can be achieved through intellectualization, an attempt to explain why in order to avoid feeling how. Mood alteration through chemical use or sexual activity is sometimes used to cope with the pain of so much loss.

THE FUTURE OF AIDS AND MULTIPLE LOSS

> This disease will be the end of many of us, but not nearly all, and the dead will be commemorated and will struggle on with the living, and we are not going away. We won't die secret deaths anymore. The world only spins forward. We will be citizens. The time has come.
> Bye now.
> You are fabulous creatures, each and every one.
> And I bless you: *More life*.
> The Great Work Begins. (Kushner, 1994, p. 148)

Having reviewed the history of AIDS, it is important to say something about the present and the future. In part, this task is addressed by reviewing the trends and forecasts in the epidemiology of AIDS, the causes and occurrences of HIV infection. The ongoing nature of the AIDS crisis means that by the time this sentence is read, current data will be out of date; but the future is observable in trends of the present.

AIDS Today and Into the Future

Major advances are being made in the treatment of HIV. Whereas all earlier treatments for HIV (AZT, ddI, ddC, d4T, and 3tc) were of the same drug family, two new classes of drugs (protease inhibitors and nonreverse transcriptase inhibitors) are now available. Combination therapy, where two or more of these drugs are taken simultaneously, is now regarded as the best approach to treating HIV (Delaney, 1996). PCR RNA viral load testing now allows persons with AIDS and their doctors to quickly judge whether treatments are effective, and the combination of drugs available allows various options. For the first time, scientists are talking theoretically about the possibility of eradicating HIV from the body. Encouraging medical results from combination therapy continue to astound those who have been disappointed by so many other potential hopes. In 1996 AIDS service organizations routinely reported decreases in their cases. One indicator of increased survival for PWAs is the sharp decline in the number of obituaries published in gay newspapers, such as the San Francisco's *Bay Area Reporter*. Whereas obituaries ranged as high as 37 for 1 week, they have recently been in the low single digits (James, 1996, p. 3)

These medical advances may have significant implications for survivors of multiple AIDS-related loss. The pace of multiple loss may lessen for survivors whose main contact is with people who have good health insurance. These combination therapies are expensive, costing between $15,000 and $20,000 a year. This level of treatment will not be available to most of those suffering from AIDS throughout the world. In the United States, Canada, and western Europe, tough choices are just beginning to be faced. For economically disadvantaged people, even in prosperous nations, these hopeful options may not be available. Disenfranchised groups will continue to suffer disproportionately. The chasm between the wealthy and poor, the higher and lower functioning, and the middle-class gay man and disadvantaged urban minorities may widen.

A lot has been learned recently about drug resistance. The HIV virus is amazingly adept at quickly developing resistance to almost all existing drugs when used alone. Multidrug therapies require strict compliance with drug regimens. Like tuberculosis treatment, those who fail to follow exact dosage and schedule guidelines are likely to develop a virus that is resistant to the drugs they have taken, and new treatments will offer less significant benefit. When this resistant virus is transmitted, opportunities for treatment are foreclosed for the newly infected, who receive an already resistant virus. Therefore, although survivors may experience much greater longevity in some of their loved ones or caseload, survivors may also experience rapid progression of the disease in others.

Although discouraging, AIDS will probably be increasingly viewed as a chronic, terrible, but accepted reality, much as we now view homelessness and violence. Although obvious benefits of a longer life ensue, a prolonged period of anticipation will precede each death. Survivors may also find themselves

knowing increasing numbers of persons dying with AIDS. The growing numbers of deaths from AIDS means that more and more people will be affected by
multiple AIDS-related loss. More people will die, and more people will notice
that they have survived multiple deaths from and other losses related to AIDS.

Throughout the world as a whole, AIDS is predominately a heterosexually transmitted illness. Heterosexual transmission through sexual intercourse
accounts for 75% of worldwide HIV infection (Brookmeyer, 1991; Novello,
1991). Ignorance of this fact and tendencies to foreignize AIDS promote the
belief system that separates the "normal" population from those affected by
AIDS. There remains a tendency among survivors to perceive their own experience with AIDS as typical. Hemophiliacs don't appreciate the experience of gay
men. Gay men don't appreciate the experience of hemophiliacs. One goal of
this book is to broaden the survivor's perspective to encompass the experiences
of other survivors of multiple AIDS-related loss. Hemophiliacs, for example,
have been hard hit by AIDS but have received scant attention. Caregivers and
volunteers, who have exposed themselves regularly to the pain of AIDS-related
loss, are an underappreciated group of survivors.

For some time, the fastest growing population of those with AIDS has not
been gay men, although this perception still predominates. Recent trends have
demonstrated a widening incidence of AIDS into more diverse populations. Four-
teen percent of all men with AIDS are bisexual, and there is concern that this
group may act as a bridge for HIV transmission from gay men to heterosexual
women (Chu, Peterman, Doll, Buehler, & Curran, 1992). Bisexuals "seem to
engage more frequently than homosexuals in AIDS-related risk behaviors"
(Messiah, Mouret-Fourme, & French National Survey on Sexual Behavior Group,
1995, p. 1544). In part, it appears that "gay-oriented prevention messages are
not reaching bisexual men" (p. 1544). Among heterosexual adults, Catania et al.
(1995) concluded that risky sexual behavior among heterosexuals increased in
23 American cities and that "movement into and out of the 'at risk pool'"
(p. 1497) is irregular and has complex causation. Heterosexuals

> with a history of risk factors for HIV seldom obtain testing prior to cohabitation or
> marriage and do not regularly use condoms after establishment of the relationship.
> Furthermore, the present study suggests that married people reporting extramarital
> sexual partners are typically the least likely to use condoms or obtain HIV testing.
> (Catania et al., p. 1497)

Rosenberg (1995) studied the rate of infection among different cohorts by
conducting a thorough and conservative analysis of HIV infection trends that
included the use of deconvolution methods known as back-calculation and
adjusted for cases that are not reported. "Only among white males was there a
marked decline over time. Rates may also have declined among younger Hispanic men. Black females showed increasing infection rates" (Rosenberg, p.
1374). "The proportion of cases among women has increased steadily during

the past decade" and "is increasing most rapidly among those infected hetero-sexually" (CDC, 1995, p. 5). For example, in the mid-1980s, male AIDS pa-tients outnumbered women 124 to 1; in 1995, the ratio was 4 to 1 (Goering, 1995). According to the World Health Organization, worldwide, women are the fastest growing group with new HIV infections, and "3,000 women a day be-come HIV infected. Around the world, 500 women die from AIDS each day" (AIDS Caregivers Support Network, 1996, p. 6).

Increasingly, Blacks and Hispanics comprise a growing percentage of AIDS cases. It has been the leading cause of death among Black men age 25–44 since 1991. Fifty-one percent of AIDS cases through Summer 1995 were Black or Hispanic (CDC, 1995). This information remains largely unknown even among those most active in the AIDS epoch. More alarming are the trends documented by national studies in the United States that reveal that Black adolescents have disproportionately higher rates of sexually transmitted diseases, even after adjusting for socioeconomic factors, than do White, non-Hispanic adolescents (Ellen, Kohn, Bolan, Shiboski, & Krieger, 1995). Studies have also shown that African American and Hispanic adolescents are becoming infected with HIV at the highest rates (Atwood, 1993). "The highest national prevalence rates were seen among minorities, and in particular among young black men" (Rosenberg, 1995, p. 1374).

Young people are at highest risk for contracting HIV and continuing this epidemic into the future. "HIV must be considered an endemic infection affect-ing successive cohorts of young adults" (Rosenberg, 1995, p. 1375). HIV con-tinues to spread among young gay men. A study by John Karon of the CDC in which 1,781 men aged 15 to 22 were interviewed concluded that one third "of these young men had anal sex without condoms in the previous six months." Five percent of the young men aged 15 to 19, and 9% of those 20 to 22, were HIV infected (Haney, 1996, p. A11).

A 1993 survey by the Department of Health found that 28.7% of 17- to 19-year-old and 34.3% of 20- to 22-year-old gay men reported having had un-protected anal intercourse within the past 6 months. A study of gay men under 30 in Amsterdam showed similar findings (de Wit, van den Hoek, Sandfort, & van Griensven, 1993). If current rates of seroconversion continue, one third of young men will have HIV by the time they are 30 years old (Van Gorder, 1994). Psychodynamic factors behind continued or relapsed high-risk behavior are explored in chapters 6 and 7. Sophisticated new tests can now measure resistance to specific drugs used to combat HIV. In western Europe and North America, 12%–35% of newly HIV-infected persons have been infected with a form of the virus that is already resistant to AZT. Therefore, "it is clear that people who know they have HIV are spreading it" (Delaney, 1996).

Early in the AIDS crisis, it was taken for granted that a person was homo-sexual if he mentioned the loss of a friend to AIDS. Gradually, death by death, the situation has changed so that it is now more common to hear that a person has experienced at least one AIDS death rather than none. However, the admission of having had several friends die is still assumed to be tantamount to saying "I am gay." The statistical evidence presented above indicates that this assumption will disappear with time, although its legacy will continue to affect the availability of support.

The world of multiple-loss survivors is mainly segregated, cut off from the regular experience of most others. Perhaps the most common lament of survivors is that family, friends, and acquaintances "don't get it." Again and again survivors complain, "I don't think anyone understands what we are going through." This book was repeatedly rejected by other publishers whose main criticism was that "there is no market for a book about multiple AIDS-related loss."

Language

An awakening awareness of multiple AIDS-related loss must begin with an appreciation for the existing language about this experience. A vocabulary to properly convey, through language, the experience of multiple AIDS-related loss is inadequate or nonexistent, although a vast vocabulary has come into being, or been popularized, by AIDS:

- opportunistic infections: Pneumocystis carinii pneumonia, PML, Kaposi's sarcoma, MAC, CMV, dementia, neuropathy
- treatments: AZT, ddI, ddC, d4t, 3TC, ritonivir, saquinavir, Crixivan, nevariapine, delavirdine, gancyclovir
- organizations and persons: Gallo, Curran, Gottlieb, National Institutes of Health, Centers for Disease Control, person with AIDS, HIV+/-, GMHC
- markers of disease status: CD4 count, PCR RNA viral load, lymphocytes, monocytes, MCV

In comparison, little language exists to describe the experience of survivors of multiple AIDS-related loss.

Some traditional words and terms apply but are inadequate: *grieve, bereaved,* and *traumatized.* What are persons who live on through this tragedy? Are they victims? *Survivor* is the term used in this book, but it lacks the clear definitiveness immediately understandable in the terms *veteran, abused,* or *widow.* Using the term survivor in a conversation with no preceding qualifier would leave the listener wondering if one meant to refer to a Holocaust survivor, natural disaster survivor, sexual abuse survivor, or something else. Least likely to occur to the listener would be what one actually meant by survivor, in part because there is no language to adequately describe families of choice.

The focused impact of AIDS on gay families of choice, a social arrangement undervalued by society (Nord, 1996c), generates a belittling and cheapening of the loss. Survivors rue the response to their loss that says "He was *only* a friend." When a person loses their significant other, for whom do they grieve? All existing terms are troublesome. *Lover* connotes a predominately sexual relationship or a sweetheart (*Webster's New World Dictionary,* 1980, p. 838) or "one who loves illicitly" (*Oxford Universal Dictionary,* 1933, p. 1172). *Significant other* is cumbersome, sounds impersonal, and is not included in most dictionaries. *Partner* is unclear, implying a business relationship. Margaret Atwood said, "The Eskimos had fifty-two names for snow because it was important to them: there ought to be as many for love" (cited in Staudacher, 1994, p. 98).

Extended families of choice have an even more limited vocabulary to describe their relationships. There is no equivalent to *aunt, cousin, grandparent,* or *niece.* "He was a friend" may be strictly accurate but utterly fails to define the depth and meaning of many relationships. As a result, many survivors use embellishing qualifiers. One hears survivors say: "He was a *really, really* close friend." Listening to survivors, one sometimes wonders how many "best friends" they have had. Survivors themselves are aware of this inadequate vocabulary and the tendency to exaggerate existing terms. When talking about his best friend John's illness with AIDS, Keith, whose story is told in chapter 4, said, "I don't use the term *best friend* lightly. He really was my best friend."

Our language implicitly minimizes the experience of survivors by assigning few adequate words. A vocabulary must be created and popularized if the experience of surviving multiple AIDS-related loss is ever to be properly acknowledged. This book is a beginning. An important goal of this book is to codify terms and create a vocabulary about the event of multiple AIDS-related loss.

Challenges

One frequently hears caregivers, whether professional or volunteer, wonder aloud if the energy necessary to sustain a proactive response to AIDS can be maintained. The threat that the public will lose interest in AIDS is heightened by new hopes in drug therapies. Two trends seem to be occurring. First, those who have been tireless caregivers from the beginning have grown tired. Those still involved are purposeful and calculating about their commitment to future work. Second, an army of new caregivers continues to rise to the challenge. Persons who choose to become involved, knowing in advance the heartache and hard work, are worthy of praise.

CONCLUSION

Not all survivors of multiple AIDS-related loss have a choice about their continued exposure to loss, although most do. The mother with sons who have HIV and hemophilia still faces a future of loss. A young man in a committed gay relationship whose partner and many friends have AIDS still faces a future of loss. To them all, and for the professionals who care for them, this book is meant to provide a resource of information and suggestions for coping with multiple AIDS-related loss. The next chapter follows this path by explaining specifically what characteristics of this disaster make it historically unique.

Chapter 3

Understanding Multiple AIDS-Related Loss

This may serve a little to describe the dreadful condition of that day, though it is impossible to say anything that is able to give a true idea of it to those who did not see it, other than this, that it was indeed very, very, very dreadful, and such as no tongue can express.—Daniel Defoe (1721/1969), *A Journal of the Plague Year*

Survivors of multiple AIDS-related loss are affected by a historically unique calamity. This assertion may seem exaggerated to those outside the event's zone of severest impact. Yet it is important because it sets the foundation for the first step in recovery from this event, normalizing the abnormal. Designating this event as unique is important for both the survivor's positive adjustment to multiple AIDS-related loss and the professional's intervention with survivors. This chapter briefly outlines the specific characteristics that distinguish the experience of surviving multiple AIDS-related loss; the implications of these characteristics are elaborated later in the book, mainly in the chapters on grief and trauma.

The reader may wonder why this book refers to multiple AIDS-related loss rather than multiple AIDS-related deaths. Although some survivors have sustained a deluge of death, all survivors have also sustained a number of other losses. This chapter outlines the various losses that arise out of this experience. Cumulative and compounding effects of loss have a synergistic impact on survivors, creating, among other things, the common experience of bereavement overload. The ongoing occurrence of loss distinguishes this disaster from most historical disasters and has profound implications for survivors' experience and hope for recovery.

Various characteristics of AIDS itself influence the survivor's experience. The age inappropriateness of its victims and survivors intensifies reactions to this experience. Protracted illness and episodic health and unhealth distinguish the process of AIDS-related illness and death from most other terminal conditions. Painful and debilitating opportunistic infections commonly arise in persons with AIDS, evoking revulsion and dread. The etiology of AIDS, combined with particularly harsh stigmatization, simultaneously magnifies the impact of loss and diminishes social support.

One survivor told the following story about a breakfast he had with his father and stepmother.

> We hadn't seen each other in 2 years, so we were engaged in a tense catching up. As a part of letting them know what had been going on in my life, I mentioned a few of my friends who had died from AIDS. I think they had even met a couple of them. Betty interrupted me to say that she too had friends who died, but from breast cancer. "It's the same thing, you know," she said. "It's just that you are dealing with AIDS and I am dealing with breast cancer." I was shocked. I couldn't say a thing; I only looked at her in disbelief. What was the same? People died. That is the *only* thing that was the same!

This survivor's story focuses our attention and this discussion on a realization that is primary to the survivor's experience, the multiplicity of AIDS-related loss.

QUANTITY OF LOSS

Quantity and quality of loss influence the survivor's experience. In the following section of this chapter, the character of loss is explored. First, a review of the quantitative amount is in order. A wide range of loss occurs among survivors, and it is useful to quantify this span. This will help those outside the population most affected comprehend the scope of loss that survivors experience while helping survivors realize that their experiences are not isolated.

The impact of multiple AIDS-related loss centers on specific communities for two reasons. First, the virus is spread by a difficult route, requiring introduction of the virus from an infected person into the bloodstream of a noninfected person. Second, because this route of viral transmission is specialized, actual infection only concentrates on groups where bodily fluids are inserted into blood. These are mainly discrete communities that existed prior to the existence of the virus. They may be communities that already have cohesive connections and interrelationships, such as the gay community. They may be communities where the majority of people hang around with each other, such as IV-drug-using communities (Stowe, Ross, Wodak, Thomas, & Larson, 1993). They may be diffuse communities that share a common risk factor but had varying degrees of relationship before the AIDS epoch, such as hemophiliacs. These groups, who are those most likely to get infected, are also most likely to associate with others most likely to get infected. This concentrates the effect of multiple loss on specific communities. Thus, it is understandable that one group would have absolutely no exposure to multiple AIDS-related loss, whereas another group would be devastated.

Little systematic study has been undertaken to determine the scope of multiple AIDS-related loss. Naturally, the quantity of loss mounts with time. Among a panel of New York gay men in 1987, each person reported an average loss of 6.7 people to AIDS (Dean, Hall, & Martin, 1988). In 1991, Boykin estimated an average range of 8–16. Shrader's (1992) study targeted at gay survivors of multiple loss showed a mean loss of 67.7 persons to AIDS. Generalizing about the amount of loss endured by any individual within groups at high risk for multiple loss is difficult. However, large quantity of loss does not seem to be a random happening. Survivors of a few AIDS losses can, and frequently do, limit their exposure to further loss through explicit avoidance. Recall Debra's observation that some hemophiliac families only stay involved with other families until their own family members die, and then they drop out. Some urban survivors choose to move into rural communities where AIDS is less prevalent. Almost one half of Martin and Dean's (1993a) sample of urban homosexuals had no loss.

> The fact that after 10 years of the epidemic, nearly half . . . had *not* lost a lover or close friend to AIDS suggests that bereavement is not a random event in the gay community but rather that losses are clustered within a specific subgroup of the gay population. (pp. 322–323)

Given the lack of objective study, one is left mainly with anecdotal accounts of quantity. It is not uncommon to hear gay survivors talk about losing more than 100 friends and acquaintances. Larry Kramer (1994) has kept a list and observed that

> I have lost some five hundred acquaintances and friends to AIDS. I realize that putting a figure to this loss is both gruesomely macabre and too Madison Avenue. It makes me sound weird: that I have for over seven years kept a record of these names. How could anyone *know* five hundred people, straight friends tell me disbelievingly. . . . Because gays live in a ghetto we know personally and generally recognize most of the people in it. (p. 218)

Two aspects of Kramer's account are heard regularly from survivors: the huge amount of loss endured and the discrediting incredulity expressed by people outside the zone of severest impact. To hear a survivor estimate more than 100 deaths is no longer unusual or, sadly, surprising. When survivors talk about their quantity of loss, they commonly hear contemptuous disbelief from family members, friends, and business associates. When a survivor receives a sympathetic response, it is usually one of numbed shock. "Really big numbers tend to have a numbing effect" (Kastenbaum, 1977, p. 315). Recall the experience of Steve Parsons presented in chapter 1, where he described his experience telling coworkers about his losses. When they mocked him, he quit speaking about those losses. This happens to many survivors. This decision has adverse effect on adjustment.

Quantity of loss matters. In his study of New York gay men, John Martin (1988) found "significant dose-response associations" (pp. 860–861) for a variety of negative outcomes. The more loss a person had experienced, the more likely were traumatic stress responses, demoralization, sleep problems, psychological distress necessitating the use of psychological services, and sedative and recreational drug use. For reasons explored in chapter 5, complicated bereavement and unresolved grief reactions are common, aggravated in proportion to the amount of loss an individual endures.

LOSSES AS MORE THAN DEATH EVENTS

Death is the central loss from which the threat and reality of all other losses arise. However, death is only one of the several losses emanating from the AIDS pandemic. Almost all death occurrences result in different levels of loss (Rando, 1984), but a unique cluster of loss types arises for survivors of multiple AIDS loss. This loss is more than the loss of *an* other. It is frequently collective as well as individual, global as well as personal. Below, some losses are presented to provide the reader a foundation for the remainder of the book. They are elaborated on in more detail later, when the context and implications of these losses are analyzed. Because these losses are interrelated and layered, survivors frequently face multiple, multiple losses.

Loss of Family, Friends, Lovers, and Acquaintances

It helps to view relationships with survivors in concentric circles (see Figure 1). The closest familial and intimate ties are in the central circle and may include a spouse, best friend, or child. The next circle out may include the few persons most relied on and loved; these may include parents, siblings, or close friends. The next circle out may vary considerably in size and composition and may include friends, family members, and important occupational and social colleagues. The next circle out may include a vast number of acquaintances, casual friends, business associates, sexual partners, and social companions. The final circle would include the varying number of persons with whom one has irregular and relatively insignificant relationships. The placement of various persons within these concentric circles of relationship varies with the individual.

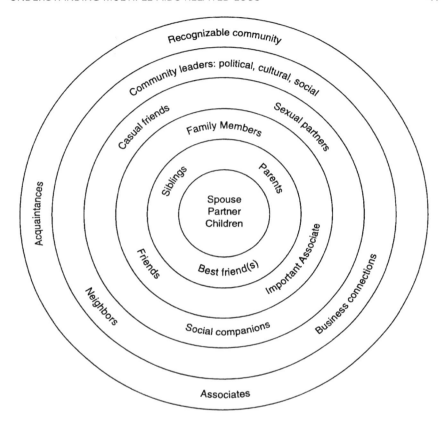

Figure 1   Circles of relationships.

The circles of relationships are an important consideration for understanding the survivor's experience with multiple AIDS-related loss. A survivor may need to adjust to losses in all these circles of relationships. This consideration is especially important in the gay community, where an individual may feel the constant impact of loss, from his closest relationships to his most distant. For example, normally the death of a hair stylist, travel agent, or florist would quickly be accommodated to because it is rare and distant. However, in the urban gay community, vast amounts of previous loss destabilize the survivor's environment. Another death serves as a chronic reminder of previous loss and provokes feelings of alienation and separation.

The loss of closer relationships provokes more severe grief and disruption. The intensity of loss is increased in proportion to its proximity to the center of the concentric circles of relationship. Survivors may lose their closest, most immediate family members, including a spouse, a loss commonly acknowledged to be among the most difficult, whether it is a spouse in a heterosexual relationship (Parkes, 1972; Zisook, DeVaul, & Click, 1982) or in a homosexual relationship (Britton, Zarski, & Hobfoll, 1993). Parents who lose children experience particularly intense grief (Rando, 1984).

Loss of Personal History

People are a crucial part of an individual's history. Lives are marked by memories and relationships. The death of the people with whom an individual shared his or her life is a loss of personal history. One survivor who had lost all his long-term friends said, "If my life is like a book, no one is left who knows more than one page of it."

Reminiscing is an opportunity that most enjoy, find valuable, and take for granted. For many survivors of multiple AIDS-related loss, the value of reminiscing is noticed when it becomes impossible because of loss. Recall Steve's observation in chapter 1 that "I can't say to someone, 'You remember in 1980. . . .' " Because memories are inexact and changing, lost mutual sources of history may foreclose an individual's ability to know part of him- or herself.

Loss of Future

A host of future plans and hopes are devastated by AIDS. Some of life's most basic expectations are undermined. Survivors are also faced with the knowledge that a huge amount of future potential is lost forever. One survivor said, "What books or stories will not be written or read? What civic and global improvements will be canceled or delayed?" The loss of dreams, the "specific hopes for something that did not or cannot now occur" (Bowman, 1994, p. 12), is one type of loss that is often overlooked. The normal dreams of parents, families, lovers, spouses, friends, and communities are dashed by multiple AIDS-related loss.

Thus, it is no surprise that high levels of anxiety are observed in survivors of multiple loss (Viney, Henry, Walker, & Crooks, 1992). Parents lose the generational continuity embodied in their children, hopes for grandchildren, and expected caregivers for their old age. In a lifetime frequently full of previous losses, many homosexuals face a wave of abandonment just at the time when life seemed to have stabilized. Gay men show increased demoralization, disillusionment, and discontinuity (Dean et al., 1988).

Loss of Security

The survivor of ongoing loss lives in a world of instability and vulnerability. A pervasive sense of hopelessness, helplessness, and despair was found among most survivors in a study by Shrader (1992). The survivor's landscape is forever altered. An event like multiple AIDS-related loss creates a profound impact on one's basic assumptions about the world. Survivors adjust to this loss of security with a range of response, from a general dissatisfaction and disappointment with life (Colburn & Malena, 1988) to a positive and purposeful redefinition of values (Carmack, 1992).

Loss of Emotional Range and Well-Being

The loss of capacity to feel a spectrum of emotions is one of the most consistent and persistent experiences of multiple-loss survivors. The "survivor's psyche closes itself off so as not to feel the onslaught of emotions that occurs as the result of so many deaths" (Boykin, 1991, p. 250). One survivor explained, "I just don't let myself feel anything anymore. It's too painful." To the extent that emotional screening is a conscious choice, the survivor's desire to screen out only uncomfortable feelings is futile. One cannot choose to feel only happy or joyful. The screening of certain feelings necessarily limits the capacity to feel others.

The emotional well-being of survivors is usually affected. A variety of deleterious consequences is noteworthy. Survivors of multiple AIDS-related loss are prone to anxiety, depression, suicidal ideation, dysfunctional anger, severe guilt, moodiness, irritability, nervousness, alcohol and drug abuse, sleep disturbances, despair, isolation, withdrawal, and self-destructive behaviors. Chapters 5, 6, and 7 on grief and trauma elaborate on this emotional impact.

Loss of Hope

Loss of hope may be the most distressing outcome of surviving multiple, ongoing loss. Shrader (1992) observed feelings of hopelessness, helplessness, and despair in survivors, and Dean et al. (1988) noted that survivors expressed disillusionment and demoralization. Looking to the future, survivors rarely dream of a cure anymore. Repeated "cures du jour" have crushed hope and provoked understandable cynicism.

One perspective that shows the depth of lost hope is the fear expressed by some members of the gay community for a world without AIDS. "The cure" is frequently discussed with less-than-hopeful anticipation. This anxiety is hard to pinpoint. Yet it seems to involve a concern about returning to the superficial, objectified relationships common before AIDS. Some survivors talk about personal growth and spirituality being gained the hard way and worry that a letdown may follow a cure.

Loss of Interest in Life

The loss of pleasure in formerly pleasurable activities (anhedonia) is frequently noted by survivors, especially in the early stages of responding to multiple loss. One frequently hears survivors ask, "What's the point?"

Rick, who has lost his lifetime partner and nearly all friends, described his life in the following terms:

I used to be the life of the party. I would walk in the room and light up. I could joke and get everyone going. Now, I don't think anyone wants to be around me. I am always depressed. My whole personality has changed. I used to laugh. I don't think I will ever be happy again.

Loss of Self-Esteem

By association, the survivor's self-regard is influenced by stigmatizing forces related to AIDS. The same internal logic that drives victims to blame themselves arises in survivors of multiple loss, who tend to believe that something intrinsic about their selves must be flawed. AIDS has created a doubly stigmatizing identity for gay men in the AIDS epoch. Homophobic attitudes are exacerbated by AIDS, which "continues to be used to rationalize prejudice, discrimination and violence against gay men and lesbians" (Appelby, 1995, p. 9). These negative attitudes may be internalized to create "a basic mistrust for one's own sexual and interpersonal identity" (Stein & Cohen, 1984, p. 61). Lowered self-esteem and internal homophobia are especially pronounced among persons who test HIV positive (Lima, Lo Presto, Sherman, & Sobelman, 1993).

Loss of Roles

Survivors lose their roles in relation to others. Parents cease being parents when their children die; lifetime partners cease being partners with the death of their spouses; friends cease being friends when one dies. The survivor occupies various roles in the lives of the deceased. These roles are displaced or entirely lost.

One lost role widely ignored or minimized is the loss of the role as caregiver. Many survivors of multiple loss have devoted themselves to caring for people with AIDS. One survivor calls himself a professional caregiver. When that role is eliminated after the death and estate disposition of those for whom they have cared, survivors report a sense of emptiness and lack of purpose: "What am I supposed to do now?"

Loss of Spirituality, Meaning, and Assumptions

On the death of his wife, C. S. Lewis (1961) said,

> If God's goodness is inconsistent with hurting us, then either God is not good or there is no God: for in the only life we know He hurts us beyond our worst fears and beyond all we can imagine. (p. 31)

If these doubts went through the mind of C. S. Lewis at the prospect of one death, how much more do survivors of multiple AIDS-related loss have reason to doubt, to have their entire foundation of spiritual belief shaken? This spiritual crisis is unavoidable and provokes an unlimited range of options. Every survivor of multiple AIDS-related loss struggles individually with questions of meaning. It is unavoidable. Existential issues are so predominant in the survivor's response that chapter 8 is devoted to these issues.

Loss of Privacy

Forced coming out is a reality for some survivors. "Coming out is no longer a private or arbitrary choice" (Kayal, 1994, p. 42). Lesbians and gay men "were forced out of the closet by the necessity of caring for sick and dying friends" (Mancoske & Lindhorst, 1995, p. 28). To receive support, survivors are forced to acknowledge their need for support and, thereby, their personal life. A simple request for time off from work to grieve is not so simple a request.

Loss of Community

The tragic irony of multiple AIDS-related loss is that the more tight-knit and supportive a community had been, the more it is devastated. The focused quantity of loss within the gay community is staggering. More than 250,000 gay men are reported to have AIDS in the United States (CDC, 1995). Although estimates about the total number of gay men and lesbians vary widely, this amount of death would be significant if concentrated in any defined community. Leaders and role models of all varieties have died, from artists to politicians.

Loss of Celebration and Sexual Freedom

The 1960s and 1970s were a time of emerging sexual freedom for heterosexual and homosexual persons. Multiple sexual partners were commonplace for many people who pushed personal and social limits of sexuality. AIDS fostered a fatal fear that dramatically curtailed sexual expression.

In the years after the Stonewall riots, which many attribute as the beginning of the gay rights movement in the United States, the gay community experienced a giddy, newfound ability to exercise freedom. This newfound freedom meant not only the ability to openly live as homosexuals, but the ability to freely and frequently engage in all sorts of sexual behavior. This "sexual revolution abruptly ended in fear of death and cautionary messages about safer sex" (Lloyd, 1992, p. 95). Among gay male survivors, Martin (1987) found a 78% reduction in sexual activity. Even kissing declined by 48%. Stulberg and Smith (1988) reported that over 50% of gay men in their study agreed with the statement "I enjoy sex less since AIDS" (p. 278).

Facing a Challenge

Multiple AIDS-related losses are vast and varied. Survivors face a challenge that extends beyond normal grief response and requires an individualized effort at resolution. Exactly what losses occur and, most important, what these losses mean to each survivor, differs. In the same individual survivor, the focus of loss and meaning will vary.

CUMULATIVE AND COMPOUNDING IMPACT

Surviving multiple AIDS-related loss means surviving a cumulative toll of deaths that has lasted for years. Judy, a caregiver to persons with AIDS, said,

> Sometimes being a caregiver is like being the front end of a car that's owned by a really bad driver. The whole AIDS experience feels like being hit, over and over again in the front end. You have more dents and creases than you can believe. Each blow puts another dent in you. (Gough, 1996, p. 1)

This sums up the experience so often heard from survivors.

In Daniel Defoe's (1721/1969) book *A Journal of the Plague Year*, the narrator notes that "towards the latter end [of the plague] men's hearts were hardened, and death was so always before their eyes, that they did not so much concern themselves for the loss of their friends" (p. 25). One consequence of surviving multiple AIDS-related loss is the emotional numbing necessitated by overwhelming suffering. Insufficient time between loss to work through grief and adjust to a new reality is the hallmark trait of surviving multiple AIDS-related loss. It has been noted in nearly every written account of multiple loss. Unfortunately, nearly all attention has focused exclusively on bereavement. Although crucial, bereavement issues do not wholly explain the various adjustments necessitated by the cumulative and compounding impact of multiple AIDS-related loss.

The experience of older people provides a useful comparison for understanding the experience of survivors of multiple AIDS-related loss. Older persons who have survived beyond most of their friends and some of their family will experience losses that are far more than death events and include "a multiplicity of losses in several significant areas" (Freeman, 1984, p. 287). The old house has been sold. The old neighborhood has been so transformed that it is unrecognizable. Prized possessions have disappeared. One's own body may become a source of grief rather than of pleasure.

> The elderly may be more likely than others to experience unrelated, multiple losses over relatively brief periods, at a time when most of their coping capacities and environmental resources have diminished. Thus, the cumulative effects of losses may have greater impact, particularly if there has not been sufficient opportunity to resolve all or some of the losses involved. (Freeman, 1984, p. 288)

A number of adverse outcomes may arise; several studies have reported that older persons may have a more difficult time with bereavement (Gallagher & Thompson, 1989, p. 459). "One might go so far as to suggest that many of the negative behavior patterns we tend to associate with old age are the result of a bereavement overload" (Kastenbaum, 1969, p. 48).

For survivors of multiple AIDS-related loss, cumulative and compounding events are more than deaths and their anticipation. The toll includes social calendars filled with memorial services, countless hospital and hospice visits, interminable discussions about AIDS, actual and contemplated suicides of friends, scanning obituary pages, and hours upon hours of pure worry. The cumulative survivor experience is one that usually leaves a permanent psychological mark that has been called a *death imprint* (Niederland, 1971). The term death imprint accurately describes the experience of ongoing, multiple loss in that nearly every aspect of a person's life is imprinted with death. Those affected by multiple and ongoing loss grieve continuously (Bidgood, 1992), as one loss reminds them of previous losses. For many gay men, "death is less an event than an environment" (Sullivan, 1990, p. 19). As Lifton (1993) noted, "Every death encounter is itself a reactivating of earlier 'survivals'" (p. 16). A study of survivors of multiple loss found that "preoccupation and searching rose with increasing numbers of losses" (Neugebauer et al., 1992, p. 1376).

ONGOING, RELENTLESS LOSS

When disaster strikes, no matter how horrible or vast, it normally ceases. At some point in time, the event ends, becoming a past occurrence. Survivors of most tragedies derive immeasurable comfort in the expectation and fact that loss does not continue unceasingly: "Things will get better."

Multiple AIDS-related loss is different. Nick, a survivor of multiple loss, said, "I feel like a tennis ball. I get hit back and forth, out of control. When it stops I'm put back in a dark can and pressure is pumped up in me." Time goes by with no cure or vaccine in sight. Losses mount; the impact broadens and hope for an end point disappears. The perception that survivors of multiple AIDS-related loss lack the control to lessen future impact hinders the potential for resolution. The reality that AIDS-related loss will continue into an interminable future is mentioned, more than anything else, by survivors as a reason for feeling hopeless and despairing. The future holds no respite, only the inevitability of additional compounding loss. This realization often dawns on survivors, causing them to reevaluate their voluntary involvement with AIDS. Margaret Anderson, a support group leader from Washington, DC, said,

> One year ago I thought that I could never leave. I wouldn't even allow myself to think of leaving because it would be like admitting defeat. Then there was this wave of new people. I realized it would never end. People left to whom I had a bond. I didn't let myself get as close to new people. I felt guilty. It was so painful to know that after seven years of this, we were still in the same situation.

Withdrawal and isolation are covered in more detail in chapter 6. Similar to the effect on survivors of AIDS-related multiple loss, the effect of multiple loss in elderly persons is to gradually isolate the older person. "A typical result is that the elderly person becomes more isolated and loses social skills that are essential for developing and maintaining a mutual support system" (Freeman 1984, p. 291).

> He might attempt to reconstitute his personal world by replacing the losses. This process often requires a great deal of time even under the best circumstances. And if there were *no* appropriate replacements available (as in the death of a life-long friend), then his response would have to take another form. (Kastenbaum, 1969, p. 49)

There are good reasons that the elder survivor of multiple loss does not re-create lost friendships and social opportunities.

> The experience of multiple losses may lead to a sense of extreme caution. "I had better not care about anybody or anything else. Sooner or later I will lose these people and things as well. And I just cannot bear to lose and mourn again." With such a sentiment in effect, the overly bereaved person may pass up opportunities to become reinvolved with life. (Kastenbaum, 1969, p. 49)

It is inherently risky to reestablish relationships, especially with peers, thus withdrawal and isolation are understandable. The older survivor may respond to the pain of so much loss with bitterness, becoming "paranoid, distrustful, unpleasant company" (Kastenbaum, 1969, p. 49), resulting in isolation. The parallels with survivors of multiple AIDS-related loss are obvious.

CHARACTERISTICS OF AIDS THAT AFFECT THE SURVIVOR'S EXPERIENCE

Distinctive characteristics of AIDS-related illness, death, and social response mark the survivor's experience. The combination and interrelation of these increase the impact on survivors while making adjustment more difficult.

Age Inappropriateness

The perception that nearly all AIDS-related deaths are premature and untimely has profound implications for survivors.

> Both society and the individual tend to behave as though death grants special immunity to the young adult. When we hear or read of a person having suffered an untimely death, it usually proves to be a relatively young man or woman. (Kastenbaum, 1977, p. 142)

Most of those dying of AIDS are younger than 40. This reality adversely affects survivors. In his last interview before his death, Randy Shilts ("Interview," 1995) explained this tragic sense of untimely waste when he said, speaking of himself,

> It's very frustrating because here I am at the pinnacle of my career. I could literally do anything I wanted to in the world of journalism. You're left with a strange feeling that your life is somehow finished without being completed.

Like much of the suffering experienced by persons with AIDS, the anguish of untimely death is shared by survivors.

So many deaths occurring in clusters of the young has an impact on surviving peers, who typically are also young and ill prepared to cope with it. "A great majority of survivors of lovers who died from AIDS are young people who have not before experienced mortal loss, making their pain all the more confusing" (Shearer & McKusick, 1986, p. 165). Age has been demonstrated to correlate with the degree of death anxiety. Studies have demonstrated that young people have greater death anxiety than older people. Heightened preexisting death anxiety is exacerbated by confronting death so vividly through AIDS.

> As AIDS most often strikes people at the prime of their life, emotions related to the meaning of life, sickness and suffering are particularly hard to endure. Normally, these are issues that are confronted gradually as people age. However the progression of HIV infection and AIDS requires that people confront and integrate these issues rapidly, even though they may not have had adequate life experience to cope with their losses. (Dworkin & Kaufer, 1995, p. 47)

Survivors of multiple AIDS-related loss commonly speak of experiences usually reserved for older persons. Survivors themselves seem to understand the developmental-stage dissonance of these tasks. In his study of survivors of multiple AIDS-related loss, Shrader (1992) found that survivors characterized themselves as not being as developmentally prepared as older people to deal with so much loss. Correspondingly, most survivors believed that they were "more mature and older than their same-age heterosexual peers" (p. 105).

Protracted Illness: Episodic Health and Unhealth

"The hardest part of AIDS is the timetable. There isn't any timetable," said a caregiver who has survived multiple loss; "It just isn't something that can be plotted out" (Gough, 1996, p. 11). The episodic nature of AIDS, including cycles of relative health and devastating sickness, are commonly referred to as a roller coaster by survivors of AIDS-related loss. Most terminal illnesses have a straightforward prognosis, with a relatively clear course of progression. AIDS does not. A person with AIDS may appear at the verge of death, only to recover. Penny, a Marin AIDS Project worker, said, "I saw a client at the hospital and said goodbye to him. When I say goodbye, I mean this person's going to be dead—I'll never see him again. Two weeks later, I saw him at the mall. AIDS is such a roller coaster. You just don't know" (as cited in Garfield, 1995, p. 4).

This continual up-and-down anticipation provokes profound anxiety in many survivors. When unpredictability is the norm, caregivers, friends, and families must plan for uncertainty, an oxymoronic task. This exacerbates feelings of helplessness. Stress is "exacerbated by the unpredictable course and episodic nature of the disease process" (Lloyd, 1992, p. 97).

These regular "near-the-brink" experiences exact a toll. They may have the paradoxical effect of producing surprise when the person with AIDS does die. Denial may be encouraged by the long period of health that precedes an AIDS death

> where from outward appearances life continues as usual. Hope is high so denial may interfere with family and friends' ability to realistically evaluate their loved one's future. Therefore, anticipatory grief work is problematic. This stance is reinforced since the person may have minimal, if any, limitations placed upon previous daily functioning. When full-blown AIDS is evident, the downhill course may be rapid. (Sprang & McNeil, 1995, p. 140)

Survivor's guilt receives more attention later in chapter 6 on grief, although its connection to the disease's episodic and prolonged nature deserves mention now. One survivor's experience illustrates this dilemma.

> My friend Charles had been close to death many times over the past few years. At each emergency, I rushed over to see him at the hospital and I would spend a lot of my time being with him. When I heard that he was hospitalized two weeks ago, I wanted to go see him but I had other things to do. Besides, I thought, what's the rush? I'll see him again as soon as I can. Well, he died, so I can't. The funny thing is that I was surprised when he died. Even though he was horribly sick for a long, long time, I guess I thought that he wouldn't die. He had recovered so many times. Now I feel badly about not being there for him in his last days. I can never fix that.

This bind between the conflicting desire to be there for a friend and to go on living for one's self is not the only one that places survivors at risk for guilt. Survivors, especially primary caregivers, may experience a double-edged guilt. The survivor may feel guilt about not having taken the person with AIDS to the hospital sooner. There may also be guilt about having encouraged or legally approved painful and prolonged medical procedures (Oerlemans-Bunn, 1988).

Sometimes there is a sense of disappointment when someone recovers from yet another opportunistic infection. Pain and dementia lead some family members and friends to wish that their loved one would go into a coma or die. A survivor may wish that the person would "get it over with" because the roller coaster ride of AIDS can be very, very long. The life span of persons infected with HIV continues to lengthen; it is no longer rare for individuals to live with the virus for more than a decade. Although this trend is encouraging for obvious reasons, it does prolong the period of stress and anticipatory grief.

The long incubation period of HIV allows those with the virus, and those around them, to be unaware of who is infected and who is not infected. This hidden, latent nature of risk increases dread (Sontag, 1989).

Opportunistic Infections

No one dies of AIDS; rather, people die from opportunistic infections to which the body is susceptible because of a damaged immune system. Twenty-five conditions, combined with HIV infection, define a diagnosis with AIDS (CDC, 1995). These opportunistic infections are often disfiguring, crippling, debilitating, and painful for those with AIDS and are, therefore, emotionally distressing for those emotionally attached to the sick.

Gary volunteers for Shanti, an organization that provides one-on-one emotional support for people with AIDS. He described an experience with one client that is not atypical for caregivers.

> I was working with a man, Howard, and I only knew him five months, but it was a very intense five months. He had what I often refer to as diagnosis of the month. Every month it seems like he had something else—he had tubercular canker sores, he had KS lesions in his gums, he had CMV retinitis, you know—every month it was some big thing. His parents, his wife, they wouldn't be in the same room with him. They were afraid of catching the disease. So he was pretty much alone. And he relied on me a lot. I was on my knees holding his hands during a spinal tap one time. I changed his diaper. I did things you don't normally do for another adult. I remember once sitting at home with my family eating dinner and the phone rang. It was Howard saying, "I'm bleeding from the rectum. Can you come and help me?" I got up from the table, put on my coat, and as I am driving over there I'm thinking, blood, infection, bleeding from the rectum. . . . But then I said, I can do this. Because if he's doing that, I can do this. (as cited in Garfield, 1995, pp. 190–191)

"The most terrifying illnesses are those perceived not just as lethal but as dehumanizing" (Sontag, 1989, p. 38). Speaking of the Black Death of the mid-14th century, Ziegler (1969) noted that "almost every account breathes the revulsion as well as the fear which the plague inspired. . . . Everything about it was disgusting, so that the sick became objects more of detestation than of pity" (p. 20). Similar outward physical manifestations of AIDS provoke dread, disgust, and stigmatization. Outward physical appearance is sometimes significantly altered by opportunistic infections: Wasting creates the skeletal look of death camp survivors. Kaposi's sarcoma lesions are most dreaded when they are visible, especially on the face. A study on the psychosocial impact of multiple AIDS loss demonstrated that "fears of bodily mutilation were common in the more bereaved community" (Viney et al., 1992, p. 159). Interestingly, this study showed a higher level of anxiety associated with mutilation than with death. Sontag (1989) analyzed the dread resulting from mutilation of the face. When the face is not affected by illnesses, the resulting dread is less severe. However,

> [t]he marks on the face of a leper, a syphilitic, someone with AIDS are the signs of a progressive mutation, decomposition; something organic. (p. 41)

It is hard to imagine a syndrome with a more terrifying and horrible cluster of potential symptoms than AIDS. Pneumocystis carinii pneumonia was the chief cause of death early in the epidemic. Though awful, Pneumocystis carinii pneumonia was relatively quick and usually killed the person with AIDS before a host of other opportunistic infections arose. Prophylactic treatments have greatly lessened its occurrence and also helped to lessen outbreaks of toxoplasmosis, cryptococcal meningitis, thrush, fungal infections, mycobacterium avium complex, and CMV retinitis. As a result of better treatment and prevention strategies, the prevalence of different opportunistic infections continues to change. Persons with AIDS are more likely today to endure a number of different opportunistic infections before their deaths.

These opportunistic infections include mental and neurological problems, such as dementia and the untreatable progressive multifocal leukoencephalopathy, that make it impossible for persons with AIDS to care for themselves. Therefore, family and friends perform tasks ranging from meal preparation to diaper changing. The capacity of the person with AIDS to function may also be handicapped by wasting syndrome, mycobacterium avium complex, and incontinence. Blindness can result from CMV retinitis. Various fungal infections, vaginal yeast infections, and skin manifestations, such as chronic herpes ulcers, thrush, candidiasis, folliculitis, and molluscum contagiosum, arise. When infections occur in the mouth, throat, or esophagus, they may impair one's ability to eat. Cancers, including three types of lymphoma, cervical cancer, and Kaposi's sarcoma, occur. The leading killer of HIV-positive individuals in the world is now tuberculosis ("New data," 1995).

The reader may contemplate this list of infection and feel overwhelmed and confused. This is an indication of how it is for the survivors, who must learn these new terms, understand their significance, keep up to date on the latest treatments, and incorporate their reality into their lives.

Etiology of HIV

The assignment of cause has affected the quality of support for persons with AIDS and survivors from the earliest days of the AIDS epoch when AIDS was first referred to as gay cancer or GRID. When a survivor decides to speak about a friend or family member with AIDS, nearly inevitably the question "How did he get it?" is asked. It is a question nearly never asked regarding other diseases.

Even where behavioral choices are directly linked to illnesses such as lung cancer, emphysema, or cirrhosis of the liver, a survivor is rarely challenged with the questions "Is she a smoker?" or "Is he a drinker?"

The survivor of AIDS-related loss understands the implication of blame in the question. Their suffering is deserved because they associate with blameable people and is, therefore, less worthy of sympathy. No other disease would evoke a comment similar to the one offered by the Reverend Willie Wilson, who said "Perhaps the fear of AIDS is just what is needed to scare these men straight" (as cited in Burkett, 1995, p. 184).

It is a relatively recent development of history to not blame the suffering for their suffering. Disasters are regularly associated with "the mood of the universe and its governing deities. A moral or divine significance is attributed to the catastrophe" (Kastenbaum, 1977, p. 110). When the enemy suffers it is "proof that the gods have taken our side and confirmation of our superior virtue" (p. 110). Sontag (1989) noted that

> Interpreting any catastrophic epidemic as a sign of moral laxity or political decline was as common until the later part of the last century as associating dreaded diseases with foreignness. (Or with despised and feared minorities.) And the assignment of fault is not contradicted by cases that do not fit. (p. 54)

Moralizing about the etiology of AIDS is common. "AIDS is the most politically controversial epidemic in human history" (Burkett, 1995, p. 191). The discomfort, if not outright hostility, people feel toward topics associated with AIDS significantly influences the availability and quality of social support. Pedro Zamora, the 22-year-old star of MTV's *Real World*, who died of AIDS in 1994, spoke to the heart of this issue when he said, "If you want to deal with my health and my life, you have to acknowledge that I take another man's penis and put it in my anus and do it because I want to. If you can't handle that, find me someone who can" (Gay City Health Project, 1995, p. 1).

Discussions about sex do not come easily for many, but it is an important issue for many survivors. For many, especially families with serodiscordant partners and gay men, it is impossible to adjust to the reality of multiple AIDS-related loss without dealing with the losses entailed in sexual issues.

When the etiology of AIDS is related to blood products given hemophiliacs, a whole different set of issues arises. Many hemophiliacs carry a tremendous amount of anger toward the blood companies, and sometimes the hemophilia organizations, for not protecting their families. This anger may be transferred onto the nursing staff that has cared for their family members over years. Bearing the brunt of that anger, on top of the grief from losing patients to AIDS, is hard for the nursing staff.

> The deaths of haemophilia patients are keenly felt by the nursing staff. The repetitive nature of the losses is common to all AIDS units or hospice programmes. However, staff in these programs have usually chosen to work with the dying while

nurses entering haemophilia care prior to the HIV era did not. In addition, haemophilia nurses have cared for their patients for many years. (Gordon, Ulrich, Feeley,
& Pollack, 1993, p. 365)

The gratitude of patients and families may be "overshadowed by their anger at
the haemophilia staff" (p. 365). The combination of these factors "makes for
one of the most wrenching experiences in medicine"(p. 365).

Stigmatization

"A person does not just die. He dies of 'something'" (Kastenbaum, 1977, p.
205). It is impossible to understand the impact of AIDS-related loss on survivors without understanding the context of stigmatization that surrounds AIDS
(Herek & Glunt, 1988). As is discussed in the chapters on grief and trauma,
social support is crucial, yet it is greatly handicapped by the effects of stigmatization.

AIDS Stigmatization   A stigma is a mark of shame, disgrace, and re-
proach. Although association with death is itself stigmatizing, a number of the
factors that potentiate stigma (Jones et al., 1984) arise in connection to AIDS. It
is deadly, incurable, and progressive; it causes immense suffering; and because
it is transmissible, those with HIV are often perceived as dangerous. People
with AIDS are frequently blamed for their condition: Gallup polls demonstrated
that half of Americans agreed with the statement "Most people with AIDS have
only themselves to blame" and that "it's people's own fault if they get AIDS"
(as cited in Herek & Glunt, 1988, p. 887). AIDS has been called "junkie illness"
and the "gay plague." Attempts to blame are always attempts to divide the
"normals" and the stigmatized (Goffman, 1963).
   Attribution theory (Shaver, 1985) provides a valuable framework for AIDS-
related stigmatization. Those with AIDS and those surviving AIDS-related loss
are judged to be responsible for their suffering based on four variables, the
extent to which (a) behavior caused the suffering, (b) the potential consequences
should have been known, (c) the person intended to engage in risky behaviors,
and (d) factors that were uncontrollable influenced the behavior. Survivors of
multiple AIDS-related loss may "violate" all four variables, increasing their
potential for social death, which is the consequence of stigmatization. Volunteer
or professional caregivers of persons with AIDS are blamed for putting themselves at risk for suffering multiple loss: "It's your own fault; you knew they
were going to die." The homosexual survivor is blamed for "choosing" to be
homosexual. A wide brush of blame stigmatizes members of minority communities who "get what they deserve."
   Symptoms of AIDS-related conditions are often visible and disfiguring.
Because AIDS vividly presents the issue of death, anxiety is inevitable. "All
individuals are confronted with death anxiety, most develop adaptive coping

modes" (Yalom, 1980, p. 110). Stigmatization of AIDS is an adaptation that allows a psychological separation from the source of anxiety. The stigmatized are different, separate, apart from. The wish to separate physically those with AIDS from the rest of society was explicitly voiced by Senator Jesse Helms when he said, "I think somewhere along the line that we're going to have to quarantine if we are really going to contain this disease" (as cited in Burkett, 1995, p. 296).

It is a mistake to think that only those with AIDS suffer the cruelty of stigmatization. The survivor often feels stigmatized by association with the victim (Shearer & McKusick, 1986). Mary Ann Perga (1995), who lives in the small community of Turtle Lake, Wisconsin, wrote,

> The sadness that it has brought me has not been the sorrow for which I had braced myself. Imagining that I would be moved by the sight of people suffering both emotional and physical pain, I thought that it would be painful watching them grow weaker. Instead, the people who have caused me anguish are ones who are not infected . . . because of their reaction toward those who have AIDS. . . . Every day, often in subtle ways, people with AIDS are treated cruelly by those who can attack the psyche more effectively than the virus is able to ravish the body. (p. A18)

Survivors suffer these indignities because the effects of stigmatization hurt the persons whom they love. Fear of stigmatization remains especially intense in rural communities where people are less familiar with AIDS.

Connection to homosexuality, drug users, and minorities greatly exacerbates its stigma. AIDS would be stigmatizing even if it were not so directly connected to groups that were "prestigmatized" (Nord, 1996a). Homophobia (Weinberg, 1972), the fearful attitude and aversion to things related to homosexuality, plays a significant role in the stigmatization (Dean et al., 1988) and social response to AIDS (Herek & Glunt, 1988). The complementary processes of homophobia and heterosexism shape social response to AIDS (Appelby, 1995). Mainly this is true because of the "homosexualization of AIDS" and "AIDSification of homosexuality" that inexorably links the two (Odets, 1995, pp. 101–105).

One does not have to be a homosexual, a drug user, or disenfranchised to be negatively affected by this stigma. "[H]emophiliacs and blood-transfusion recipients, who cannot by any stretch of 'blaming logic' be considered responsible for their illness, may be as ruthlessly ostracized by frightened people" (Sontag, 1989, p. 26). Association with these groups represented potential discrimination, violence, and vulnerability to hemophiliacs (Whitney, 1989).

Parents often feel the sting of stigmatization through the absence of support they receive. A woman who lost her son to AIDS said that everyone at her company knew about Evan's death "but not one person has said anything. They all look at me funny and avoid me. They seem embarrassed when they are around me." Foster parents who courageously take on the responsibility of raising children with AIDS face the effect of stigmatization. Some foster parents are shunned by neighbors, family, and friends. They may find their children and themselves isolated. "The result of this caution is an isolation of the foster parent from natural support networks" (Anderson, Gurdin, & Thomas, 1989, p. 48). Hemophiliac survivors report a fear of disclosing their losses (Brown & DeMaio, 1992). IVDUs are less likely to tell family than friends if they have HIV, fearing nonsupportive reactions within their family (Stowe et al., 1993). Even before AIDS, it was more difficult for gay men and lesbians to receive support while they mourned their losses (Siegal & Hoefer, 1981). AIDS has made disclosure even more difficult (Houseman & Pheifer, 1988).

One might imagine a lessening of stigmatization as familiarity and knowledge increase with time, but evidence has instead suggested an increased amount of stigma in the second decade of the AIDS epoch (Herek & Capitanio, 1993). Survivors may be subjected to "courtesy stigma" (Goffman, 1963), which is acquired by simple association with the victim. Garfield (1995) observed that "in an odd application of 'guilt by association,' more than one AIDS caregiver has felt the sting of social and even professional disapproval for working with people with AIDS" (p. 5).

Black and Hispanic Stigmatization Issues   Stigmatization of those with AIDS and those surviving AIDS-related loss is rampant in Black and Hispanic communities. Although the rate of HIV infection in these communities is disproportionately higher than in the White community, chronic denial is common. The survivor faces a troubling dilemma, fed by culture and history, that fosters stigmatization marked by fervent denial and judgmental blame.

Hispanics and Blacks suffer AIDS-related loss at a rate far higher than Whites. Seventeen percent of all AIDS cases are among Hispanics, and 34% are among Blacks (CDC, 1995). Rosenberg (1995) analyzed CDC statistics and back-calculated other data to determine, in Neergaard's words, "the most precise look at HIV prevalence to date" (Neergaard, 1995). He determined that among men 27 to 39 years old, the rate of HIV infection among Whites is 1 in 139; among Hispanics, 1 in 60; and among Blacks, 1 in 33. Among women 27 to 39 years old, the rate of HIV infection among Whites is 1 in 1,667; among Hispanics, 1 in 98; and among Blacks, 1 in 222. Nine out of 10 children with AIDS in New York City are Black or Hispanic (Atwood, 1993). Most Black community members are not aware of this extremely high rate of HIV incidence despite the fact that AIDS has been the leading cause of death among Black men aged 25–44 since 1991. Rosenberg (1995) concluded, "It is sobering to consider that 1 of every 50 black men in the United States aged 19 to 59 may be infected" (p. 1374). Thirty-two percent of all deaths among Black men and 22% of all deaths among Black women are AIDS related.

Given these extreme rates of HIV infection, it is astounding that so little awareness of multiple AIDS-related loss exists in the Black and Hispanic communities, but proof of denial abounds. The fact that the statistics offered above are surprising speaks to the rejection and neglect that underlie stigmatization. Although these statistics are alarming, they are also certainly understated. CDC literature observes that AIDS-related cases and deaths for Hispanics are understated by at least 30%. Damian Pardo, the president of the board of Health Crisis Network said, speaking of AIDS in the Hispanic community, that "the numbers are not accurate—that the actual cases are far higher. Everyone in the community lies about HIV" (as cited in Bardach, 1995, p. 27).

Among Blacks, AIDS brings up the most embarrassing issues for the community, including drug use, prostitution, and teen pregnancy. Black people have felt blamed for the disease because of its origins in Africa and its early prevalence in Haiti. Conspiracy theories have flourished in fertile ground in the Black community. These have included alleged plots by Whites to destroy Blacks and conspiracies to ignore the AIDS "cure," Kemron (Burkett, 1995). In a 1990 study by the Southern Christian Leadership Conference, more than one third of Blacks agreed that AIDS was a form of genocide against Blacks; another third were unsure. More than a third believed that HIV was produced in a germ warfare lab (Rosin, 1995). Hostile attitudes toward homosexuality, often fueled by Black church leaders, further contribute to ambivalence and stigmatization toward infected persons and survivors.

No more telling fact could support the extreme stigmatization that permeates Black and Hispanic attitudes toward AIDS than the fact that AIDS is ignored and denied. Drug use, crime, high rates of Black male imprisonment, out-of-wedlock pregnancies, and irresponsibility among Black men are regularly discussed; AIDS is not. The shame surrounding AIDS in Black America is evidenced by its denial and by the fear of becoming a pariah when one tells the truth. One reason for this, cited by Rosin (1995, p. 21), is "uneasiness in the community about open homosexuality, still closely associated with the disease." Rosin quoted Frank Oldham, a former director of Washington's Agency for HIV/AIDS, as saying that among Blacks there are "a huge number of bisexual men who don't identify as gay. It's fascinating: they go to church, to the park with their families, then at night you'll see them cruising the gay bars" (p. 21). Rosin observed that open homosexuality is viewed as something imposed by the gay White culture (p. 21). Thus, AIDS stigmatization is doubly exacerbated by connection to homosexuality and White culture. Blacks may feel estranged from AIDS support networks because of their color and from Black support networks because of perceived connection to homosexuality (Roberts, 1995).

Hispanics also face historic and cultural issues that provoke stigmatization surrounding AIDS. Bardach (1995) quoted a person who has worked in East Los Angeles for 21 years and was a case manager for HIV patients as saying, "Nothing is ever said. The entire community is in denial. They just don't believe it is happening. They think that AIDS is about gay white males" (p. 31). Cultural considerations, especially those surrounding the machismo ethic, strongly condemn homosexuality. Men who have sex with men often do not identify themselves as gay. That is how they avoid discrimination, according to Freddie Rodriguez, a Health Crisis Network worker, who said, "Ours is a culture of denial" (cited in Bardach, 1995, p. 27).

Family and community are vitally important to most Hispanics. To speak of AIDS, as a victim or survivor, is to pay a "huge price—a shattering loss of esteem within the family and community" (Bardach, 1995, p. 28). "Latino families tend to regard homosexuality as a source of shame and dishonor" (Morales, 1995, p. 93). The connection between AIDS and homosexuality serves to stigmatize those affected in a way that is more debilitating than the stigmatization affecting other communities. Grief is mainly handled within the Hispanic family (Shapiro, 1995), but AIDS-related grief may often remain a closely guarded secret. When stigmatization prevents the expression and work of grief, survivors are injured.

CONCLUSION

The phenomenon of multiple AIDS-related loss is new. This chapter has laid the foundation for understanding the survivor's experience by outlining the characteristics of this disaster and describing common survivor responses. The next chapter presents the stories of two more survivors. In their stories, the reader will be able to identify a number of the issues raised in this chapter.

Chapter 4

Survivors' Experiences: II

The thought that we are enduring the unendurable is one of the things that keeps us going.—Molly Haskell (1994, p. 4)

This chapter presents the stories of two more survivors of multiple AIDS-related loss. It is placed after the preceding chapters because the reader now has a better conceptual understanding of the experience of surviving multiple, ongoing loss. Keith is a gay man who tested HIV positive several years ago. Besides losing several friends and lovers to AIDS, Keith has struggled with some of the common issues faced by survivors, such as drug and alcohol abuse, subintentional suicide, and spirituality. Terry is a heterosexual woman who tests negative and continues a long period of multiple-loss exposure through professional and volunteer work. She observes much change and growth from her experience.

KEITH ARNETT: A SURVIVOR OF MULTIPLE LOSS, LIVING WITH AIDS

> **Keith:** *The first loss that I had personally was in 1984; my best friend John was diagnosed with AIDS, and I don't use the term* best friend

lightly. He really was my best friend. He got sick and he fought like hell. He stayed alive, but he was very sick. He was pretty miserable. He died in 1987, and that was the first memorial service that I ever went to. I remember being pretty devastated.

His loss was devastating to me emotionally, especially after I found out that I was positive also. I remember him being the first person I talked to about being positive. We spent hours and hours and hours on the telephone. So, his death was a pretty big loss for me.

I was battling depression at the time, and it seemed insurmountable. I was feeling alone and depressed and that was tied into hopelessness. I was not able to be present with him in a physical way through his illness. On the telephone I was able, but very rarely could I see him in person. Partly because that was the way he wanted it because he didn't look very good anymore, and partly because my partner at the time was terrified that I would get something. He was not very rational about that. He was fearful of contagiousness. It was a real point of frustration for me because I couldn't be there for him physically. I really wanted to go by, say "hi," and give him a squeeze.

In 1989, I started going to the Seattle AIDS Support Group [SASG is much more than a support group. It is a big house with many activities, including volunteer opportunities.], *and I met a man named Alfy; his real name was Jim Thorne. We hit it off pretty good. I became his last boyfriend, his caregiver–boyfriend. He was very important to me, and looking after him was the bright spot of my life. It was painful and it was hurtful. Part of the reason I wanted to be there for Alfy was that I hadn't been able to be there for John.*

I was crazy about him. I really was. I was crazy about him. He wasn't perfect at all. He was a recovering person and so was I. It was a good friendship, a real good friendship. It was quite a great thing. He died within 6 months of my having met him. Again, it was really tough. I felt like I would fall apart for a while. I moved into SASG because I didn't know what to do with myself. I would come home alone. I couldn't see my therapist every day. I wasn't going to meetings at the time. I just wasn't connected.

While I was camping out at SASG, I met Skip Wright. From all outward appearances, Skip was as healthy as a horse, totally involved in life and just having a great time. We started dating in very short order. On our second date, or something incredible like that, I promised him that I would always take care of him. And I did that for the next 6 years. He was such a creative spirit and always on the go, just a real doer. He wouldn't lie around and be sick even though sometimes he was, at times, terribly ill. He would usually rise to the occasion and manage to have a pretty good time. He was good for me. He told me once, a few months before he died, that he really had need of a rock, and I could admit that I had really needed a kite. It was a great match; we were opposite from each other in most every way except that we cared a lot for each other.

He died this past July and had AIDS for 7 years when he died. He never knew how long he had been positive. He was an amazing person. He was incredible. I miss him terribly. I still miss him terribly.

The other day a friend and I were in a restaurant. He told me that he had seen Skip's name on a plaque at Rainbow Lodge, and I just lost it. We were in a public restaurant having dinner, and I just lost it. All these months later it came out. I don't mean that I teared up a little bit, I mean I cried. Because I still miss him terribly, and I kind of wonder if this really happened. But it was a Sunday, and those are typically the worst days for me around grief and loss.

While Skip and I were together, in 1993, my ex-partner Gene took a turn for the worse. He was happily remarried to somebody who was healthier than him. He had AIDS also. His new partner was my age, and they were getting along pretty good. Gene was needing a lot of looking after. All of a sudden his partner died. So it was like "Oh my God, who's going to take care of Gene?" having no idea that it was going to be me.

Within a month or so he was placed in Bailey Boushay house [a hospice for people with AIDS]. *He had nobody. He had absolutely nobody. He was not exactly a friendly person who had a support system. He kind of just had me. So, I took my focus off Skip for a while. I was Gene's pretty much everything. I was his liaison at Bailey Boushay, his power of attorney, his executor.*

He lived there from December to April; then, he finally let go. It was a healing time because we had parted on very bad terms. That was a 5-year relationship.

David: *What other losses have you had?*

K: *Of course, there's been a lot of friends. My first boyfriend, when I moved to Seattle, is dead. I looked after him a bit, not as much as I would have liked to but it was just too difficult at the time. I finally accepted that I just cannot be there all the time for everybody. That has been an ongoing realization. I am still learning it because I want to be there all the time for everybody, but it doesn't mean that I can. Right now my friend Chris is at Bailey. He moved in the week after Skip died. He's been like a little brother to me. It's been really tough to see him. I tell him that I will be there at a specific time, and I am always late because I just do not want to go. I don't want to go there. I don't want to go there. It is so . . . hard sometimes that I'd rather scour the bathroom than go there. I could pick my least favorite thing to do, and most days I would rather do that than go there.*

I have never seen the physical depths in anybody that Chris has gone to. He is 80 pounds; he is unrecognizable. It's . . . the KS [Kaposi's sarcoma] has gone crazy and. . . . No one has any idea what he is still doing here, but his spirit is not ready yet, I guess. I'm still seeing him twice or three times a week and that's as much as I can do.

He has a partner and, I think, some other friends that stop by. He can't really determine reality from fiction. He's on a lot of morphine, and I'm pretty sure that he has dementia. The other night he was watching something on television. It didn't seem like he was watching it. It was all about prison, death row and all that stuff. He sort of put himself in that place. That's where he was. He wasn't at Bailey anymore, he was someplace else. He says, "They put me in here to die." So, he's hearing all this stuff about death row and executions. His eyes got as big as half-dollars, and he said, "What are they going to do to me? Do you think they will hang me?"

It's so heartbreaking that I just have to laugh, otherwise I'd just cry all the time.

[Keith interrupted his account to ask David to emphasize that his sense of humor has been a source of strength and perspective.]

K: *I've been present at the time of death for, I can't remember how many folks.*

D: *Is there one overshadowing death?*

K: *Skip.*

There was a period of numbness. I don't know how long, but I would go from numb to really knowing he was dying, feeling all that pain, and then I would go back to numb. I didn't feel like I was in control of that. When I was busy at the task at hand, I didn't have to deal with the grief or loss. So I kept absurdly busy.

Closing up his apartment and selling things and giving things away and hanging onto things that I just couldn't part with. . . .

I felt like I lived in a storage locker with a view. There was a lot of stuff that I just couldn't give away. I don't believe in storage lockers, especially if you know you are never going to move into a larger place. What's the point? In a large way, I still feel like I'm living in the Skip Wright Memorial Museum. It could have been a lot worse. I could have hung onto absolutely everything he ever made or did.

At this point, Keith points out a number of beautiful stained-glass objects around the apartment and speaks proudly of Skip's works that are displayed in SASG and Bailey Boushay.

K: *Of course, his picture is up all over the place, but little by little a lot of the memories have gone into drawers.*

Me and some of my friends went to Hawaii and scattered his ashes at his favorite beach. We managed to have a pretty good time despite our reason for going there.

D: *When did you first realize the extent of loss that was occurring in your life?*

K: *I'm not sure that I remember, but I recall knowing in my innermost self that there was no relief in sight. Except, I think that I will have a personal reprieve because there is nobody that I'm really close to who is very ill and on the wait list for Bailey. It may be quite a while.*

I know there's no end in sight, and so I try to keep optimistic about my own health, but every once in a while the reality bleeds through. I've been incredibly lucky; it will be 11 years this January. Just some infections and discomfort, nothing disabling, nothing immobilizing.

With each person's illness and passing, all through their illness and all through their dying process, I have at times visualized myself in their place, not for long, it's not the kind of place I like to go very often, but I find myself going there. It's actually too awful for me to consider for too long, so I try to focus in on something else, but it's scary. I do know that I want to fast forward through the parts at the end.

D: *Have you kept track of your losses?*

K: *I can't keep track anymore. I used to remember everybody's death-day. Some I still remember, but some, it's all gone. I had quite a fat file before I quit cutting out obituaries and memorial service programs. I still have a lot of things, but I haven't added to them in a while.*

D: *Are there particularly difficult times during the year?*

K: *September is difficult. September 2nd was the anniversary of our first date. That didn't go by unnoticed, I can assure you. Skip's memorial service was August the 20th. That was the day we picked in advance for our marriage. We had the date all picked out, we worked on that together. That didn't go by unnoticed.*

And December, I am dreading December. His birthday was December the 14th. He was a big Christmas kid. Whereas I don't *want to be home for Christmas!*

D: *Are your parents supportive about your multiple losses?*

K: *They don't get it. They don't show any recognition of the relationship with Skip. It was 2 weeks before I even found it necessary to pick up the phone and tell them that Skip died. I just don't rely on my parents very much for that sort of thing. They're just not there. It's really too awful for them to bear because of the disease that I have.*

A gay relationship doesn't really command the type of respect that a heterosexual relationship does. I've learned that again, and again, and again. I don't like that.

My Mom is as supportive as she humanly knows how. Sometimes it doesn't seem like enough but I think she's trying. She walked in the walk! The AIDS Walk L.A. I am quite proud of her for that.

My grandmother knew. My grandmother knew, and I knew that my grandmother knew. Because I could relate to what she was going through with the loss of all of her friends. I know that she spent the last 10 years of her life in grief paralysis. She couldn't even speak of a friend without bawling. She would stand and just cry for a while. Very sad.

D: *How would you describe your family of choice?*

K: *It is actually AIDS that gave me my family of choice. Most of the people I consider family today I met at SASG through groups, volunteering, whatever. I've been there for 6 years. Now it might only be 1 day a week, but it is a constant. It is the only constant in my life. If it's noon on Monday, I should be there. That's how it's been since August of '89. That was right after Alfy died, and I did not know what to do with myself.*

The big picture of my life is pretty terrific. It's probably better than it has ever been, but some of the close-up individual frames are. . . .

There are some low periods during some days that really seem insurmountable.

D: *Of what value is your volunteer work to you?*

K: *It is very important. It keeps me out of my own quagmire. It's helped me to be more social. Before I went into treatment, this last time, I had pretty much been a vegetable in a recliner. As I got more and more addicted to pills, not knowing what was happening at first, but then knowing and then keeping it very secret. I used to say that my favorite thing was to sit in that chair and stare out the window. And I had most everybody convinced that I was actually happy.*

It's really helpful to be more social. Even during my heavy, heavy pill-taking years, SASG was the one constant thing I did.

You know there are some people I just won't talk to about this because they don't understand. They say stupid things that annoy the hell out of me and so, I don't talk about it. Fortunately, there are those who I can talk to about it with. They know because they are in this too, and they know exactly what I am saying and I know exactly what they are saying. I hang out with a lot of widows; we get it.

Keith describes a way he gains support from supporting others.

K: *Being present for others and listening to them say "ouch" when it hurts. Why does that help? I don't have any idea why that helps me. All I can be is a good listener at times. If I can just listen and try to imagine what it is that they are living with. For at least that moment in time, I am not thinking about me and my shit, my problems, myself.*

That's what I've mainly done with Chris. And especially once they have gone to Bailey. It's the last stop! Everyone knows that. With him, I remind him that this is the final chapter and that pretty soon he will find out.

D: *Did your use of alcohol and drugs have anything to do with your grief?*

K: *Yes, it was all about numbing out; it was all about numbing out, all about numbing out. The greater the pain, the greater the desire to mellow out.*

I set out in a drunken rage to get infected, and that's what happened. That's what happened. I wear a lot of political buttons. One you almost always will see me with is "High Equals High Risk." That's exactly my story. I wouldn't have it if not for some of the stupid things that I did when I was loaded and hating myself.

It was January of '85. There were four guys, three of them in one night at the old Dave's whorehouse [a gay bathhouse]. I was all fucked up. I intended to just go throw myself off the bridge after it was all over because I was so upset over John. I was upset about life. I hated everybody, especially myself. But I had such a good time at Dave's whorehouse that I decided that I didn't want to jump off the bridge. Then I freaked out. So, I know when and where.

D: *You said this was in response to John. Do you think if you had known a healthy way to handle your grief and get support that you might test negative today?*

K: *Yeah, I do. I do. I think that's highly possible. I willfully and self-ishly, in a long pattern of self-destructive decisions, set out to give myself the ultimate insult. I have lived to regret that, and I have also lived long enough to forgive myself, to a large extent. I no longer judge myself as harshly as I did then.*

D: *What has helped you cope with multiple loss?*

K: *Probably this ever-growing, little, tiny bit of faith I have. Some kind of plan that I do not get at all. I am not privy to that information just yet. It makes no sense to me at all, but I try not to have contempt about it, about the plan, not knowing the whole scheme of things. I just accept and accept and accept and accept and accept. There is so little I can do.*

During the past 12 or 13 years, they have learned much about the human immune system, and I think also they have learned much about the human capacity for caring and grieving. America doesn't like to grieve. Human beings don't like to grieve, but especially not Ameri-cans. It's just not OK. Somebody, sometime will tell you that "You just got to get over this now." I don't. I still have a big ache in my heart for John.

D: *Do you ever think you will ever reach a sense of resolution or acceptance?*

K: *I have no idea.* [There is a long pause.] *No, I expect that I won't have to think about it every single day and that I won't be immobilized by it all the time, but I still hurt for the ones that were the first to go.*

D: *What about the impact on the gay community?*

[Keith is quiet]

K: *It's been huge.* [Again, he is quiet.] *I sense that through the loss there is a unity that seems to happen. The emotional bonding that's taken place among gay men and lesbians. Collectively, as diverse as we all are, a positive unity has come out of it, a united front to lobby.*

There's also a tremendous amount of cynicism that's come into life in general in the gay community. The inevitability of getting HIV that a lot of guys feel. That's absolutely horrifying to me. I am one of those guys.

D: *Do you have any rituals, other than memorial services, that help you?*

K: *The AIDS Vigil I can do. The Quilt absolutely just sends me over the edge, at least the last time that I saw it. I don't want to see the Quilt again. I am not making a panel for Skip. I don't know if his mom is either. For myself, I don't want one. I think it's a wonderful thought, but there is nowhere on earth that's big enough to set up the whole quilt. Let's just move on.*

So, I have some of my own cynicism, don't I? It's just too much for me. I was such a wreck for the next several days after I saw it. I saw just a partial display at the Convention Center here a few years ago. It was absolutely awful. It was way too much for me.

I don't know how we live with all this really, all this grief. I just don't know how we do it.

D: *What do you envision for the future?*

K: *Well, I am pretty optimistic with scientific promises for those of us who still have some semblance of an immune system. In terms of curing AIDS, I don't think that's going to happen in my lifetime.*

I hope that as the whole country becomes more and more involved in this disease and others that take the lives of children and young people, merciless diseases that bring on so much guilt, and so much hurt. I hope collectively, as a country at least, as a result of AIDS, we can learn how to grieve.

D: *You just mentioned guilt. Have you had any experience with survivor's guilt?*

K: *Huge. It's not a rational thing. That doesn't mean it doesn't harm us. Sometimes I am angry that I am still here and the others. . . .*

I don't think I entered adolescence with abandonment issues, but I certainly have them today. [laughs] *You know its just like, please don't leave me. I'm real over being left. I'm really over it. People get sick and die or move away. I can accept a lot, but I still don't like it.*

D: *What positive experiences have resulted from all this?*

K: *I know that I will never be the same again, and in a sense, that's good. With every person's death that I have been a part of, their health care and their death, as they passed on, and if I happened to be there during their passing, it is absolutely a life-changing experience that I can't explain. Any fear that I once had about death has been greatly relieved from being a party to some very lovely passings. Skip's passing was textbook wonderful. It was everything he wanted. It was swift. It was dignified. It was private. It was just us. He just went to sleep, went into a coma, within 11 hours. . . .*

He was beautiful.

Some of my friends knew, some I called, some called others. A small group of us were there with him at Bailey for quite a while. They asked me if I wanted to call the mortuary, and I said, "No, no, not at all." We didn't ignore him or anything. We were still there. He just wasn't using that particular body anymore, but he was still there.

I put my sunglasses on his face. It was like the Blues Brothers, or something. We chuckled about that. I don't know; it was a very good day.

It's a very emotional, life-altering experience to be present and love someone while they are in their passing. I wish that none of my friends would go, but they are. In some way I know that I helped ease them through that in my own small way.

I know that this has not always been unselfish. I think that all this care-giving stuff that's happened over the past few years is like insurance that someone will be there for me. I don't know who. I just know that I will be taken care of, so I don't obsessively worry about that.

When I was first diagnosed, I spent the next 2 years planning my memorial service, selections of music, every dirge that I could dig up. I was just insane; I was just totally sure that each month was my last. That's been a very important thing to work through and get past. We always seem to change when we are not looking, maybe especially when we are not looking.

Widows, traditionally, travel extensively. Do you know what a crone is?

D: *No.*

K: *A crone is generally applied to an old woman who helps people die. It's like the opposite of a midwife, sort of like the wise old woman. Sometime, I feel like a crone. But sometimes I just feel angry that I am deserted.*

There's that plan again. I don't know the whole scheme of it. After being very angry for a long time, I find that really useless. To remain angry all the time just doesn't serve me well. My fondest remark these days is "I don't know." I have some theories but who doesn't? Anyhow, they're cheap.

TERRY JOHNSON: A HETEROSEXUAL CAREGIVER

Terry and I first met in 1990 during a training for Shanti, a volunteer organization that provides emotional support for persons dealing with AIDS. When Bailey Boushay, a hospice and day health care facility for people with AIDS, began, Terry volunteered for a while and was soon hired as a staff person in the day health facility. Terry alerted me, right away, to strong emotions she was feeling the day we met. Our interview took place

right on the heels of a client's death who I was very, very close to. Not being at work for the last week, last night I went and saw the Passage Board with eight new names on it. It was unsettling. When you are there every day and names are put up every day, its different. So, I'm feeling just a little emotional.

Terry's first contact with AIDS came in 1990.

I had two adult children who were sexually active. AIDS was getting a lot of press. I was fearful about AIDS. I didn't know anything. I knew the cursory stuff, but I didn't know if I needed to be concerned about my children, so it was important for me. Knowledge counters fear in my mind. So, getting the knowledge about AIDS helped. The other aspect was that I wanted to give some time volunteering. It was either battered women or AIDS. I thought it would be easier for people to volunteer in the battered women's area because of so much of the stigma around AIDS, the perception that it was a gay disease. I felt that I could be of service. So, I took the chance that I could make a difference. It's such a cliché to say that AIDS has changed my life, but I really don't think there's any other way to say it. AIDS has changed my life.

Prior to getting into AIDS in 1990, I would categorize myself as pretty white-bread America, middle class, a circle of friends that was not as diverse as it could be, certainly they were more like me than not like me, and Republican, and so was I. My views have evolved and changed. My experiences now have exposed me to people from a very wide spectrum of social and economic backgrounds: people who are homeless, prostitutes, and drug addicts, people with a history of crime, people with a history of far more dysfunctional families than I come from. People have experienced physical abuse that I cannot even repeat. And lifestyles that are much different than mine. From that perspective, it has enriched my life. I consider each experience to be a gift, such as interacting with a prostitute. In the past I don't think I would have reacted as caringly and lovingly towards an individual who, in my perception, made those choices. I've now come to realize that sometimes people do what they have to do to survive. My approach to survival might differ and it doesn't mean I'm better. It's taught me a lot about judgment, about being judgmental.

At first Terry kept a list of people she knew who died of AIDS. "I had a fear of not being able to remember them." After 6 months and 68 names, she realized that she couldn't keep doing that. Now she says, "I don't want to know the numbers. I remember a face, a name."

T: *I have pictures. I have a lot of pictures. Pictures that were given me, or pictures that are taken of the two of us together or pictures that were taken at work. I have some pictures on my board at work.*

A lot of people with AIDS seem to have a gift for the written word. I am so blown away by it. A lot of clients have given me poems, and those are really treasured.

Sometimes, they bring me a flower and I will dry and press the flower. I have a box and every so often, not very often, but every once in a while, I will take out the box. What I will do with it, I don't know.

I think that working in this environment, day after day, with people constantly dying around you, is bizarre. When I started working at Bailey there were 33 clients; right now I think there are only 4 clients left, maybe 5, that were there when I got there.

I am around them all day long. I see them at their best and at their worst. I am with them day in and day out. I think it's a very abnormal environment. So much work is done around normalizing what is abnormal. I have learned how to normalize the chaos.

I was recently asked by someone in my old circle of friends, "How do you do it?" Sometimes I feel that there is a sense of awe, a sense that "I couldn't do this." But I don't happen to believe that. I think

that anyone could do this because it sort of gets under your skin. You can't be around people that you begin to really care about, that you see with so many challenges, and not feel compassion.
D: *Is there an overshadowing loss for you?*
T: *Yes, a person who I let get to me. I didn't keep my boundaries: Levy. He was an enigma to me. At first I thought there was very little about this person that I will be able to identify with and connect with him on. He was homeless, and had been living that way for years, a crack addict, had a history of crime, a sort of arrogant air about him and a hustler. But our relationship did evolve and despite all those challenges in his life, he had an incredible thoughtful and caring side to him.*
D: *Do you recall the day he died?*
T: *November the 6th, 1994. I didn't anticipate that the death of Levy would be so hard or that the anniversary would be so difficult.*

She also remembers another date: March 20, the date of Steve's birthday. Some years she sends a card to his mother; other years she visits his grave and leaves a rose.

T: *April is hard, it's the month my first Shanti client died. October and November are always hard because I remember Levy dying.*
Actually, around March, March 20th to be exact, is a difficult time for me. It reminds me of the time of Steve's birthday [chokes up and softly cries], *and I think a lot about him and that's one of the real hard times. Something around those times, I remember.*
Sometimes it's not the client who just died that I am grieving over. It's something about someone else. In this case it was clear.
D: *Are there losses, other than deaths, for you?*
T: *There are a lot of other losses, besides death, that I've experienced: friendships, loss of confidence in the government, and personally, my own loss of control. Control has been a big thing in my life, and I have had to grieve my lack of control in this situation. Oh, I am still a bit of a control freak, but I have learned what I can and cannot control.*
I think I've become enlightened about the government and the politics of AIDS. Certainly it has changed my views and which way I tend to lean now.
It's impacted my values systems. I am far more accepting and forgiving and less judgmental around people.
It's also helped me on my own spiritual journey. In the past, I was too busy or it was too easy to avoid it. So, it's given me an opportunity to really, sort of look at my own spirituality, and I feel blessed because of that because I feel that I am much more spiritual than I was 5 years ago. I am still evolving. My views on death have changed. I don't want to say that I am more blasé, but I do see it as a part of life and living.
I have learned a tremendous amount about unconditional love and

*the building of community. I never believed that love could make such
a difference.*

D: *Have your relationships with other people changed?*

T: *I like to be around people who are nonjudgmental. I like people
who don't care what the rest of the world thinks about them.*

*In terms of new relationships, I don't tend to get as close to clients
as I would have in the past. I maintain, for me, a somewhat safe emotional distance. I don't make myself available all the time.*

*In terms of my relationship with people, I tend now to be more
attracted to people who I see as willing to go the distance, step up to
the challenge, people who are compassionate and caring people. I'm
not sure I would have gone that direction in the past. I also find myself
more attracted to people who are willing to talk about what they are
feeling and willing to look at life's issues and talk about those in a
sharing sort of experience, a mutual experience.*

D: *It sounds like there are a lot of positives arising from your experience.*

T: *I have given a lot, in the work I do, but it doesn't compare to all
that I have gotten back. At some level, I feel a little guilty about that.
Mostly I feel grateful. I continue to marvel about the men and women
I work with who have given so much of their life to helping others with
AIDS.*

D: *How have you changed since your early work with AIDS?*

T: *Well, being a recovering codependent I can certainly say that my
earliest experience was wanting to love every one of them. But, I had
to learn. I am getting better at limit setting and boundaries and being
more clear about what I can do and can't do and knowing the difference. In the beginning, I thought that I could help someone; I could
make their life better. I have come to find out that none of that is true,
really. I can be there for someone, I mean really be there, as a good
listener to the degree they want to share. I can't take away their pain.
I can't fix their dysfunctional families. My expectations are different
from what they were.*

*When I first got involved, I did a tremendous amount of visiting
people in the hospital. I went to the hospital and visited almost every
single client whether they were on my caseload or not. There was a
piece of me that felt like someone needed to maintain that connection
so they would know that someone cared. That is an example of me
overstepping my boundaries. I had to learn to let go of that. I became
more selective about the memorial services I attended and the hospital
visits. Now, they are either with someone I have a very solid connection with or someone whom I felt that nobody, no one would be there
for them. So I would stop by with a magazine or something. Oftentimes
the look on their face made it all worthwhile.*

D: *What are your experiences with memorial services?*

T: *The memorial services, I think, are more for the people attending
than they are for the person who has died. For most people, it is a time
of closure.*

Terry had just attended a memorial service the day before. She quietly cries.

> **T:** *What is making me emotional is that he lived in the same building that my friend Levy lived in and he died on the same day that Levy died and I attended the memorial service, yesterday, in a chapel that was in the same building where they both lived. It brought up a lot of stuff. So, I think it was more about my ongoing grief about Levy than it was for that particular client.*
>
> **D:** *Do you ever notice yourself shutting down or becoming numb?*
>
> **T:** *You know, it's interesting. Sometimes when a client passes that I was particularly close to, I don't cry, and I'm a very emotional person. I tend to cry easily. I have wondered what that's about. At other times, it's a person who I didn't really have a connection with at all, but it brings on a floodgate. I am not sure what that's about but it does and when it does, I let it be. Sometimes I feel very sad, very vulnerable, and it is a challenge to be emotionally available for others.*
>
> *I am not as emotional. At other times, I have to step back and be OK with it, but I don't think I've developed any kind of callousness. I think if I started feeling callous I would not continue with this work.*
>
> **D:** *What else have you learned?*
>
> **T:** *I have learned something very important about community, about unconditional love and acceptance. It's very powerful; it brings people back. Oftentimes it is the only time they have ever felt that love, that acceptance in their life. That gives me a tremendous sense of it being the right thing to do. I want to be a part of this. This is powerful. This is giving some increased quality of life to people at a time when. . . .*
>
> *But that can be a challenge because people can be absolute assholes. Some of the people we deal with come from tremendously challenging backgrounds, preexisting psych diagnosis, so they can act very unloving, unfeeling, uncaring. But that never changes the way we treat them. That person is still as cared about as the person who wouldn't give you any grief at all, who wouldn't complain about a thing. There seems to be no change in how that love is shared. There is power in that. I think it helps people live longer.*
>
> **D:** *Do you ever encounter any attitudes of what I call narcissistic entitlement in your clients?*
>
> **T:** *When people have been denied most of their life, at some level, when they start getting it, they feel that sense of entitlement. A good example are street people; about 10% of our population are street people. When they first start coming in, we have food available all the time and you can eat as much as you want. They will take platefuls and platefuls of food to their table. There is no way that they can eat it all in one sitting, but they are afraid that they will not get what they feel they are entitled to. We have to work with them to help them see that there is as much food as they want, it's available, they don't need to do that. We have to help people learn those skills.*

Certainly our community meetings are a challenge because it is a time for people to be able to speak out about things as they perceive them in the community. Some people do have that strong sense of "This is owed me." "The food is lousy here." Well, as one staff member said, "The last time I checked it was free." But there is that sense. I don't find myself getting angry about it. There is no point in getting angry about it. There is an inability on those individuals' part to see the reality as it is. You just learn to be forgiving. If that kind of behavior came from my children I would respond differently. I look at people who haven't had, or who have experienced things so far beyond my imagination. Who am I to say, you don't deserve it? There is no sense of being angry about their sense of entitlement.

D: *What about anger?*

T: *We see anger, sometimes rage, especially in our clients who have preexisting psych issues. Prior to ever getting AIDS, they already have psych challenges. I think AIDS exacerbates it. It makes them more angry. It makes them more fearful. So, I see that played out. We do spend a significant amount of time talking about safety in the community to be able to temper that rage, not to squelch it, but to be able to handle that rage in a positive way, to help people express that rage. "What is that rage really about? It's not about the food here. It's not about the person who sat down at the table next to you when you didn't want them to sit there. It's not about the fact that your care manager said 'no' to a request. That's not what it's really about." We spend a lot of time helping people work through that rage so they can feel that it's OK to be angry but it's about how you act.*

D: *How do you cope with multiple loss?*

T: *Some times better than others. I talk about my feelings, seek some ritual of closure, pray and cry. The main thing I do is give myself permission to grieve, experience it, talk about it with others and know that this too shall pass, in time.*

I see so many [people with AIDS] *that have no family or friends. I am able to give something back, to leave my mark by making a meaningful contribution to the world and a few people in it.*

D: *As of today, do you think you have reached some point of resolution, and, if not, do you think you ever will?*

T: *No, and I hope not. I feel grief is a process. My work has exposed me to that process. I think it has given me a lot of comfort because in the past I saw it as something to get over. Sometimes I believe "yes," then for some unexplained reason, something will happen that will trigger a thought or memory of someone who is no longer here. Sometimes it makes me feel very sad, but often I feel grateful that I have these recurring periods to remind me of the special people who have touched my life. That is probably the message; "don't forget me." I hope I don't ever fully resolve my grief, but certainly it takes on a different look.*

Because I am constantly working in an environment where there are multiple losses, where I feel more connected to some people than to

others, that will be constantly evolving. I feel more accepting about one client while, with another, I will be more angry or disbelieving.
D: *What do you envision for the future?*
T: *I am not a future tripper. I tend to have a positive outlook about things.*

I am disappointed in the government's lack of response. Lack of government support and cutbacks in funding when the numbers keep growing. I tend not to have a lot of hope for the future around AIDS issues. There are good things happening out there. I really try to focus on the present so I don't spend much time thinking about the future. I wish that I could say that I was positive about the future, but I don't feel that way. I think it's going to get worse.

A lot of people who think this will never affect them, the "It won't happen to me syndrome," sadden me because it is something they are unprepared for. It's going to be really challenging for them.

I don't think I walk around with a dark cloud over my head. I don't feel sad. I don't feel sad. I think certainly that there is a component of that but if I sat around and thought about it all the time or got obsessed with it, I would get mired in it. I accept death, grieving, and loss as natural parts of living. They are as much about living as life itself. So, you lose things and you just learn to deal with it. You have to come to a sense of acceptance. That doesn't mean you ever learn to like it. It doesn't mean that the pain ever really goes away.

Keith and Terry come from very different backgrounds but experience some similar effects of multiple AIDS-related loss. They both observed that AIDS had dramatically changed their lives. Their relationships with other people have been affected by AIDS, and they report a deepening in the value they place on their relationships with others. Keith's story demonstrated the potential for unresolved grief and survivor's guilt to lead to self-destructive behaviors. Terry sees a distinction in her life "prior to getting into AIDS" and the way her life is now. Both of their stories help to explain the impact of AIDS on survivors' lives.

Part Two

Theoretical Perspectives on Multiple AIDS-Related Loss

This part explains the experience of surviving multiple AIDS-related loss through different theoretical perspectives. Chapter 5 analyzes the grief that naturally arises and presents a new definition of grief necessitated by the realities of the experience. Chapter 6 reviews common psychological complications that survivors face when grieving and adjusting to multiple loss. Chapter 7 carefully outlines the factors that legitimize naming multiple AIDS-related loss as a form of traumatization. In chapter 8 the impact of AIDS on families of origin and choice is looked at. It makes the argument that the extreme nature of this experience proves that families of choice are just as valid as traditional families.

Chapter 5

Grieving Multiple Losses

I wish I could translate the hints of dead young men.—Walt Whitman

Existing grief theory provides a foundation for understanding the experience, and treating the complications, of surviving multiple AIDS-related loss, but it has limitations. Because traditional grief theory and practice tend to focus on an individual response to a single event of loss, they fail to explain a loss sequence that is multiple, ongoing, and community wide. The traditional bereavement model is inadequate (Bidgood, 1992). Further, the interrelated characteristics of AIDS-related loss—including the quantity of loss, cumulative effect, relentlessness of loss, age inappropriateness, protracted and episodic nature, grueling illness, etiology, and stigmatization—distinguish this experience from most other grief experiences. This chapter assesses how these unique characteristics influence the grief experience of survivors.

Limitations of existing theory combine with the extreme nature of multiple, ongoing loss to offer an opportunity to augment existing theory and discover novel approaches to treatment. This chapter, and the next, are meant to broaden perspectives on grief and bereavement. This is necessary, in part, because as "the manner in which humans live and die has changed, so must our conceptualization of 'normal' mourning behavior change as well" (Sprang & McNeil, 1995, p. viii). As Sprang and McNeil (1995) concluded, "To apply traditional models of grief across all populations, irrespective of the manner of dying, is injudicious and limits the clinician's ability to appropriately assess and intervene" (p. viii).

Grieving multiple, ongoing loss is a fundamentally different experience than grieving other types of losses. Both individual and global losses must be considered when assessing and adjusting to multiple AIDS-related loss; failure to account for both will handicap the adjustment process. If, for the survivor, "the grief may never end" (Colburn & Malena, 1988, p. 23), as the majority of survivors in Shrader's (1992) study believed, survivors must adjust to an environment of chronic grief.

GRIEF THEORY

Definition of Grief

Grief is the Process and Work of Adjusting to Irrevocably Lost Objects, Relationships, and Dreams   This definition acknowledges responses arising spontaneously in the survivor as well as those that are chosen. It realistically emphasizes the necessary perspective that these various losses are irrevocable and, therefore, necessitate acceptance and adjustment. This definition acknowledges that grieving arises as a natural response to more than dead people. Grieving also arises from lost communities, dreams, material goods, and expectations. Multiple AIDS-related loss makes this distinction important in a way that single-loss events do not. Previous definitions of grief arose from singular loss events, usually deaths, that do not include the ramifications of multiple loss. To encompass the truth of grief, a definition of grief must explicitly state that grieving is work, does involve irrevocable loss, and arises from various losses. A definition declaring grief simply a response (Kastenbaum, 1977; Martocchio, 1985), reaction (Crow, 1991), or process (Rando, 1984) implies to the survivor and professional the erroneous perspective that grieving is a passive happening. Worden (1991) explained this point:

> Phases imply a certain passivity, something that the mourner must pass through. Tasks, on the other hand, . . . imply that the mourner needs to take action and can do something. Also, this approach implies that mourning can be influenced by intervention from the outside. In other words, the mourner sees the concept of phases as something to be passed through, while the tasks approach gives the mourner some sense of leverage and hope that there is something that he or she can actively do. (p. 35)

Empowering the survivor of multiple AIDS-related loss to purposefully approach the necessary work of grief is a cornerstone to adjustment suggestions offered later in this book. Adjustment provides a more culturally sensitive and inclusive perspective on grief than detachment ever could. Shapiro (1995) commented that detachment as a pathway to healthy mourning has continued to be influential in large part because it mirrors several underlying assumptions in modern Western and North American culture: death severs all ties to the deceased; the grief process is fundamentally individual and private; within a specified period of time, the grieving individual "lets go" of the relationship to the deceased and accepts the finality of death. (p. 160)

An example of a perspective of death that conflicts with the idea of detachment was recounted by Joseph Campbell (1988). In Africa,

the "living dead," that is the remembered dead, are the principal intermediaries between the living of the tribe and the Invisibles. For, though themselves now invisible, they are still engaged in the world of the living . . . they constitute an enclosing, familiar company of favoring powers. (p. 14)

Experiencing the presence of the deceased is a common response across cultures and is highly relevant to the experience of many survivors of multiple AIDS-related loss who tell of being surrounded by ghosts, having departed loved ones return in their dreams and provide guidance in their waking. Adjustment is also incorporated into this definition to highlight the inevitable process of adaptation to loss that must occur in response to every loss. Healthy grief always requires the survivor to conform to the realities of loss.

Loved ones provide "for us the center of the universe, the place where all the threads forming the web of our life, of our world, come together," according to Ortega y Gasset (1961, p. 89). Love binds us to things. What we love "appears to us as something indispensable. The beloved object is, for the moment, indispensable" (p. 33). This is precisely the challenge of irrevocable loss, the necessity of adjusting to the loss of someone, or something, that was previously indispensable.

Ignoring the irrevocable nature of aggrieved losses allows the survivor to remain stuck in a place of bargaining (Kubler-Ross, 1969), chronic confusion, or, in Erik Erikson's (1959/1980) paradigm, despair. The healthy personality will accept losses that permit no substitutions as a part of "one's own and only life cycle" (Erikson, 1959/1980, pp. 104–105) When these losses are not accepted and integrated, despair and disgust ensue. This is particularly important in the process of grieving global, collective losses, which are harder to define and concretize. In work with survivors of the 1972 Buffalo Creek flood disaster in West Virginia, for example, Titchener and Kapp (1976) emphasized the need to encourage "active recall and working through of painful memories" (p. 299) that resulted from both individual and community-wide losses.

Kastenbaum (1977) defined grief as a response to bereavement but differentiated it from other possible responses to loss such as anger or indifference (p. 242). The definition of grief presented here includes anger, indifference, guilt, and many other responses. The variety, range, and plenitude of valid grief responses are dramatically evidenced in a one-sentence chapter written by

Joseph Bess (1969), "Grief Is"; in this chapter, he details 233 descriptions of grief. The process and work of grief includes an entire spectrum of responses and options available to survivors.

Applying Existing Grief Theory to Multiple AIDS-Related Loss

Characteristics of AIDS and ramifications of multiple loss stretch traditional theoretical assumptions related to grief and bereavement. Rando (1993) observed,

> Even in the field of clinical thanatology, in which terminal illness, stress, loss, grief, pain, suffering, and death are routinely confronted, AIDS-related bereavement is perceived as a scourge. . . . AIDS is the archetypal dread disease because it contains all the worst elements of the great pandemics (e.g., the bubonic plague), which devastated entire communities, and the shameful stigmas (e.g., cancer and leprosy) associated with an insidious and painful process of individual death. (p. 632)

In the title of her book on AIDS, Elisabeth Kubler-Ross (1987) called AIDS the ultimate challenge. Surviving is influenced by features associated with AIDS that "affect the bereavement process" (Worden, 1991, p. 112) and "complicate the issue of care" for survivors (Colburn & Malena, 1988, p. 20).

Grief theory and treatment strategies are almost exclusively an outgrowth of single-event bereavements. Multiple loss has received scant attention. Rando (1993), a foremost expert on grief, wrote a book focusing on the treatment of complicated mourning but devoted only five pages to multiple deaths and admitted that her discussion "will concern only situations in which all of the loved ones die in a common experience" (p. 563). That is not the usual experience of survivors of multiple AIDS-related loss. Worden (1991) devoted only three paragraphs to multiple loss. Kubler-Ross offered none. To find an analysis of similar issues and concepts raised by multiple AIDS-related loss, one is forced to go back to an article written in 1969 by Kastenbaum, related to multiple deaths in elderly persons. Experts have ignored multiple loss because it was extraordinarily rare until AIDS.

Below, the distinctive issues confronting survivors of multiple AIDS-related loss are reviewed in the context of existing grief theories. Where these distinctive experiences expose a limitation in existing theory, suggestions are offered. Although some implications for treatment are addressed below, for the most part issues of treatment are discussed in chapter 9.

GRIEVING MULTIPLE AIDS-RELATED LOSS

Grieving is never pleasant or easy. The survivor of multiple AIDS-related loss usually confronts a number of factors that make grieving even more painful and difficult to resolve. The issues presented below are common influences on the grieving process and factors that make unresolved grief and complicated bereavement likely.

Community-Wide, Collective Loss

The gay survivor of multiple AIDS-related loss who lives in a community of gay people faces a staggering amount and depth of loss for which there is no equivalent in nongay communities (Klein, 1994, p. 15). More than the accumulation of sometimes massive individual losses that one survivor likened to Chinese water torture (Shrader, 1992, p. 88), collective losses irrevocably disrupt the survivor's environment. Gay survivors consistently lament that the gay community, as it once was, is gone forever and will never be the same. This includes the social, cultural, political, sexual, and spiritual aspects of community. The massive individual and collective loss endured by the gay community means that the entire community reels under the impact of loss.

High-density networks, in which members of a social group maintain close relationships, produce bereavement that is marked by greater symptomatology, poorer mood, and lower self-esteem. Stylianos and Vachon (1993) noted that high-density networks increase the chance that stressful life events involving loss will concurrently affect many group members. "In such situations network members may not have the emotional energy to deal with one another's needs" (p. 398).

Individuals who are survivors themselves are less able to support other survivors. The impact on grief is circularly devastating. At the time when support is most needed, it is likely to be least available. Recovery from grief is hampered, not only by the cumulative and ongoing occurrence of loss, but also by the absence of the very people previously relied on for support. "When multiple deaths occur, the people to whom the mourner would ordinarily go for support are gone" (Rando, 1993, p. 565).

Cumulative and Compounding Loss

"Grief becomes not only a backdrop, but a backlog in one's life" (Garfield, 1995, p. 263). *Overwhelming* is a word used regularly by survivors to describe their experience. Survivors of multiple loss "have difficulty grieving because the losses are too overwhelming to contemplate or deal with" (Rando, 1984, p. 65). Survivors lack the time necessary to complete a normal bereavement process. Kastenbaum (1969) noted that "other deaths may intervene before the mourning is completed," leading to bereavement overload (p. 47). In cases of such extreme loss, such as the Holocaust, Cohen (1991) observed that survivors are in constant mourning (p. 228) and that successful grieving may never occur (p. 229).

Survivors regularly say that they do not know for whom they are grieving. Recall Terry saying that sometime a person dies "who I didn't really have a connection with at all, but it brings on a floodgate." All of their grief gets rolled up in one collective grief. Shrader's (1992) study of survivors of multiple loss concluded that "the losses were connected and that they accumulated, adding up to one big loss" (p. 88).

Krystal (1981) observed that "there is an absolute or lifetime limit to what individuals can absorb either in terms of loss or of accepting negative qualities in themselves" (p. 179). When cumulative loss passes the individual's threshold of tolerance, blocking or muting of emotional affect ensues in the form of chronic denial, withdrawal, numbing, and anhedonia (the absence of pleasure in activities previously found pleasurable). "Effective grieving requires total emotional responses, which are felt and recognized as such" (p. 186). Overwhelming cumulative loss forecloses this necessary emotional response in some survivors, and this is the point where traumatic response overlaps with grief in survivors of multiple AIDS-related loss. As chapter 7 demonstrates, traumatic response in the form of "numbing of general responsiveness" (American Psychiatric Association, 1994, p. 428) commonly arises in survivors.

Anticipatory Grief

The extreme nature of multiple AIDS-related loss offers a perspective that challenges the meaningfulness of the term *anticipatory grief.* Traditional grief theory arose almost exclusively from single-event deaths, permitting and fostering a dubious distinction between pre– and post–death-event reactions. This distinction is unmaintainable in an atmosphere of multiple, ongoing loss.

The term anticipatory grief is meant to divide genuine grief reactions from anticipatory grief within the normal grieving process (Lindemann, 1944, p. 147). Rando (1986b) justified the study of, and presumably the distinction of, anticipatory grief for "its unique ability to provide an arena for primary prevention" (p. 4). Although the goal of facilitating a healthy grief process is admirable, whether before or after the death event, artificially dividing the process and work of grief serves no useful purpose. Grievers certainly may have different concerns before death and after death, but grief is always an individualized process. All grievers have different concerns.

The division between pre- and postdeath grief is probably harmful for two reasons. First, to divide genuine grief from anticipatory grief overtly minimizes the survivor's experiences (i.e., "Your grief is not yet genuine") and serves to discount the emotions and cognitions necessary for adjustment. Second, the distinction between predeath and postdeath grief is artificial and inaccurate. Increasingly, science and philosophy recognize the continuum between life and death, matter and nonmatter. Distinguishing one type of grief from another reverts back to fundamentally discredited ways of viewing life and death.

Lindemann (1944, p. 147) acknowledged that the anticipatory griever "goes through all the phases of grief." The range of grieving that is an inherent part of surviving multiple AIDS-related loss makes the term anticipatory grief untenable because the only distinction is the moment of physical death. Many survivors of multiple, ongoing loss deny the distinction. One survivor said, "I see the line between life and death as blurred. At the same time I am surrounded by ghosts, I am surrounded by walking cadavers."

It is vitally important that survivors and professionals properly view grief as grief and avoid making false and minimizing distinctions between grief simply because it arises prior to or after a given death event.

Another way the concept of anticipatory grief is traditionally used is to assume that early grief prepares the eventual survivor for grieving after the death event. One might imagine that the long period of illness that typically precedes a death from AIDS helps prepare the survivor for the actual death event. However, evidence has suggested otherwise. Kastenbaum (1977) concluded that an early introduction into the grief process did not reduce the impact of the actual death: "One could not pay the emotional suffering in advance . . . in return for an easier time at the moment of impact" (p. 246). To the extent that grief occurs in anticipation of a death event, it is simply more grief.

The survivor who believes that early completion of some grief work prior to death will result in less work after the death event may instigate a series of emotional and physical withdrawals that prove damaging. Survivors of multiple AIDS-related loss regularly observe themselves detaching from loved ones prior to the death event. One survivor said, "I won't let myself get close to anyone. Especially when they have HIV I start thinking about them as though they are already dead." Inevitably, predeath detachment is a part of grieving when a death is foretold. What, however, are the implications for the survivor when withdrawal and distancing become a deliberate choice? A survivor who detaches too soon and too much, emotionally or physically, is likely to suffer negative consequences, including a lack of closure with the deceased, regret, and guilt. Odets (1995) observed,

> The consequences of premature grieving are experienced routinely in the AIDS epidemic. Familiarity with death and loss does not make the process easier, but more difficult. . . . The ill person may be abandoned precisely when he most needs intimacy and support, and the survivor may be left with troubling guilt about his premature withdrawal after the death actually occurs. (p. 87)

Hospice programs have identified variables that tend to predict a survivor's difficulty with grief. Physical or emotional withdrawal from the dying person is one such variable (Lindstrom, 1983). When a survivor chooses to withdraw and detach from dying friends and family, even when the reasons are ostensibly justifiable, there is a cost to the survivor. This is one of the delicate balances that the survivor of ongoing loss must maintain.

The amount of anticipatory grieving demanded of survivors of multiple, ongoing loss takes a toll. Martocchio (1985) made this point when he wrote of only a single death: "Too much anticipation and a repeated cycle of anticipatory grief may leave the survivor with no energy to complete the grieving process" (p. 335). Imagine, then, the toll of many anticipated deaths, all in different stages, from early infection, to first symptoms, to serious opportunistic infections, to institutionalized care, to death, to planning memorial services.

Anniversary Reactions

Anniversary reactions are "regrief" experiences. They arise in connection to special events that the deceased and survivor shared. These may include anniversaries of marriage, commitment, or first date. Birthdays and deathdays are frequently recalled. Holidays, especially Christmas and Thanksgiving, because they remind survivors of social gatherings, reignite both individual and collective losses. Special events that recur each year provoke memories of past years when loved ones were still alive. In the gay community, Gay Pride Day, summers at Provincetown, Massachusetts, the Folsom Street Fair in San Francisco, or special summer parties (e.g., the White Party) may refresh memories. Summer camps for hemophiliac children have a similar grief-inducing effect for parents and children.

The survivor of multiple AIDS-related loss is prone to having anniversaries scattered throughout the calendar. Although anniversary reactions are to be expected (Rando, 1984, p. 115), the survivor experiencing them may be unaware of the connection between them and their heightened sense of grief or depression (Musaph, 1990). Professionals or friends may help survivors understand the context of their regrief experience by normalizing its occurrence.

Ongoing, Relentless Loss

Survivors who continue to involve themselves with AIDS live under a persistent shadow of death. A tremendous amount of loss and grief are ever present simply from living amid the constant drum of death and suffering. This loss of a carefree, untroubled, secure, at-ease life may be totally alien to nonsurvivors, who consequently fail to understand. When David's partner seroconverted, a whole new dimension to ongoing loss confronted him:

> I always expected that when I died of AIDS, the suffering would be over for me. I knew others would keep on dying but for me personally, the pain would be over. When Kurt tested positive it blew my world away. My hope that this would end with me collapsed. Even after I die, the person I love most of all in the world will suffer, then he too will die. Lots of my friends have died, and I have AIDS, but nothing has ever hurt this bad!

Survivors of multiple AIDS-related loss know that there will be many more who will die from this disease and that there may never be a cure for AIDS. Parents may feel particularly stung by this realization of grief projected into the future.

Ongoing, fresh bereavement significantly affects grieving. Martin and Dean (1993b) found a difference between survivors who had only recent multiple loss and those who had chronic multiple loss. Chronic loss was particularly stressful and resulted in elevated depression and drug use. All stage theories of grief presume an orderly progression that begins at the moment of a loss and continues to some end point of resolution, recovery, or acceptance. This model is wholly incapable and unfit to describe the grief experience of survivors of multiple, ongoing loss. Grief is continuous and, with no end in sight to the barrage of loss, survivors may ask, "What is the point?" when deciding whether or not to engage in the purposeful work of grieving. Survivors may live under constant fear and anxiety. Even when a survivor is committed to doing the grief work and begins the process of systematically grieving each individual loss, new losses may disrupt those efforts. Fresh losses will affect even the most purposeful, well-intentioned efforts to resolve grief.

Etiology and Stigmatization

The effect of stigmatization was discussed in chapter 3. In this chapter, three ways in which stigmatization adversely handicaps the grief process are reviewed.

1   The effect of stigmatization intensifies the grief experience, leading to a heightened propensity for unresolved grief and complicated bereavement.
2   The fear of stigmatization reduces the potential for support during the grieving process by causing survivors to adopt conservative attitudes and behaviors in regard to seeking support.
3   The fact of stigmatization limits support during the grieving process by deeming the cause of suffering justifiable and therefore unworthy of sympathy.

AIDS Stigmatization Intensifies Grief   AIDS-related loss is apt to provoke grief reactions intensified by stigmatization. AIDS is an illness that causes terrible suffering, inevitable death, direct association with prestigmatized groups, and connection to socially disapproved behaviors. One mother described the added pain that her son's AIDS illness and death caused her:

> It was bad enough that he was dying, but did it have to be from AIDS? I couldn't tell anyone. Seeing my grown-up son with diapers and mumbling incoherently was just too much to bear. I wished he had died of something simple, like brain cancer.

Grieving an AIDS death is more difficult than grieving most other forms of death. Deaths from AIDS are more difficult to endure because of the reasons outlined in the previous chapters. Although grief is usually more pronounced, it is less supported.

Survivors feel the stigmatization of AIDS (Houseman & Pheifer, 1988; Klein & Fletcher, 1987; O'Neil, 1989). AIDS-related stigmatization may provoke feelings of blame, guilt, or shame in the survivor, complicating grief. A hallmark of the AIDS epoch is the number of obituaries that never mention AIDS as the cause of death. Survivors in urban areas who regularly read obituaries learn to piece together the clues: young age, no wife, and no cause of death.

> Even if survivors merely wonder whether the disease is a form of punishment, such questioning means that they must struggle not only with the death itself but also with the additional burden of the loved one's having been "bad" in some fashion. (Rando, 1993, p. 638)

Fear of Stigmatization   Legitimate or not, fear of stigmatization initiates a conservative stance toward seeking support. Of the factors that may portend complicated grief, a loss that is socially unspeakable is paramount (Lazare, 1979). A suicide death is similarly socially unspeakable and provides a parallel. "When someone dies in this manner . . . there is a tendency for the family and friends to keep quiet about the circumstances surrounding the death. This conspiracy of silence causes great harm to the surviving person" (Worden, 1991, p. 69). Social support, which is essential for coping with multiple loss, is unavailable for survivors unwilling to disclose their loss because of fear related to stigmatization, leading to a silent sorrow (Doka, 1987).

This fear of unsympathetic or disapproving response is understandable and likely in survivors who were prestigmatized. Those most affected by AIDS frequently have a history of secrecy resulting from social stigmatization before the emergence of AIDS, including hemophiliacs (Brown & DeMaio, 1992), homosexuals (Doka, 1987), and IVDUs (Stowe et al., 1993). Individuals in these communities are likely to be conservative about choosing whether to reveal their grief. Already aggrieved, a person is extra vulnerable, so the fear of being hurt is even more pronounced.

The Fact of Stigmatization Affects Bereavement   Multiple AIDS-related loss is often negated or minimized by society as a whole. A loss that is socially negated is one where those around the aggrieved "act as if the loss did not happen" (Worden, 1991, p. 69). Benign neglect of issues important to homosexuals, hemophiliacs, and IVDUs rather than outright hostility is usually responsible for survivors feeling socially negated. Even an issue as traumatic as multiple AIDS-related loss is ignored in a climate distinguished by unawareness.

Stigmatization can take forms far more hurtful to the bereaved, and harmful to the grieving process, than those wrought by neglect. These attitudes and behaviors are most likely at the very time when a survivor is most vulnerable. Those who know survivors of AIDS-related deaths will have heard heartbreaking stories about families of origin who excluded lifetime partners and friends from the hospital during the last days of the deceased's life, then ignored them at the memorial service. Neither of these hurtful occurrences are uncommon

(Doka, 1987; Houseman & Pheifer, 1988). Religious symbols and clergy are usually a source of solace and support during times of bereavement. Because of the strident judgmentalism often accompanying fundamentalist Christian dogma, the survivor may feel ostracized and condemned rather than supported. Lack of support from religious beliefs puts the survivor at high risk for problems with bereavement (Switzer, 1970).

Survivors of multiple AIDS-related loss regularly face layered circumstances that simultaneously aggravate the pain of grief while hindering the process of adjusting to a world without their loved ones and dreams. Not surprisingly, unresolved grief and complicated bereavement are normal in survivors. Factors that make these responses normal in multiple-loss survivors are explored next.

UNRESOLVED GRIEF AND COMPLICATED BEREAVEMENT

Complicated bereavement, abnormal grief, unresolved grief, and *pathological grief* are all terms that refer to a grief process that does not follow the regular course (Worden, 1991). Far from being abnormal, symptoms indicative of complicated bereavement may be the normal human response to the overwhelming amount of grief and loss faced by survivors of multiple AIDS-related loss.

Unresolved grief has the characteristics of being chronic, absent, delayed, or distorted. Chronic grieving is extended or excessively intense (Martocchio, 1985), and mourning fails to draw to its natural conclusion (Rando, 1984). Absent grief is marked by fending off the usual emotions associated with grief. Survivors may take pride in carrying on as though nothing has happened (Bowlby, 1980). Delayed grief occurs when normal symptoms of grief arise after a long period of absent grief (Lindemann, 1944) and may become apparent when other complaints, or presenting problems, surface (Parkes, 1972). Distorted grief presents itself interpersonally, evidenced in isolation, excessive irritability, avoidance, and other alterations of relationships with family and friends (Lindemann, 1944).

Kastenbaum (1977) identified characteristics of poor outcome in bereaved persons. These are similar to the experience of many survivors of multiple AIDS-related loss and include

- social withdrawal
- preoccupation with detail of the death
- more difficulty accepting the reality of the loss
- more disorganization through life
- anxiety
- pessimistic future outlook

Survivors of multiple AIDS-related loss are tragically well positioned to be at high risk for unresolved grief and complicated bereavement because they are likely to face multiple high-risk factors. "The existence of more factors increases the risk of complications" (Rando, 1993, p. 454). Various factors are identified to predispose survivors for developing symptoms of unresolved grief or complicated bereavement (see Krupp, 1972; Martocchio, 1985; Parkes, 1972; Rando, 1984, 1993). A number of these factors are common in the experience of survivors of multiple AIDS-related loss; therefore, the likelihood of unresolved grief and complicated bereavement is high. In addition to the primary risk factors identified earlier in this chapter, these factors include the following:

- lack of social support
- disenfranchised grief
- characteristics of AIDS-related illness and death
- history of loss
- preventability
- concurrent stressors
- mental health concerns
- ambivalent relationships
- types of losses

Lack of Social Support

Bereavement is not exclusively an intrapersonal issue, it "is a social network crisis" (Stylianos & Vachon, 1993, p. 397). Social support is traditionally and constantly viewed as crucial to positive outcome in bereavement for a variety of reasons. Sympathetic response provides the bereaved person an opportunity to reconnect or reattach to individuals and community. Social support provides a survivor an opportunity to identify and express feelings. Acknowledged survivors are given latitude to express emotions and avoid some responsibilities. In addition, a number of tangible, physical benefits are available, including help with meals, time off from work, and assistance with planning for life after a loved one's death.

Social support, or its lack, is a crucial variable in the adjustment process of survivors of multiple loss. "Grief is a social process and is best dealt with in a social setting in which people can support and reinforce each other in their emotions to the loss" (Worden, 1991, p. 69). This is especially important for survivors of multiple AIDS-related loss whose experience is atypical, therefore difficult for nonsurvivors to appreciate and support. Most of the sources of support available to the grieving are sources that were in place prior to death; when these are limited by previous loss, available support is limited. Repeatedly and consistently, "lack of social support has been demonstrated to increase the risk of adverse outcome following stressful life events, while the presence of good social support may decrease risk" (Vachon et al., 1982, p. 783). One of the best predictors of recovery from grief is a trustworthy source of emotional support (Crow, 1991, p. 118).

"The type of support the griever will receive will be based on how the griever and the deceased are valued by members of the social system and the manner and circumstances of the death" (Rando, 1984, p. 54). Multiple AIDS deaths are devalued by society. Bereavement and support are usually reserved for the immediate family; "external persons are prevented from adequately expressing and sharing their grief" (Fudin & Devore, 1981, p. 135). Among those typically excluded are the playmates and friends of children and young adults. Hemophiliac deaths often leave mourning children and playmates. Nursing staff who develop close relationships through devoted, long-term care of patients and regular contact can be left bereft. Any sign of emotion is viewed as unprofessional, and nearly no provision is made for their mourning (Fudin & Devore, 1981, pp. 135–136).

The varieties of loss typically experienced by survivors of multiple AIDS-related loss are likely to be unrecognized and underappreciated. Because thinking about grief tends to assume single, discrete death events, survivors are unlikely to receive support for the multiplicity of losses pervading their lives. To the extent support, even when available at all, focuses exclusively on the death of *a* friend, *a* spouse, or *an* acquaintance, the survivor's experience is necessarily minimized and devalued.

Disenfranchised Grief

AIDS is a disease of the cultural and social ghettos. Bereavement is mainly confined to high-risk groups or those who choose to associate with them. As explained in the second chapter, the foreignization of AIDS allows the general public to remain physically and emotionally separate from the culpable other.

Grief experienced by the survivor of multiple AIDS-related loss may be disenfranchised as a result of social strictures, but it can also be disenfranchised by the bereaved. Kauffman (1989) explained that

> in self-disenfranchised grief the source is one's own lack of acknowledgment and recognition of it. The specific psychological phenomenon operating in disenfranchised grief is shame. . . . In self-disenfranchisement the source of the shame and inhibition of the grief process is not in the actual views of others, but in the imagined views of others or the intrapsychic dynamics of the individual. (p. 25)

Fear that motivates survivors to deprive themselves of the opportunity to receive support for their grief is common in survivors of AIDS-related loss. It is especially prevalent among lesbians and gay men who suffer from ingrained shame and are accustomed, by their history, to fear of disclosing personal concerns. A man whose partner is dying may be unable to reach out to his coworkers for support. Often, this disabling fear is worse than the reality, but the effect is the same. Survivors are inhibited to express grief. Both shame and the effects of stigmatization serve to provoke fears of abandonment in survivors. The disenfranchised griever is alienated, cut off from community (Kollar, 1989). Unfortunately, as survivors attempt to lessen the risk and fear of abandonment, they may self-abandon by blocking their own expression of grief. Fear is a powerful motivator. Not surprisingly, tendencies to withdraw and isolate are common in survivors of multiple AIDS-related loss (Carmack, 1992) who believe they must hide their grief. Bell (1988) called this "the hidden epidemic of grief" (p. 25), describing his grief reaction when his last friend died of AIDS:

> He suffered for 10 months and died in January 1987. That was it—the last brick. All my losses caught up with me. My grief could no longer be hid in abeyance. The pain and the grief swept over me—it was the beginning of my dark night of the soul. His death cut the last thread to the past; I no longer had any old friends. The pain of my grief hit hard. It was as though I was floating in darkness, on a sea of pain blown by the winds of rage. There was no hope, no light. I pulled into myself, cutting myself off from the world to protect myself from more pain. (p. 29)

Survivors withdraw, seeking protection from two potential sources of pain: the risk of future relationships that might be terminated by AIDS and the pain of antagonistic response from family, friends, and acquaintances. Survivors may experience an extreme and deep sense of persecution, thus "grief may have to remain private" (Doka, 1987, pp. 459).

Some survivors of loss from AIDS are less likely to receive necessary support. Those in secret relationships with the dying and deceased often are not given support and cannot seek support because of the need for secrecy. Secret survivors, persons who are involved in relationships that must remain secret, such as homosexuals in long-term clandestine relationships, receive little or no support from professionals, families, or friends. Secret survivors may not be notified as death approaches and miss the opportunity to say final good-byes. At the time when honest catharsis is most necessary, the secret survivor may "need to 'act,' so as not to reveal the true nature of the relationship" (Weinback, 1989, p. 58). Partners in "illicit relationships hold no status as mourners" (Fudin & Devore, 1981, p. 137). Normally available sources of support are not available, including the opportunity to reminisce, mourn at a funeral, or keep special personal mementos. Secret survivors may avoid professional help because professionals are "seen as possessing traditional family values and generally unapproving and unable to understand the depth of their relationship" (Weinback, 1989, p. 59).

Foster parents of children with AIDS are "discounted for not being the child's 'real' parent" (Anderson et al., 1989, p. 52). The volunteer who becomes personally attached to people with AIDS is sometimes devastated by losses that friends and family minimize with comments such as "You were only his Buddy; you knew he would die. I don't understand why you are so upset." Or they may be overtly criticized for their grief: "It is your own fault. You are the one who chooses to help those people. Maybe you should quit volunteering for AIDS."

Characteristics of AIDS-Related Illness and Death

Four characteristics of typical AIDS death and illness make complicated bereavement more likely: the length of illness prior to death, the likelihood for painfully distressing illness, the episodic cycles characteristic of AIDS, and the age of those dying. The survivor's "perception about the meaning of the death" and "the particular circumstances surrounding the death affect the grieving process" (Martocchio, 1985, p. 335). Both the meaning attached to AIDS-related death and circumstances around the death process increase the grief arising in multiple AIDS-related loss. Death after a long illness and painful death affect the survivor's grieving process (Martocchio, 1985, p. 335) and is nearly always the case with AIDS. A long period of illness tends to heighten guilt feelings and hostility toward the deceased (Uroda, 1977). In her book on complicated mourning, Rando (1993) lists "death from an overly lengthy illness" as likely to "predispose any individual to complicated mourning" (p. 5) and specifically mentions HIV as giving "new meaning to the notion of stress in both the individual with infection and in survivors" (p. 9).

When a young person dies, grief is felt, not only for the death, but also for the lost potential inherent in the terminated life, and so it is defined as tragic. Kastenbaum (1969) compared a young death to an older death when he noted that "we mourn for what he was and what he might yet have become. This time, however, there might be a different quality to our sense of bereavement. We grieve for the premature termination of a promising existence" (p. 28). Perception of an untimely death has a more devastating effect on the survivor (Kohn & Levav, 1990).

History of Loss

Fresh losses remind the survivor of multiple loss of previous losses. Each new "loss resurrects old issues and conflicts for the mourner" (Rando, 1984, p. 21). Losses other than deaths are also provoked. "It is commonly believed that loss reminds people of other losses; thus, when gay people deal with the grief of someone dying, they are reminded of the grief of coming to terms with their own self-identity" (Biller & Rice, 1990, p. 283). Shrader (1992) observed that "these multiple losses have also triggered many of the other losses these men have suffered in their lives, or recycle other loss feelings" (p. 116). Shrader quoted one survivor who says, "I found . . . that I started grieving for losses I didn't even know I had lost" (p. 119).

A history of loss influences the survivor's response to new loss. In grief reactions, "the number and the nature of previous grief experiences have an impact. Unresolved feelings and conflicts related to earlier losses in the person's life are likely to resurface" (Martocchio, 1985, p. 335). When previous losses are "not worked through, it can hinder effective mourning" (Rando, 1993, p. 459).

Research findings appear inconsistent with regard to whether prior loss helps or hinders the survivor's grief process. Previous losses are found to correlate with poor bereavement outcomes (Maddison & Walker, 1967; Parkes 1975, 1987), although coping well with previous loss is demonstrated to predict better outcomes with contemporary grief (Shanfield & Swain, 1984; Vachon, 1976). One consistent theme emerges from the literature regarding the impact of prior loss: How well the previous loss was grieved predicts how a current loss will be grieved.

Certain types of previous loss increase the risk for adverse effect on contemporary loss. Various qualities of previous loss also "influence the type, intensity, and duration of grief" (Worden, 1991, p. 65). The quantity of previous loss matters; better bereavement outcomes tend to be associated with fewer previous losses (Rando, 1993). A history of loss that includes multiple losses, especially the loss of a very close person or losses in rapid succession, increases the impact of prior loss (Stroebe & Stroebe, 1983). "Only the mourner can determine the degree of difficulty inherent in either type of crisis" (Rando, 1993, p. 457). When factors that predispose unresolved grief or complicated bereavement occur in the context of prior unresolved loss, the survivor faces a compounded problem. This situation is typical in survivors of multiple AIDS-related loss whose poor prior loss experiences adversely affect contemporary experience.

Groups suffering the most impact of multiple AIDS-related loss are at high risk of having suffered previous losses throughout life. Those suffering AIDS-related loss who live in severely impoverished circumstances face a history of loss related to finances, safety, education, social status, and hope. The hemophiliac family has inevitably endured a number of losses directly related to hemophilia before AIDS. Even with recent medical advances, it is unlikely that parents will see their hemophiliac male children live into late mid-life or have children. Gay men and lesbians regularly face abandonment by members of their family of origin and rejection by friends and acquaintances at some point in their lives. Loss of dreams regularly arises, including loss of a traditional family, loss of political aspirations, loss of social connections, and loss of a "normal" life.

These losses all evoke grief-related pain. Each requires the process and work of grieving. When previous losses have not been successfully grieved and adjusted to, problems with grief arising from multiple AIDS-related loss are likely to be more severe. Rando (1993) observed,

> A mourner's prior experiences with losses and stresses may establish expectations regarding future loss and influence the coping strategies and defense mechanisms adopted. If previous experiences with losses and/or stresses have been negative or have not been accommodated, this can adversely affect the present experience of loss. (pp. 459–460).

Preventability

Perception of preventability predisposes survivors to complicated bereavement (Bugen, 1979) because the notion presents survivors with options for finding meaning in the death that implicitly attach an element of bargaining into the grief process. Rando (1993) noted,

When a death is perceived as having been preventable, the individual experiences additional complications in mourning. This was a death that did not have to happen—it could have been avoided. Carelessness, negligence, or maliciousness perceived to have caused the death brings anger, feelings of victimization and unfairness, the need to assign blame and responsibility and mete out punishment, obsession and rumination, attempts to regain control, lack of closure, significant violations of the assumptive world, and the search for reasons and meaning. All of these sequelae complicate mourning and interfere with coping. (pp. 9–10)

Grief is complicated because it is stuck in a stance that is patently not the process and work of adjusting to a world without the lost object, relationship, or dream. The attention of the bereaved person is not on grieving a loss; the bereaved person is essentially trying to prevent the loss by finding rationalizations that interfere with acceptance of the irrevocable nature of the loss. Rather than adjustment, attention is focused on bargaining by the survivor's "what-if" fantasies:

- If the government had forced blood companies to guarantee clean blood, Christopher would not have AIDS.
- If I had only known the truth about Pablo's promiscuity and drug use, I would have made him wear a condom.
- If Tom's father had not been so distant and his mother so overly protective, he would not have been gay and gotten AIDS.
- If Kyle had stayed in Iowa and not moved to San Francisco, he never would have gotten AIDS.

To the extent that something can still be done, even if it is only revenge, developing an attitude of bitterness, or a quest for responsibility, then the survivor avoids dealing directly with grief as an irrevocable loss.

Preventability assumes expectations. Something that should not have happened is responsible. The survivor's expectations and assumptive world are violated. The survivor's constant lament is the unfairness of this experience. New infections with HIV are particularly prone to provoking problems with grief. When the HIV test was new, survivors were accustomed to receiving news that another friend had tested positive. Today, newly discovered HIV infection presumes recent infection. The person was infected after high-risk factors were well known, after prevention education was available, and after a period of time when culpability for infection could be denied. The division between innocent and not-innocent victims is fostered anew with the "you should have known better" syndrome (B. Brennan, personal communication, 1996). Inevitably, the survivor experiences strongly ambivalent feelings toward the person with HIV. Simultaneously held, conflicting feelings toward newly infected people may include compassion and blame, support and hostility, understanding and confusion, pity and rage.

Concurrent Stressors

Stressors that preexist or arise at the same time that a survivor struggles with grief are a recognized high-risk variable for developing problems during bereavement (Parkes, 1975). Multiple losses are themselves concurrent stressors. Among these are the bereaved person's perception that his or her grief is not recognized.

Concerns with money can produce tremendous stress. Low socioeconomic status is a high-risk factor for psychological and physical illness during bereavement (Martocchio, 1985). Many survivors of multiple loss, including inner-city minorities and homosexuals, are likely to be financially disadvantaged persons with the concurrent stress of poverty. Hemophiliac families, even when they have insurance, often must pay 20% of enormous medical bills.

Poor health on the part of the bereaved (Martocchio, 1985), especially when the bereaved has tested positive for HIV (Martin & Dean, 1993b), will result in both intensification of grief responses and greater difficulty recovering. Concurrent stress leads the survivor to be overwhelmed in a way similar to the effect of compounding, cumulative multiple loss, which leads to bereavement overload. There is simply too much to bear. Secondary loss or stress may arise in survivors of multiple loss who are confronted with difficulties that simultaneously arise with the central AIDS-related loss. For example, when the family of choice and the family of origin are in conflict, financial matters and personal property ownership concerns may augment the stress inherent in grieving the loss of a loved one. The survivor's ego strength may reach a point of depletion, leaving an insufficient amount of ego available for current grief work (Deutsch, 1937).

Mental Health Concerns

Survivors of multiple AIDS-related loss seem more likely than the general population to be struggling with preexisting mental health concerns that complicate bereavement. Environmental factors, including social stresses, contribute to the development of mental disorder. These factors and stressors are more likely among survivors of multiple AIDS-related loss, who may struggle with issues recognized to influence mental health, including early attachment problems; exposure to unstable and violent environments; physical, sexual, and emotional abuse; and factors that stunt psychological development. Some of the more common preexisting mental health issues faced by survivors are depression, anxiety, adjustment disorder, posttraumatic stress disorder, personality disorders, and psychoactive substance abuse (covered in detail in the next chapter). Rando (1993) observed that

> the mourner's mental health will influence the mourning process because, inasmuch as it describes the mourner, it will also define mourning. No other factor so accurately describes and delimits who is affected by loss, how loss is experienced, or what is available for the response to it. (p. 461)

Ambivalent Relationships

Ambivalent relationships with the deceased may be "the most frequent type of relationship that hinders people from adequately grieving" (Worden, 1991, p. 65). Unfortunately, ambivalent or overtly hostile relationships frequently characterize the family relationships of parents with IV drug using or homosexual children. Houseman and Pheifer (1988) observed that

> Conflicts regarding choice of lifestyle can be a fertile ground for developing ambivalent relationships. Families of origin may love their members, but hate them for selecting values related to the drug culture or gay lifestyle. These conflicts may not be overcome at the time of death and may contribute to unresolved grief. (p. 299)

These survivors are at high risk for complicated mourning, especially when the "premorbid relationship was markedly angry or ambivalent" (Rando, 1993, p. 6).

Ambivalent relationships between the survivor and deceased adversely affect grieving when the survivor is unwilling to acknowledge negative emotions, especially anger. In the case of AIDS-related death, anger may be buried for a variety of reasons. Other highly charged ambivalent feelings may seem "unspeakable." Examples of these issues include the following:

- "Was I a bad parent? What did I do to make my son a drug addict (or gay)?"
- "Was I responsible for infecting my partner?"
- "He deserved to get AIDS: the homo!; the junkie!"
- "How can I live with myself knowing that I passed HIV on to my children?"

Unresolved feelings of hostility may contribute to guilt. A surviving loved one may have lived through years of wishing the deceased "would just die," especially when strong judgments about drug abuse or sexual behavior persist. The survivor who suppresses these thoughts and feelings, which are natural and necessary to the grieving process, becomes stuck in a past-focused stance that inhibits the work of adjustment to an irrevocable loss.

Types of Loss

Survivors of multiple AIDS-related loss regularly face, as part of their expanse of loss, at least one of three types of loss most likely to increase grief and inhibit adjustment. The death of children, especially adult children, is particularly difficult (Rando, 1986b). This is a regular occurrence for parents whose children die of AIDS and are hemophiliac, gay, or IVDUs. Death of a spouse, whether heterosexual or homosexual, is particularly difficult for the survivor because of the myriad losses inherent in this type of lost relationship. A growing phenomenon is the loss of a parent, or parents, to AIDS (Chachkes & Jennings, 1992), especially among the fastest expanding population of HIV transmission. These children face a staggering array of problems, which are explored in chapter 8 on families. In addition, these children regularly face concurrent stressors related to finances, living conditions, and stability (Doka, 1992).

CONCLUSION

Surviving multiple AIDS-related loss commonly presents a number of factors that are recognized to create a situation in which complicated bereavement and unresolved grief are likely. This combined number of high-risk factors is extraordinary and may be unique to this phenomenon. It is difficult to think of other events that regularly arouse such a number and combination of these predisposing factors. Knowledge of these risk factors increases the opportunity for survivors and professionals to understand the high risk that survivors face for troubling responses. This understanding is particularly important in the context of multiple AIDS-related loss for two reasons. First, the phenomenon itself is new and barely recognized. Second, many of the symptoms that arise in survivors are easily mistaken as primary rather than secondary; the connection between multiple loss and the symptom is missed.

Chapter 6

Problems Grieving
and Adjusting to Multiple Loss

Only people who are capable of loving strongly can also suffer great sorrow, but this same necessity of loving serves to counteract their grief and heals them.—Leo Tolstoy

Survivors of multiple loss must cope with a very difficult set of circumstances. This chapter focuses on coping responses that are viewed as problematic by most survivors who experience them. In chapters 9, 10, and 11, coping responses that are less likely to be described as problems and more likely to be described as positive growth opportunities are reviewed. The preceding chapter outlined factors that dispose a survivor to suffer from unresolved grief and complicated bereavement. This chapter begins by reviewing symptoms related to those factors that arise in survivors. Although the problems presented in this chapter are mainly presented in the context of grief, realistically they may also be said to arise in response to trauma (which is discussed in the next chapter) and in response to surviving an extreme set of circumstances related to multiple, ongoing loss. For example, survivor's guilt commonly arises in survivors; does it matter whether that response is classified as a grieving, traumatic, or coping response?

COMPLICATED BEREAVEMENT RESPONSES

Grief responses in survivors of multiple AIDS-related loss are characteristic of symptoms commonly associated with unresolved grief and complicated bereavement. Survivors and professionals may benefit from this analysis for two reasons. First, symptoms of surviving multiple loss may mask the underlying issue of multiple unresolved loss. Survivors of multiple AIDS-related loss may be unaware of the relationship between their multiple losses and their presenting difficulties. Second, because a critical step in the recovery process involves "normalizing the abnormal" (Nord, 1996c), survivors are helped by understanding that their responses, although they seem extreme, are shared by other survivors. These symptoms are presented to help survivors and professionals understand the survivor's experience. The survivor's experience may be consistent with Rando's (1984) assertion that "Grief is a 'craziness,' but grievers are usually not crazy" (p. 35).

Traditionally, *symptoms* refers to signs of illness. *Pathology* refers to results of a disease or abnormal variation from a sound condition. Distinguishing between normal and abnormal, pathological and nonpathological in the area of bereavement is difficult (Middleton, Raphael, Martinek, & Misso, 1993). The *Diagnostic and Statistical Manual of Mental Disorders* (*DSM–IV*; American Psychiatric Association, 1994) is of no help regarding the distinction between normal and pathological grief (Sprang & McNeil, 1995). Delineating normal from abnormal is imprecise because no objective criteria exist to determine the distinction (Rando, 1993). Pathological grief has been defined as "the intensification of grief to the level where the person is overwhelmed, resorts to maladaptive behavior, or remains interminably in the state of grief" (Horowitz, Wilner, Marmar, & Krupnick, 1980, p. 1157).

The extreme circumstances of multiple AIDS-related loss evoke extreme but common responses that, in the traditional sense, would be labeled pathological. Symptoms of unresolved grief and complicated bereavement are appropriate, normal, and expected. Frankl (1959/1984, p. 38) quoted Lessing as saying, "There are things which must cause you to lose your reason or you have none to lose." He concluded that "an abnormal reaction to an abnormal situation is normal behavior" (p. 38). The same symptoms that would indicate a pathology when they occur in the context of a traditional single-event–related bereavement may be entirely appropriate to the experience of multiple-loss survivors (Nord, 1996a). Surviving multiple AIDS-related loss could justifiably, though oxymoronically, be called normal abnormality or normal pathology. Perhaps, in a situation of multiple, ongoing loss, the distinction is unnecessary and futile.

In traditional theory and practice, symptoms of unresolved grief or complicated bereavement are reasons for clinical intervention by a professional. They indicate that something more than counseling by an amateur or peer support from a group is necessary (Worden, 1991). Though these responses may be normal, in the sense of their common occurrence, in survivors of multiple, ongoing loss, they are still serious and suggest the value of professional help.

"Tearless grief bleeds inwardly," said C. N. Bovee (as cited in Staudacher, 1994, p. 141). The occurrence of masked or absent grief reactions are another reason to spell out the symptoms that commonly arise in survivors of multiple AIDS-related loss. By recognizing the symptoms, one can be directed toward the cause. In her classic article on the absence of grief, Helene Deutsch (1937) observed that grief that is not expressed with overt feelings common to bereavement will be manifested in some other way. "Death of a beloved person must produce reactive expression of feeling in the normal course of events . . . [U]nmanifested grief will be found expressed to the full in some way or other" (p. 13). Although survivors "experience symptoms and behaviors which cause them difficulty," they often "do not see or recognize the fact that these are related to the loss" (Worden, 1991, p. 73).

Survivors of multiple AIDS-related loss are a diverse group of people, so responses to multiple loss are inevitably diverse. Likewise, grief is an individual process. Each individual copes with loss in a uniquely personal way. Nevertheless, a number of common responses are observed in survivors of multiple AIDS-related loss. The forthcoming discussion does not imply that any or all of these symptoms necessarily arise in all survivors or that negative outcomes are the sole response of survivors to this extreme experience. In the discussion that follows, intrapsychic responses are separated from interpersonal responses to multiple AIDS-related loss for the sake of organizational clarity.

INTRAPSYCHIC RESPONSES TO MULTIPLE LOSS

Intrapsychic responses are those that are primarily self-focused and, sometimes, narcissistic. These responses certainly may affect relationships with others, but they are marked by their individually centered focus. Prevalent among survivors of multiple AIDS-related loss are chronic denial, depression with notable anhedonia, anxiety, and mood-altering chemical abuse.

Chronic Denial

Denial takes a variety of forms, showing many faces. "Denial or postponement of emotion is one of the most frequent defense mechanisms" (Krupp, 1972, p. 430). It can serve a valuable purpose by acting as a buffer, allowing the bereaved an opportunity "to collect himself and, with time, mobilize other, less radical defenses" (Kubler-Ross, 1969, p. 39). After a time, however, denial will block the normal grief process and result in symptoms of complicated bereavement in survivors of multiple loss.

When denial continues, grieving cannot occur because there is nothing to grieve. As Worden (1991) noted,

> There is always a certain sense of unreality—a sense that it did not really happen. Therefore, the first grief task is to come to a more complete awareness that the loss actually has occurred—the person is dead and will not return. Survivors must accept this reality so they can deal with the emotional impact of the loss. (p. 42)

Even the counterproductive use of denial is understandable in the face of so much devastating loss. The survivor may need to fend off emotions that seem unbearable or dangerous. One survivor of multiple AIDS-related loss said, "If I even allow myself to think about it I will explode. It is simply too much to bear. I will kill myself before I let myself think about it." Multiple losses are more likely to be denied than are single-death events because of the intense fear associated with the threat of ego disintegration.

The survivor may not have the ego strength necessary to cope with accumulated loss. To remain functional, a pervasive shutdown of emotional response or a fervent hyperactivity may defend the ego against a perceived threat of psychic obliteration. Adjustment to loss requires reconnection to others that necessarily involves trust and vulnerability. The inherent risk in this process may be too much for the survivor of multiple, ongoing loss.

More chilling is the assertion by some survivors of multiple loss that they are not affected: "It is not that big of a deal. People die. So what?" Others claim to have gotten used to it. Odets (1995) observed that

> There are many who expect not to be affected by the losses of the epidemic and who feel they are not. Such assertions, at best, express the desire not to be affected, and, at worst, a loss of the capacity for any feelings because life in the epidemic has been overwhelming. (p. 76)

This denial is supported by a society that devalues many of the relationships lost to AIDS.

Bowlby (1980) described survivors who take pride in the superficial fact that they can carry on as though nothing happened. They keep busy and appear, on the surface, to be doing splendidly. In a single-event bereavement, a survivor can flourish behind a burst of activity associated with planning a memorial service, arranging details subsequent to death, and keeping busy with other tasks. Scott, a survivor of multiple loss, spoke about his response to his lover's death:

> I have never grieved my lover's death even though it was 4 years ago. For the first 2 years, I kept busy and avoided thinking about it. In the last year and a half I am angry at everyone and everything. I have absolutely no resolution about Steve's death.

For the survivor of multiple loss, however, this initial burst of activity is difficult to maintain. Long-term denial requires more effort or more severe methods. These survivors engage in a fanatic effort to avoid all references to

AIDS. Yet, "the expediency of the flight from the suffering of grief is but a temporary gain, because, as we have seen, the necessity to mourn persists in the psychic apparatus" (Deutsch, 1937, p. 22).

Chronic denial manifests somatically and behaviorally as well as psychologically. Survivors of multiple AIDS-related loss sometimes manifest somatic complaints. Anais Nin said that "when one is pretending, the entire body revolts" (as cited in Staudacher, 1994, p. 115). When pain cannot be expressed outwardly, because of denial, pain may be expressed inwardly. Some members of groups at high risk for HIV infection have avoided the test despite medical advances that make early knowledge of HIV status prudent. Boykin (1991) found that between 13% and 18% of gay men in his study had avoided an HIV test, which he interpreted as a "strong indication of denial" (p. 256).

Depression

In common usage, *depression* refers to feeling sad, gloomy, discouraged, hopeless, dispirited, melancholic, blue, low, or down in the dumps. The term depression arose from the word *depress*, to lower, sink, press, or force down. In its earliest use (in the early 17th century), depression signified dejection and low spirits (*Oxford Universal Dictionary*, 1933). These descriptions precisely describe the way many survivors of multiple AIDS-related loss feel. One survivor said, "I am always sad now; there is no more happy." Another said, "I feel like I keep getting punched in the gut and pushed down. It's like I am laying in the mud and people keep walking over me, pushing me down deeper into the dirt."

Professional psychological language defines depression in a way meant to include objective observations with the subjective experiences of the persons suffering. The *DSM–IV* (American Psychiatric Association, 1994) requires at least five of a list of nine symptoms that must include either depressed mood or loss of interest or pleasure. The symptoms most common in survivors of multiple AIDS-related loss arise in connection with reactive depression rather than endogenous depression and are reviewed below. This partial list does not infer that the other symptoms of depression do not arise in survivors. In fact, other symptoms of depression—including weight fluctuation, psychomotor agitation or retardation, fatigue or loss of energy, diminished ability to think and concentrate, and indecisiveness—are observed. Martin and Dean (1993a) studied AIDS-related bereavement among gay men. They discovered that

> bereaved men experienced elevated levels of . . . depression including "feelings of hopelessness, helplessness, sadness, cognitive impairment, somatic complaints, and problems falling asleep, staying asleep, and waking early; suicidal ideation, including thoughts about taking one's life, plans for doing so, and actual attempts." (p. 325)

Grief, even persistent and intense grief, is not depression, though unresolved grief can transform into depression. Freud differentiated mourning and melancholia. With mourning, the world appears poor and empty; with melancholia, the person feels poor and empty. This fall in self-esteem distinguishes depression from normal grief. Worden (1991) noted that "in a grief reaction, there is not the loss of self-esteem commonly found in most clinical depressions" (p. 30). Freud (1917/1957) came close to connecting survivor's guilt to depression when he noted that "self-reproaches and self-revilings culminate in a delusional expectation of punishment" (p. 125). Friedman (1985) further explained the connection between severe depressive reactions as a form of self-punishment that arises in response to survivor's guilt.

Depressed Mood   The *DSM–IV* lists depressed mood first as a symptom of depression.

> Depressed mood most of the day, nearly every day, as indicated by either subjective reports (e.g. feels sad or empty) or observation made by others (e.g. appears tearful). Note: In children and adolescents, can be irritable mood. (American Psychiatric Association, 1994, p. 327)

Depressed mood is regularly felt and observed in survivors of multiple AIDS-related loss. Shrader's (1992) study of survivors found "a profound sense of depression" (p. 113).

Tearfulness can become so pronounced that it becomes embarrassing to the survivor. Mitch, a survivor of multiple AIDS-related loss, said he is embarrassed every time "I cry on the bus, but that is the only quiet time in my life and sometimes emotions overwhelm me." Another survivor described himself as

> oozing. I am always ready to burst out with tears but I am not able to have a strong, cathartic release. Instead it is gradual and persistent. Last week I went to the Oregon coast to get away, but I sat looking at tide pools crying.

The reason for the prevalence of depressed mood appears obvious: So much grief is bound to produce intense sadness, gloominess, hopelessness, and melancholia, yet other, less obvious reasons considered below also contribute to depressed mood in survivors. One of the ironies of current theory is the supposed mutual exclusivity of depression and grief. The *DSM–IV* diagnostic criteria for a major depressive episode explicitly exclude symptoms related to bereavement, which it defines as "the loss of a loved one" (American Psychiatric Association, 1994, p. 327). One wonders where survivors of multiple loss fit into this scheme. A diagnosis of depression is ruled out because their symptoms are bereavement related, yet their symptoms do not arise from the loss of *a* loved one.

Unresolved grief directly contributes to depressed mood. The emotional flood that hovers over the grief process for a survivor of multiple AIDS-related loss understandably encourages avoidance of grief work. Those times when feelings of grief leak through the defenses are so painful that any attempt to deal with the accumulated toll of grief seems daunting and dangerous. So, the survivor chooses to avoid grieving. Bowlby (1980) observed that depressed mood is common among those who avoid conscious grieving.

Emotional shutdown is common in survivors and is discussed in more detail in the next chapter in the context of traumatization. Lindemann (1944) observed an "absence of emotional display" (p. 145) in survivors of acute grief. To the extent such a stance is consciously constructed, emotional shutdown is meant to eliminate uncomfortable feelings. Although the survivor might wish to only depress "negative" emotions, the inevitable result is the depression of a spectrum of emotions. It is impossible to have only happy, joyful, cheery emotions. Erich Fromm concluded, "To spare oneself from grief at all cost can be achieved only at the price of total detachment, which excludes the ability to experience happiness" (as cited in Staudacher, 1994, p. 147). Paradoxically, the survivor of multiple AIDS-related loss must face and feel a range of emotions that includes sadness, anger, frustration, and despair in order to feel more pleasant emotions.

Two characteristics of depressed mood in survivors are discussed later in more detail. The *DSM–IV* indicates that some persons with depression "report or exhibit increased irritability (e.g., persistent anger, a tendency to respond to events with angry outburst or blaming others, or an exaggerated sense of frustration over minor matters)" (American Psychiatric Association, 1994, p. 321). The next chapter discusses diffuse anger in survivors. Survivor's guilt, a condemnation directed inward, is widely manifested and discussed later in this chapter. Introjected guilt is widely acknowledged to contribute to depressed mood.

Anhedonia   The second symptom listed by the *DSM–IV* is anhedonia, "markedly diminished interest or pleasure in all, or almost all, activities most of the day, nearly every day" (American Psychiatric Assocation, 1994, p. 327). Anhedonia is common in survivors of multiple AIDS-related loss. The sense that nothing is worthwhile goes beyond the attitude of many people who struggle with depression, becoming a fundamental question of meaning whose only answer seems to be that there is no point in anything. Carol Staudacher (1994) wrote,

> For some survivors, grief does more than encompass sorrow and sadness; it produces deep depression. During this depression life seems as if it is too much trouble. The smallest task appears to be insurmountable. Nothing interests us. We don't want to have to think or act—or even be. (p. 109)

Activities that were meaningful or enjoyable no longer inspire enthusiasm. Camus (1948, p. 104) observed that the "plague had killed all colors, vetoed pleasure." In Shrader's (1992) study of survivors of multiple AIDS-related loss, he found that they "had become a great deal more serious and less fun-loving and spontaneous" (p. 102). A death pall permeates the lives of many survivors, making every activity assume the flavor of death and dread. For example, enjoyment of sex is frequently diminished in survivors (Stulberg & Smith, 1988). The connection between death and sex has been explored by Freud and others, although it takes on special salience in the context of AIDS. The act of sex can be viewed literally as an act of killing.

Anhedonia restricts future planning by constricting the survivor's vision. One survivor said, "I used to have a lot of dreams. Now, I have none." Among aging survivors of the Holocaust, Krystal (1981) observed a similar outlook: "These losses force a shift from doing to thinking, from planning to reminiscing, from preoccupation with everyday events and long-range planning to reviewing and rethinking one's life" (p. 176). Some survivors observe a loss of productivity in themselves and others. "Grieving takes up all my energy so I don't have any left to be productive."

Sleep Disturbances   The *DSM–IV* includes "insomnia or hypersomnia nearly every day" (American Psychiatric Association, 1994, p. 327) as a symptom of depression. Sleep disturbance is widely reported in survivors of multiple AIDS-related loss. The survivor may overuse sleep in a way common to depression, as a means of escaping the pain of wakefulness. Other survivors have great difficulty sustaining a whole night of sleep because of worries, memories, and preoccupation. Dreams may focus on AIDS so that the survivor is offered no escape, even through sleep. Although sleep disturbance is an indication of depression, it also arises in response to trauma. Among survivors of the Holocaust, for example, "research has shown that 85% of the survivors" (Kaminer & Lavie, 1993, p. 335) suffered some type of sleep disorder for many years. Some type of sleep disturbance seems inevitable in survivors of multiple AIDS-related loss. In a study of gay men who had survived multiple AIDS-related loss, Martin (1988) found a correlation between the severity of sleep problems and the number of losses.

Excessive and Inappropriate Shame or Guilt   The *DSM–IV* includes as a symptom of depression "feelings of worthlessness or excessive or inappropriate guilt (which may be delusional) nearly every day" (American Psychiatric Association, 1994, p. 327). This criterion for depression is actually specifying two things, shame and guilt. These two psychodynamic forces deserve to be addressed separately. Because of its endemic and dynamic effect, survivor's guilt is addressed in more detail later in this chapter.

Shame inhibits the experience and expression of grief. Kauffman (1989) concluded that "the shame-prone personality is likely to feel overwhelmed in grief by feelings of self-consciousness, failure, inadequacy, inferiority, abandonment, and exposure. He is even more likely to feel ashamed of his shame, and sometimes to disenfranchise himself profoundly" (p. 28). Shame is the belief that "one's being is flawed, that one is defective as a human being" (Bradshaw, 1988, p. vii). Guilt, however, is the belief that one has behaved wrongly. Shame is a recognized part of depression in many individuals (Beck, Rush, Shaw, & Emery, 1979). Shame is a frequent companion of grief. Death creates a sense of horror and feelings of disgrace. These are reinforced by people around survivors who may fear, patronize, or shun them (Staudacher, 1994).

At least three factors beyond those normally correlated with depression contribute to the development of shame in survivors of multiple AIDS-related loss. First, the nature of stigmatization presupposes shame. Second, perceptions of powerlessness and helplessness—which are inevitable among survivors—evoke a sense of inadequacy. Third, preexisting shame is frequently aggravated by AIDS. Homosexuals who previously internalized homophobia and hetero-sexism, which create "a basic mistrust for one's sexual and interpersonal iden-tity" (Stein & Cohen, 1984, p. 61), now internalize a diseased identity that mutilates and kills, evokes dread, and is linked to homosexual intimacy and pleasure. Likewise, hemophiliacs and addicted IVDUs who feel shame over their condition must simultaneously take on a diseased identity.

Depressed people believe themselves to be more ineffective than they actu-ally are. This is one of the areas in which the effect of grief and trauma overlap in survivors of multiple AIDS-related loss. Traumatization usually results from an experience that cannot be controlled. It is a mind-set that undermines moti-vation to initiate. "Depression is not generalized pessimism, but pessimism specific to the effects of one's own skilled actions" (Seligman, 1975, p. 86).

Suicidal and Death Thoughts   Another symptom of major depression that arises in survivors of multiple AIDS-related loss is "recurrent thoughts of death (not just fear of dying), recurrent suicidal ideation without a specific plan, or a suicide attempt or a specific plan for committing suicide" (American Psychiatric Association, 1994, p. 327). Recurrent thoughts of death permeate an environ-ment characterized by the death imprint (discussed in the next chapter). Know-ing others "who are sick, dying, suicidal or who died from AIDS increases risk" for suicide (Lippmann, James, & Frierson, 1993, p. 75). Substance abuse (Faulstich, 1987) and various AIDS-related brain diseases (Cohen & Weisman, 1986) con-tribute to suicidal risk.

Persons struggling with depression are at higher risk for suicide. Surviving multiple, ongoing loss exacerbates the risk, for a number of reasons. Sprang and McNeil (1995) suggested that "the increased incidence of attempted and com-pleted suicide found in this population is related to the anxiety and fear of death, bodily mutilation, separation and fear of loneliness, isolation, ignominy, and rejection" (p. 154). Suicidal ideation occurs in survivors who lose interest in life ("What's the point of living?"). Moreover, the future holds the certainty of more pain ("I can take no more!"). O'Neil (1989) compared the higher risk of suicide in survivors of AIDS-related loss to that of elderly persons:

> Certainly, it is well documented that the older widow and widower are at great risk for suicidal thinking and actions (Berardo, 1970). Thoughts of suicide come from a wish to join the deceased, a sense that life without the deceased is too overwhelm-ing and not worth living. Research on AIDS-related grief and suicide is new and is just beginning to be identified and documented. However, the mother whose only

son has died from AIDS and the surviving partner who is in poor health and
lacking adequate social support are both at high risk for suicide. (p. 82)

Higher than usual rates of suicide in homosexuals predate AIDS. Among gay
men, Stulberg and Smith (1988) found that more than 20% had considered
suicide because of AIDS. It is sometimes difficult to distinguish between a
suicide that is rationally thought out and planned in response to the prognosis
and pain of AIDS and a suicide that is motivated by depression and despair.
Both regularly occur in the AIDS epoch. Russ Berst, a gay man who lives with
AIDS, was devastated when his brother killed himself after discovering that he
tested HIV positive. Russ still cannot make sense of it, especially when he
compares his brother's decision with his own determination, which has allowed
him to live with HIV for over a decade. Now, as Russ lives with opportunistic
infections that threaten his eyesight, cause continual pain, and threaten a horrifying death, he is reluctant to commit rational suicide because of the pain it
would cause his family in light of his brother's suicide.

George, a survivor of multiple loss, told of his experience with AIDS-
related suicide.

> I had a good friend with AIDS who had been having symptoms of mild dementia.
> I had been away at a week-long conference, and when I returned I couldn't reach
> him by phone. I went over to his apartment and found him dead. He had taken his
> life. He had been dead several days. It really was the most devastating death I've
> experienced. . . . And the way he died—I couldn't get over it being a suicide. That
> he died alone. That he'd been dead in his apartment for days. The whole thing was
> horrific. I felt, if life can do this to him, what's it going to do to the rest of us? (as
> cited in Garfield, 1995, p. 172)

Raleigh, who has devoted his professional and personal life to work around
AIDS, called suicide "the hidden killer of AIDS. No one talks about it."

Anxiety

Mark, one survivor of multiple AIDS-related loss with HIV, said, "Who wouldn't
be anxious? I'm watching all of my friends go blind, lose their minds, wither
and die around me." Anxiety is widely observed among survivors of multiple
AIDS-related loss. Rando (1986a) noted that anxiety is a "normal accompani-
ment to the uncertain, sometimes mutually exclusive demands of the terminal
illness [and] can be exacerbated as continual changes and losses occur either
unpredictably or as part of an unstoppable process" (p. 112) that survivors are
powerless to prevent. Most survivors live with ongoing reason for worry. Loved
ones continue to sicken and die while memories of other losses reverberate.
Among communities where risk of new HIV infection persists, apprehension
about seroconversion is especially troubling. "Who will be next?" is a commonly voiced concern. Uncertainty pervades thoughts about the future.

The degree and depth of anxiety experienced by survivors of multiple AIDS-related loss, especially when they live amid ongoing dread, cannot be over-stated. Many liken their experience to "what it must be like to live in a war." Some survivors fear psychological disintegration. Witnessing dying and death provokes anxiety related to one's own mortality. Threats to one's basic beliefs about meaning, life and death, responsibility, relationships, and sense of identity are inevitable. Hardly any part of one's life remains untouched by anxiety.

A study of gay survivors of multiple loss in Australia found an increased rate of anxiety associated with "anticipating their own possible death, mutilation to their own body, and separation from many of the people important to them" (Viney et al., 1992, p. 160). Not surprisingly, those who test HIV positive experience heightened anxiety as a result of their own vulnerability to disease and death (Hays, Chauncey, & Tobey, 1990). More important, "HIV-positive men experience a global state of anxiety in which death anxiety and more general distress are not easily separated" (Hintze, Templer, Cappelletty, & Frederick, 1994, p. 197). Although Hintze et al. make no mention of it, the observed global state of anxiety might have more to do with the participants' overall experience with multiple AIDS-related loss than with worries about their own mortality.

Mood-Altering Chemical Abuse

Substance abuse is not uncommon among survivors of multiple AIDS-related loss (Nord, 1996a). Two factors account for higher than average rates of alcohol and drug abuse. First, a number of survivors began experiencing multiple loss with a preexisting chemical dependency or abuse history. Second, the stresses of surviving multiple loss lead some survivors to use mood-altering chemicals as a coping mechanism.

Needless to say, survivors in the IV drug-using community are prone to be coping with abuse. Preexisting alcohol and drug abuse among gay men and lesbians was inflated; a review of incidence studies in the United States and Europe has indicated that about 25% of gay men and lesbians "suffer from definitive drug and alcohol abuse problems, while an additional percentage experience 'suggestive or problematic' abuse patterns" (Bickelhaupt, 1995, p. 5). Homophobia significantly contributes to chronic stress that contributes to substance abuse in lesbians and gay men (Kominars, 1995). A complexity of issues related to being gay hinder recovery efforts (Pohl, 1995).

Use of alcohol and other drugs offers a route of escape from painful feelings. In a situation marked by lack of control, mood-altering chemicals provide a sense of control. Survivors of multiple loss with a preexisting pattern of drug use may increase use of this familiar method of coping. Martin and Dean (1993a) found that the use of drugs, other than alcohol, among gay survivors of AIDS-related loss was "significantly elevated among the bereaved" (p. 326). In his research on AIDS-related bereavement in gay men, Martin (1988) demonstrated a "significant dose-response relationship between the number of bereavements and recreational drug and sedative drug use" (p. 860).

The abusive use of mood-altering chemicals impedes the healthy resolution of grief (Rando, 1993). Using alcohol and drugs as a means to alleviate pain of loss is akin to drinking salt water to alleviate thirst. At first, it may seem to work, but in the end the problem is compounded. Abuse of alcohol or other drugs complicates bereavement by restricting the normal range of emotions and experiences that are the essence of grief process and work. Much of the pain and anguish of grieving is cathartic because it is genuinely felt and remembered. Psychoactive chemicals that interfere with this process inevitably interfere with grief. "Drugs become the instant defense against the pain and resolution of the mourning process" (Skolnick, 1979, p. 285). Research has consistently correlated past and present substance abuse with poor bereavement outcome (Zisook & DeVaul, 1983). This is demonstrated among families struggling with addiction (Coleman, 1980), spouses of those with alcoholism (Blankfield, 1989), and in families with unresolved grief (Raphael, 1983). The connection between psychoactive chemical abuse and complicated bereavement is so strong that Rando (1993) asserted that addiction "not only indicates but actually perpetuates complicated mourning" (p. 196).

Many survivors face up to problems with mood-altering chemical abuse, taking steps to recover from abusive or addictive patterns. Recall the personal story of Keith Arnett presented in chapter 4. Multiple loss sometimes provides the clarion call needed to convince the survivor of the need to address chemical dependency problems. Chapter 9 explores the many ways that survivors are awakened to look at existential issues. This results in survivors observing that they have grown through an experience that provided them with an impetus to live a more authentic life.

INTERPERSONAL RESPONSES TO MULTIPLE AIDS-RELATED LOSS

Surviving multiple AIDS-related loss is an interpersonal crisis. Loss and threat of loss pervade the survivor's connections to others. The risk involved and repeatedly demonstrated in relationships with others leads some survivors to withdraw and isolate themselves, although others derive great comfort from fostering relationships and increasing social involvement. Some develop a cynical attitude marked by pessimism and hopelessness. Diffuse anger presents itself as both an attitude and a way of being. Survivor's guilt is pervasive and multilayered. To complicate matters further, all of these interpersonal styles may alternatingly exist in the same survivor.

Withdrawal and Isolation

Much grieving is withdrawing. The bereaved person is hurt and vulnerable. In a way analogous to covering a wound with a bandage, the injured person withdraws to protect her- or himself. "Grief is a very antisocial state," according to Penelope Mortimer (as cited in Staudacher, 1994):

> All survivors tend to avoid gatherings. We don't want to be looked at. We don't want to have to hide our feelings. We don't want to listen to conversations that seem inane. We don't want to have to try to concentrate on something that doesn't interest us in the slightest. (p. 122)

Normal withdrawal impulses tend to subside with time, but time is measured by its distance from the loss event. When multiple, ongoing losses accumulate, time cannot provide a normal healing respite.

"Progressive social isolation" was identified by Lindemann (1944) and many others as a sign of complicated bereavement reaction. Parkes (1975) noted the tendency to isolate among those suffering complicated bereavement. Kastenbaum (1969) connected the tendency to withdraw to "a sense of extreme caution" (p. 49) in multiple-loss survivors. New relationships involve risk. Although this may always be true, survivors of multiple, ongoing loss are particularly conscious of this risk. Participants in Shrader's (1992) study "reported withdrawing and feeling extreme isolation" (p. 114).

Survivors of multiple AIDS-related loss are liable to find themselves with choices about whether to establish relationships that are likely to produce future losses. Characteristics of being a survivor increase the potential for future loss that is only avoided by withdrawal and isolation. Caregivers of people with AIDS may have a professional or voluntary involvement that heightens their investment. Choices to avoid connection must be deliberate and usually require a multilevel decision. Those unfamiliar with the world of multiple-loss survivors are sometimes taken aback by choices that seem callous and cold. One nurse chose to move to a small, rural community in central Oregon to avoid the pain of loss that he described as unbearable, but he first had to make an agonizing decision to sever relationships with persons for whom he cared deeply. Volunteers face a similar dilemma. All must confront the dilemma of self-care versus the tremendous needs of the AIDS epoch.

Persons with AIDS, because of their involvement with AIDS-related services, are likely to have contact with others with AIDS and have choices to make about relationships that will expose them to additional loss. Mainly, however, long-term survivors of AIDS prioritize the importance of personal relationships (Remien, Rabkin, Williams, & Katoff, 1992). One of the most effective coping skills many people with AIDS use is to volunteer their time helping others with AIDS, as is discussed in chapter 10. Although socializing with other people with AIDS "can be empowering and helpful," such relationships "can mean setting themselves up for more loss in the future" (Jue, 1994, p. 329).

Two parallel processes occur. Along with withdrawal, survivors confront isolation as their support system is eliminated. The survivor, faced with the loss of existing friends and family, either replaces them or grows increasingly isolated. The only way to avoid ongoing loss is for the survivor to neglect existing friends, social activities, and sometimes family while avoiding new relationships. This attempt to control future loss through isolation and withdrawal occurs among some survivors of multiple AIDS-related loss. A similar tendency was observed among survivors of the Holocaust, who experienced the fear of loving someone (Cohen, 1991). Other survivors realize the risk involved but choose to establish new relationships anyhow. One survivor said, "I know that I am exposing myself to more pain but what is the choice? I will not live in a shell!"

Withdrawal occurs at a psychological as well as a physical level. Survivors may distance themselves purposefully, preventing close attachments and avoiding existing relationships. Avoidance behavior is undertaken to reduce anxiety but more likely produces the opposite outcome. In a study of gay men with AIDS, reliance on avoidance techniques actually resulted in higher anxiety, more pessimism, and greater psychological distress (Kurdek & Siesky, 1990).

Ross moved to Seattle after his partner died in Los Angeles. "I have quit calling anyone in L.A. The first thing they always say is 'Did you here that so-and-so died?' Well I'm sick of it." One survivor explained how he protects himself from the shock of loss: "I imagine that they have already died before they die." Odets (1995) concluded, "In the face of familiar and repeated death, intimate relationships become distant, perfunctory, asexual, hostile, or fall apart; and the friendships evaporate" (p. 87). To the extent that there is value in close relationships, this value is foreclosed. The survivor also puts him- or herself at high risk for regret and guilt.

Survivors who have lost the capacity to attach may also lose the capacity to detach effectively, a critical element of successful grieving. Speaking of the difficulty that Holocaust survivors had with grieving effectively, Krystal (1981) wrote that

> they do not experience love, nor do they have the kind of empathy that would permit them to sense their object's affection for them. One has to feel love to be able to believe in its existence. Most of all, one has to feel love to be able to accept one's own self and one's own past. (p. 187)

The same shell that the survivor of multiple AIDS-related loss builds to protect him- or herself from further loss may also be a shell that walls in the emotional discharge necessary to adjustment.

Contrary Attitudes and Diffuse Anger

Francis Bacon said, "No man is angry that feels not himself hurt" (as cited in Staudacher, 1994, p. 46). Survivors of multiple AIDS-related loss live in a world permeated by hurt, sickness and death, mistrust and betrayal, and cycles of raised and dashed hopes. Friends and family await the coming of new infection, painful agonies, and the near certainty of death. For hemophiliacs, an "incredible sense of betrayal and resentment" (Goss, 1994, p. 1) is felt by those who are certain that infections through the blood supply could have been prevented or that earlier efforts at education could have saved tens of thousands. Countless hopes for treatments and cures never pan out. The most basic assumptions pertaining to social stability and life expectations are dashed.

Cynicism and pessimism are understandable and common responses, yet these attitudes are scarcely acknowledged in published material pertaining to multiple loss or AIDS. Attempts to discuss this survivor response are strongly criticized: "How dare you say that?" Three reasons may account for the tendency to ignore these attitudes. First, pity for the survivor or person with AIDS restricts forthright assessment of critical characteristics. Second, the survivor's experience has received scant attention; analysis of survivor issues is immature. Third, there is risk in appearing to criticize any part of the gay community. In Randy Shilts's last interview ("Interview," 1995), he spoke of the bitter attacks he endured within San Francisco's gay community because of his reports about continued high-risk, promiscuous sex behaviors. Some who have publicly discussed recent high-risk sexual behaviors have similarly been denounced.

Some authors have observed contrary, antagonistic attitudes in survivors. Klein (1994) noted "pervasive expressions of pessimism, cynicism, fatalism and insecurity" (p. 15). Her connection of these attitudes to insecurity is insightful. Insecurity combines with an understandable siege mentality in the face of continuing overwhelming loss. It is the psychic equivalent of a good offense making the best defense. Shrader (1992) observed that certain emotional reactions in survivors of multiple AIDS-related losses were another outstanding characteristic of this population. The most palpable of these emotions were the intense anger, rage, fury, bitterness, hostility, cynicism, sarcasm, and frustration that these men expressed (Shrader, p. 108).

Anger is common in grief. Nearly all authorities on grief have discussed it, but survivors of multiple AIDS-related loss will likely experience more than the normal range and intensity of anger. First, they have multiple grief events, and thus multiple angers. Second, the characteristics of surviving multiple AIDS-related loss provoke an unusual amount of anger. Survivors may encounter anger from a variety of directions:

- anger that values and beliefs seem empty and unhelpful
- anger that losses are beyond any normal expectation
- anger at being left alone
- anger at the family of origin or family of choice
- anger at those dying and deceased for becoming infected
- anger at medical personnel and caregivers for being ineffectual
- anger at AIDS and opportunistic infections
- anger at society for ignoring and mistreating those with AIDS
- anger arising from personal helplessness

Anger may be normal during grieving, but it is typically not well accepted, understood, or handled by either survivors or those closest to them. The belief that anger is not supposed to be expressed exacerbates the tendency of multiple-loss survivors to express their anger indirectly and diffusely. If it will not be accepted in its pure, direct form, the survivor does not cease feeling angry. Rather, she or he may express anger indirectly, generally, and irrationally. Anger becomes a way of being more than an expression of emotion. Survivors frequently have insight about their anger. "I *am* angry. That's who I am. I am Jonathan the angry."

Anger may also become a justification for survival. The passion to bear witness includes anger. Among Holocaust survivors, Krystal (1981) observed that many viewed their justification for survival as being an "angry witness against the outrage of the Holocaust" (p. 178). Some survivors of multiple AIDS-related loss, especially those who are themselves struggling with AIDS, strike a perpetually angry, even hostile, stance. These angry activists are encountered time and again in AIDS policy meetings. Perhaps Larry Kramer (1994) personifies anger as justification. He commented on his own style of addressing issues. "When I am asked why I write at such a high pitch of invective, my response is that this seems to be the only way I can get anyone there to hear me" (Kramer, 1994, p. 117).

This attitudinal stance makes it challenging for friends, family, caregivers, and professionals. It is often those to whom the survivor feels closest and safest who receive the harshest treatment. Despite understanding the root causes for this negativism, those in close contact with survivors who express this mindset usually find relationships with these survivors difficult. The effect is sometimes to further isolate the survivor.

Survivor's Guilt

It is the rare survivor of multiple AIDS-related loss who does not experience a significant amount of survivor's guilt. Because the issue of survivor's guilt is so prevalent and critical to the survivor's experience, a thorough discussion is necessary. Various preexisting factors combine with unique characteristics of surviving multiple AIDS-related loss to predispose survivors to guilt. The widespread devastation of a particular community heightens the sense of guilt felt in those who seem singled out to survive. Again, the extreme nature of this phenomenon provides an opportunity to illuminate and expand theoretical understanding. Unresolved survivor's guilt indicates and hinders resolution of unresolved grief. Also, it may contribute to a number of potentially dangerous behaviors.

"Why Not Me?"   "Intimately connected with the experience of loss is the feeling of guilt" (Mogenson, 1992, p. 65). Traditional grief theory has consistently linked guilt and grief. Rando (1993) defined guilt as "the feeling of culpability deriving from perceived offenses or a sense of inadequacy" and connected it to "regret, remorse, negative self-evaluation, and feelings that one should atone" (p. 478). Survivors of multiple losses, especially those related to disasters, regularly question why they survived while others died. Survivor's guilt arises as a potential defense against feelings of helplessness in trauma survivors (Lindy, 1985). There is a sense that their survival was bought by the other's death. Survivors of the Holocaust, for example, frequently developed severe survivor guilt (Krystal, 1981) and were "haunted by the question 'Why did I survive when others better than me perished?'" (Cohen, 1991, p. 228). In survivors of multiple AIDS-related loss, guilt is often expressed as sorrow for the survivor's survival. This guilt does not need to be rational or accurate; the important part of guilt is the "person's *belief*" (Friedman, 1985, p. 529).

Helplessness and Blame   A paradoxical psychic paradigm of helplessness and blame mark the survivor's experience. The survivor suffers a perplexing and contradictory internal blame of inefficacy arising from helplessness. Some nurses treated patients with hemophilia in the early 1980s when the blood supply was contaminated. When these people return with AIDS, especially when they are angry, nurses may be particularly vulnerable to guilt for being involved in the treatment that led to AIDS (Gordon et al., 1993). The survivor has limited capacity to respond to the ongoing threat and invokes self-blame to account for that inadequate response. Lifton (1993) referred to this as the paradoxical guilt of victimized survivors. There is always a moral meaning attached to suffering. "We have no choice but to make judgments" (Lifton, p. 18) about suffering and one's relation to it. Lifton's observed that the survivor's fundamental inner question is

> "Why did I survive while letting him, her, or them die?" It is a relatively simple step to feel that by having so failed in one's image actions at the time, "I killed him," or that if I had died instead, he, she or they would have lived." This last feeling may in part reflect the psychic death one did actually undergo. . . . Death guilt ultimately stems from a sense that. . .one has no right to be alive. (pp. 17–18)

The circular, downward spiral of shame is engaged.

With multiple, ongoing loss, survivors continue to experience their own pain as victims while continuing to witness the pain of those they love. They struggle constantly with the need to master and find meaning in the ongoing disaster. "There must be something I can do!" Yet, survivors are powerless to stop the continuing suffering of themselves or others. Their fundamental incompetence is laid bare; they are to blame.

Frankl (1959/1984) discussed the mental state of those in Nazi concentration camps who were frightened that any decision might put them at odds with fate. Should I volunteer for a chore detail? Should I go to the left or right? Should I look or avoid looking at the guard? One (perceived) slip-up could mean death. Although the death camp survivor lived in an environment marked more by randomness than control, a natural human response to master and find meaning dominated. A magical sort of thinking pervades the survivor's attempt to make sense of his or her survival and others' nonsurvival. One survivor of multiple loss accompanied his partner to the doctor's for the results of his partner's HIV test.

> When the doctor told Kurt that he had tested positive I couldn't believe it. The last time he was tested I had prepared myself, telling myself that he would test positive. Then, he had tested negative. This time I was sure he would test negative. In fact, I remember resenting the bother of having to go to his doctor's office when I knew that he would test negative again. Then, he tested positive! I guess that I should have believed he would test positive. Then he would have tested negative.

This survivor has causally linked two unrelated facts: his cognitions about his partner's HIV test and his partner's actual HIV test results. The desperate need to find an explanation, any explanation, outweighs all rationality in an otherwise intelligent person. Looking at this type of thinking from the outside, the objective observer is tempted to deride it disdainfully: "It makes no sense!" Yet, it need make no sense. The confusion and pained anxiety behind this magical thinking deserves more sympathy than criticism. Still, at some point in the adjustment process, the survivor must be able to separate the rational from the irrational that underlies guilty magical thinking. This is the proper function of psychotherapy.

To this end, it helps to see this thinking in the context of B. F. Skinner's theory about superstitious behavior (Seligman, 1975, pp. 18–20). In 1948, Skinner dropped grain for hungry pigeons at regular and brief intervals. Whatever the pigeons did had no control over the delivery of grain. By the end of the training, Skinner noticed that all of the birds were doing something. One bird pecked incessantly, another hopped around. Skinner concluded that whatever the pigeon happened to be doing when grain arrived would be reinforced, thereby increasing the behavior's frequency. He called this superstitious behavior akin to people walking around ladders instead of under them. Humans (and some other animals) need to make sense of their environment, find order, and derive control from the ability to understand. As Seligman (1975) and others have demonstrated, uncontrollable events produce more distress than controllable ones. More about helplessness and survivors of multiple, ongoing loss is presented in the next chapter.

These judgments are made to avoid the seemingly more dreadful alternative conclusion about suffering, which is that it has no meaning. Frankl (1959/1984) observed that "it is not the physical pain which hurts the most; it is the mental agony caused by the injustice, the unreasonableness of it all" (p. 42). The same point can be made about the grief endured by survivors of multiple, ongoing loss who report that the unfairness of it all is the hardest to bear. The implications of that uncertainty and randomness so horrify survivors that meaning must be found. Faced with no frame of reference adequate to this challenge, the ego reverts to its earliest developmental frames of reference. The survivor may regress to the simple frame of narcissistic cause and effect: "I caused the disaster. I am to blame. If I had done something different, this never would have happened." Prior conflicts about trust and separation resurface.

When the true nature and meaning of the survivor's helplessness settles into the survivor's conscious and unconscious interaction with life, a horrifying fear related to nonbeing is inevitable. This is an anxiety worse than any fear, including the fear of death, because it is an anxiety with no definable target. One's identity, if it exists, is buffeted by forces utterly beyond both control and comprehension. When both legs on which humans stand—the capacity to master and find meaning—are cut off, the survivor is adrift without foundation, without tangible existence. This conclusion is utterly terrifying, so the survivor dreads the dread that threatens disintegration of his or her self-identity. This anxiety is more potent than any fear of death. Yalom (1980) observed that "a fear that can neither be understood nor located cannot be confronted and becomes more terrible still: it begets a feeling of helplessness which invariably generates further anxiety" (p. 43). The connection between helplessness, culpability, and guilt is complete: "I am too inadequate to live; I am nothing." Guilt, however, provides a grounding, a sense of control.

Although this anxiety is inevitable, it is easily transformed into a fear of something. Survivors may displace their anxiety of nothing into fear of something. Then, a purposeful, if frenetic, effort to combat fear can commence. Once an object or concept is feared, it can be challenged. Fear of death and fear of AIDS are obvious targets. Death and AIDS may be taunted; risks may be undertaken, as if to say, "See, I'm not afraid." The opportunity to negate the connection of guilt, culpability, and helplessness combines nicely with the opportunity to confront death and AIDS. Now, even self-destructive attitudes and behaviors are explicable. Control of AIDS and death contradicts helplessness, culpability, and guilt. The survivor's identity is preserved.

The Problem with Survivor's Guilt   Guilt, like denial, offers benefits to the survivor when its effects are temporally appropriate as an ego defense. It becomes dysfunctional when used persistently. First, guilt provides a defense against helplessness. Control counteracts helplessness. Guilt implies a manner of control, albeit a negative one. The survivor's fault caused harm; without the survivor or his or her fault, there would be no harm. Second, guilt provides meaning to an event that appears senseless. Therefore, guilt lessens anxiety. Guilt defends against anxiety (Friedman, 1985). It is better to live as a villain in an orderly world than to live as a helpless pawn in a world of chaotic disorder. Third, guilt keeps the memory of the loss alive by keeping it potent. To these can be added a fourth provision of guilt: The bargaining stage of grief work is fostered by the continuation of the lost object, relationship, or dream through guilt. Fundamentally, guilt seeks to negate the loss in a manner conceptually similar to the bargaining characteristic of predeath grieving in which the survivor attempts to suspend the inevitable. Kubler-Ross (1969) called bargaining "an attempt to postpone" (p. 83). Guilt is an attempt to suspend. In the short run, these provisions of guilt may benefit the survivor by shielding him or her from overwhelming exposure to pain and despair.

Guilt is always harmful to the grief process when maintained as a primary stance toward loss because it focuses attention back upon the mourner himself, thus preventing objective contemplation of the loss. Sorrow is felt for the survivor's survival, not for the lost object, relationship, or dream. This unfinished nature of guilt, its past-tense focus, and the continuing attachment it engenders obscures and defends against the process and work of adjusting to the irrevocable loss. An unconscious attempt to internalize the loss through guilt is an attempt to prevent the loss (Odets, 1995). Similarly, the death cause is readily internalized by taking HIV inside one's self.

The interrelation of guilt and ambivalence as a hindrance of normal grieving is particularly acute in the scenario of surviving multiple AIDS-related loss. Psychoanalytic theories have indicated that guilt and ambivalence disturb the normal course of mourning. Writing about absent grief, Deutsch (1937) concluded that "the degree of persisting ambivalence is a more important factor than the intensity of the positive ties" (p. 12). The working out of ambivalence necessary in grief work is stymied by the self-directed focus of guilt. (The guilty feel anger directed at themselves, not at the deceased.) Adjustment to loss necessitates detachment from what is lost, as Freud (1917/1957) noted:

> Just as the work of grief, by declaring the object to be dead and offering the ego the benefit of continuing to live, impels the ego to give up the object, so each single conflict of ambivalence, by disparaging the object, denigrating it, even as it were by slaying it, loosens the fixation of the libido to it. (p. 130)

When this process does not occur, attention is focused on the self in self-denigrating ways characteristic of guilt, and in Freud's conceptualization, of melancholia. Anger, turned inward, becomes depression. The increase of depression, isolation, and psychiatric illness were observed by Parkes (1972). These interrelate in survivors of multiple AIDS-related loss, circularly aggravating grief and hindering resolution.

Scott has advanced AIDS and survived his partner's death 3 years ago. He readily admits that he has never gotten over Stan's death. Occasionally he cries, but mainly his emotional and cognitive expressions are blunted and marked by denial. He regularly speaks of the anguishing guilt he feels about his survival and Stan's death. Scott finds reasons to feel guilty over the most innocuous events. Even decisions that were made to benefit Stan are sometimes spoken about as though they were the heinous deeds of a hateful man. Inevitably, Scott's self-criticism is matched by glowing praise for Stan, who "was perfect." Listening to Scott, one would conclude that Stan was the most giving, generous, loving, intelligent, sociable man who ever lived. "He was a far better person than me. I should be dead and he should be alive." There is no capacity for ambivalence in Scott's view of his life as a survivor or in his partner's life and death. He was good; I am bad. Thus, there is no way to sort out the ambivalence that is a part of all grief work.

Guilt and feelings of helplessness are sometimes sublimated into excessive AIDS-related service work, sometimes at burnout levels. This work conforms with society's prioritization of work, provides a sense of gratification, and paradoxically defends the psyche by allowing avoidance of focus on AIDS-related loss. This tendency seemed more prevalent earlier in the AIDS epoch before so many caregivers burned out and when overwhelming need for caregiving predominated. Many caregivers trace their earliest involvement back to feelings related to guilt.

Gay Guilt   Prior losses that remain unresolved predispose one to complicated bereavement, particularly when guilt surrounds the loser's losses. Guilt is a type of loss, a loss of identity, a failing to live up to personal expectations. The guilty see their interaction with the world as inadequate, prone to incompetence. Mainly, guilt is an interpretation of the past: "I did it wrong." A guilty stance predisposes future guilt. Guilt becomes a built-in tendency in the individual's interpretation of life events. This tendency is especially likely when major life developmental stages and transitions have been interpreted through the prism of guilt. Prior losses that were interpreted as an individual's fault will predispose a survivor of further losses to contextualize the experience guiltily. These losses are likely to be unresolved. The more an individual's response to loss is imbedded in guilt, the more likely are responses of guilt to future losses.

Gay men are uniquely poised to assume guilt in the context of multiple AIDS-related loss. Although guilt has been well studied and analyzed in traditional, single-event, heterosexual bereavements, "there is a paucity of research" (Boykin, 1991, p. 250) on gay grief in general and gay survivors' guilt in particular. Their personal histories are frequently marked by guilt, especially in relation to major life development and transition. Walt Odets (1995), a clinical psychologist who works in San Francisco with gay survivors of multiple loss, concluded that survivor guilt has a central position among gay men living with the AIDS epidemic partially because "gay men as a group suffer inordinate problems with guilt, beginning very early in life" (p. 51).

> Among the developmental circumstances that make survivor guilt a significant issue in the lives of many gay men is being homosexual itself. Very often the simple fact of a homosexual son introduces survivor guilt into family relations. The son's homosexuality is experienced by the family as an abandonment, and by the son himself as the reason he must abandon others to survive as himself. . . . Abandonment is often made literal by the son's leaving home in order to live

homosexually. . . . Because abandonment of the family may be integral to being homosexual, survivor guilt may be too. (Odets, 1995, pp. 52–53).

Although Odets speaks mainly of the gay male experience, this familial experience and guilt apply equally to lesbians. Their nature may be an affront and injury to their parents. Early experience with blame "is a central experience leading to guilt" resulting "in a profound conviction of one's culpability and unworthiness and leaves one extremely vulnerable to blame in later life" (Friedman, 1985, p. 533). Not a few lesbians and gay men have heard something similar to "If you tell your grandmother that you are homosexual it will kill her!" or "Our family line will end; you are killing the family!"

AIDS offers the perfect opportunity to feed the guilt cycle that began early. The gay sexual act kills. Gays kill other gays. These ideas are explicitly reinforced by any public statements that assign blame for AIDS to gay men. New infections with HIV are particularly susceptible to this guilt-induced reasoning. Those with HIV often make explicit efforts to communicate the fact that they were infected before the mid-1980s. Those infected after educational prevention efforts began are treated with disdain because they are at fault. "How could you let yourself get infected?" This attitude is in the same vein of reasoning that distinguished innocent victims earlier in the AIDS epoch. The reality is that "no group in society has demonstrated the ability to sustain change in their sexual behavior like those achieved by gay men" (Van Gorder, 1994, p. 3). Yet, instead of pride, guilt accompanies the low rate of infection.

The disease's impact has focused on gay men. Widespread perception persists that the primary defining characteristic making a person homosexual instead of heterosexual is sex (Cass, 1984). It is this sexual identity that readily transmits the virus. Public attention has embedded the idea that AIDS is a gay disease. The public that views homosexuality as a choice must also see AIDS as a choice. Those with AIDS become culpable; homosexuals are to blame. To suffer the impact of multiple AIDS-related loss is the consequence of avoidable fault. It is a small step to guilt in gay survivors. To be a member of the gay community is to be blamable. The reasoning—"The community is guilty. I am part of the community. Therefore I am guilty."—need not be conscious.

Gay grief may exacerbate guilt about sexual preference, according to Siegal and Hoefer (1981), who observed that "conflicts regarding one's sexuality may resurface" (p. 520) as a result of grief. Self-doubts and insecurities about being gay are restimulated. In large part, this occurs because of the normal tendency of one loss to provoke memories of previous losses. A gay identity involves many losses, which may resurface in the survivor of multiple AIDS-related loss.

Lack of social recognition for gay relationships fosters guilt. Chapter 8 discusses the importance of relationships, including families of choice and friendships, that are affected by multiple AIDS-related loss and devalued by society. The lack of recognition and support these relationships receive leads directly to a lack of recognition and support for their loss. Survivors may easily conclude that their relationships are wrong, invalid, and somehow unreal. Thus, survivors may doubt their feelings of grief, including guilt, thereby feeling guilty for feeling guilty. Survivors may feel guilty for feelings that other, "normal" people tell them that they should not have: "He was only a friend; what are you so upset about?"

Gay men who test negative for HIV often face an intensified form of grief. The same question is heard in a variety of forms: "Why did Steve and Ron and Brian and Mark and Paul and Pedro and Joe get it while I didn't? I did exactly the same things as they did!" Sometimes a guilty comparison is explicit: "John was a better person than me. I should have died, not him." These thoughts are regularly ridiculed and belittled by those who expect that a gay man testing negative for HIV would, and should, feel only gratitude and relief. Yet, these gay men have often lived the majority of their lives as outsiders. Having accepted their sexuality, they are no longer outsiders to themselves. Having disclosed their sexual orientation to family, coworkers, and friends, they are no longer outsiders in their world. Having established meaningful interpersonal relationships by living among other gay men, they are no longer outside a community. Then, AIDS came along, and these men have found themselves outsiders again. Rachel Schochet works in San Francisco, where she is investigating the incidence of stress disorders in gay men who test HIV negative. She wrote that

> some men find it difficult to disclose a seronegative antibody status because they fear friends who are positive will reject them. In order to gain social acceptance, some men may lie about their serostatus in an effort to join with seropositive friends and avoid their potential rejection. This may be particularly true in communities where social and political activities focus on AIDS, and where people with AIDS may be the greatest folk heroes and receive the most attention. (Schochet, 1989, p. 3)

Worse than feeling like the odd man out, they are physically left as the odd man out when their friends have died. It is not surprising that many gay men report a decrease in anxiety when they test positive or receive an AIDS diagnosis (Tartaglia, 1989).

Gay men who test negative have a difficult time asking for and receiving support for these and other issues. Without any way to work through the issues of chronic survivor's guilt, some gay men express their guilt through irrational self-destructive behaviors. Living in a world where so many have died and continue to die is not an appealing prospect. Odets (1995) observed that for those who are guilty, depressed, anxious, and living a life that often seems not worth living, the self-destructive aspects of unprotected sex are incentives to practice it.

Survivor's guilt plays a significant role in many forms of self-destructive behavior. This discussion on the psychodynamics of survivor's guilt and self-destructive impulses is presented here as one explanation of high-risk gay sexual behavior. However, it applies equally well to others who experience survivor's guilt as a result of multiple AIDS-related loss, including the IVDU who continues to share needles and the hemophiliac who is not careful about preventing bleeds.

Friedman (1985) traced this self-destructive impulse, which may be "properly termed self-punishment" (p. 535), back to the child's experience with punishment from a blaming parent. Early experiences with punishment instill guilt for the perception of wrongdoing and suggest reparation through punishment. Repeated experience of blame and culpability early in life "leave one extremely vulnerable to blame in later life" (p. 533). When the actual parent is no longer available to mete out punishment, the individual's superego can enforce justice.

Self-punishment serves a number of useful functions. It becomes a way to mediate anxiety associated with guilt. By sharing the fate of the person or group who suffers, the empathic component of guilt is diminished. One feels less guilty when suffering the same fate. By contracting HIV, the survivor identifies with those who have died, ameliorating guilt about survival. The cognitive component of guilt is also diminished. "By inflicting suffering on one's self, one can more easily deny that one has caused another to suffer. By a process of magical thinking one becomes the victim and therefore not the offender" (Friedman, 1985, p. 535).

It is easy to see how each of these functions is important to, and used by, the survivor of multiple AIDS-related loss. There is much anxiety to mitigate, not the least of which results from helplessness. Self-punishment effectively provides a sense of control and a tangible response. The survivor who physically suffers the effect of HIV, another disease, or somatic complaints becomes less of an outsider and less of an offender.

CONCLUSION

After reading this chapter and chapter 5, it should be clear that the survivor of multiple AIDS-related loss faces many issues that complicate the normal course of bereavement. Although some generalizations apply to all survivors of multiple AIDS-related loss, the survivor's grief experience is notable mainly for its individuality and the complexity of interrelated factors that affect it. Normal bereavement is not the norm for survivors of multiple AIDS-related loss. This conclusion may help by encouraging a more refined approach to conceptualizing grief, including the interrelationship of various factors that influence the survivor's experience while discouraging the forced application of stage theories or viewing the "proper" accomplishment of grief as necessitating detachment. This realization should bolster a recent theme in thanatology, namely that "bereavement does in fact have many faces" (Sprang & McNeil, 1995, p. 181).

The survivor of ongoing, multiple loss confronts the process and work of grief in an environment that greatly handicaps adjustment. Although this discussion has focused on AIDS, many of the concepts might also apply to survivors of other multiple, ongoing loss scenarios such as those who are living amid war, the violence of some inner-city neighborhoods, and persistent abuse.

Grief is the process and work of adjusting to irrevocably lost objects, relationships, and dreams. Grieving must not be viewed as simply a process or sequence of stages. Neither should grief be associated only with death events. The challenges posed by multiple AIDS-related loss provide an opportunity to better understand normal grief by pushing the edges of grief concepts. In the next chapter, traumatization is reviewed in the light of surviving multiple AIDS-related loss. Traditionally, grief and trauma have been studied separately, usually as two distinctly different responses. AIDS forces a unitary approach to grief and trauma. Traumatic grief is a regular occurrence among survivors of multiple AIDS-related loss.

Chapter 7

Multiple AIDS-Related Loss as Trauma

> If only he could put the clock back and be once more the man who, at the outbreak of the epidemic, had only one thought and one desire. . . . But that, he knew, was out of the question now; he had changed too greatly. The plague had forced on him a detachment which, try as he might, he couldn't think away, and which like a formless fear haunted his mind.—Albert Camus (1948), *The Plague*

A psychologist with extensive experience working with clients affected by AIDS said that "the traumatic effects of multiple AIDS-related loss are usually ignored. These people have suffered trauma and show symptoms of [post-traumatic stress disorder] but hardly anyone has recognized it" (C. Tollfree, personal communication, 1996). In thinking about multiple AIDS-related loss, grief and bereavement issues easily come to mind. The potential for traumatization is less obvious. In books, scholarly articles, and seminars about AIDS, the topic of trauma is rarely mentioned in connection with surviving multiple AIDS-related loss. Nevertheless, traumatization does arise out of the experience of multiple AIDS-related loss.

TRAUMA DEFINED

In common, day-to-day use, the word *trauma* connotes a shocking or painful emotional experience. A number of negative experiences, including a single death, lost job, or relationship breakup can be considered traumatic, given this definition. Indeed, the term trauma is greatly overused, which is unfortunate. The haphazard application of the term dilutes its authentic meaning and leads some to scoff when it is applied. This book uses the term trauma carefully and deliberately outlines the professionally accepted characteristics of trauma, applying them to multiple AIDS-related loss.

When used as a descriptive term in psychology, trauma connotes something more than misfortune. A traumatic event is something outside the normal range of human experience. The *DSM–IV* (American Psychiatric Association, 1994) defines trauma as a confrontation with an event that involves actual or threatened death or serious injury, or a threat to the physical integrity of self or others. Events traditionally viewed as producing this type of trauma have included war, violent personal assault, and disasters but are expressly not limited to these.

The traumatic experience is one that produces lasting injury to the traumatized individual. Symptoms cluster in three categories: persistent avoidance of stimuli associated with the trauma or generalized psychic numbing, recurrent distressful recollections associated with the traumatic event, and persistent symptoms of increased arousal.

Therefore, according to a psychological perspective, deaths that are normal and expected are not considered traumatic events. Even when a death seems particularly terrible, such as the death of a child or spouse, it is not a traumatic event in the context of the psychological definition of trauma. The person suffering such a loss would certainly be experiencing grief, but not trauma.

MULTIPLE AIDS-RELATED LOSS AS TRAUMATIZATION

The realization that surviving multiple AIDS-related loss can be traumatic is important for survivors, caregivers, and professionals for a number of reasons, including the following:

- Defining multiple AIDS-related loss as a form of traumatization provides a context for understanding the experience of survivors.
- There is little theoretical or clinical information available for treating the multiple-loss survivor's response. Previous experiences of treatment with survivors of other forms of traumatization may provide a foundation of treatment options.
- Viewing the experience as traumatic allows a framework for normalizing this abnormal experience. The survivor is helped by knowing that his or her experience is extraordinary.

Surviving multiple AIDS-related loss has not been previously identified as traumatic for a variety of reasons. First, the phenomenon of multiple AIDS-related loss is relatively new. In the early years of AIDS, single deaths were tragic but not traumatic. Only in the past decade, as the number of losses have mounted, have people begun to realize the impact of multiple losses from the AIDS pandemic. Second, the experience of multiple loss has been largely confined to populations that are undervalued in society, namely homosexuals, IVDUs, and minorities. Therefore, in keeping with the lack of attention that these groups traditionally receive, the focus of traumatic impact on these groups has been minimized or ignored. Third, no existing diagnostic category is appropriate for survivors of multiple AIDS-related loss. The closest psychiatric diagnostic category that could apply, posttraumatic stress disorder, does not apply to the occurrence of multiple AIDS-related loss because this experience is ongoing. It is not *post*traumatic, it is presently traumatic. Fourth, secondary traumatic stress arises in many survivors, especially caregivers, but only recently has it received attention.

Commonly accepted indicators of trauma are reviewed next to provide a foundation of knowledge about trauma that can be compared with the experience of surviving multiple AIDS-related loss. The survivor's individual experience of trauma is variable, and these variables influence the intensity of traumatization. Therefore, this chapter begins with a review of commonly accepted variables that influence the degree of traumatization and discusses their influence on survivors of multiple AIDS-related loss. Then, because experts in trauma have conceptualized the event of experience of trauma in various ways, these various frameworks in connection with multiple AIDS-related loss are reviewed, including the shattering of assumptions, the death imprint, helplessness, and the alternating experience of numbing and intrusions.

CHARACTERISTICS OF TRAUMA

Dramatically different events of trauma may cause identical reactions (Janoff-Bulman, 1985, p. 16). Common psychological experiences, among a wide variety of victims, allow the identification of trauma from its effects. The consequent behaviors and emotions of traumatic stress reactions are often the first indication of the presence of trauma (Figley, 1985a, p. xix). A traumatic event "contains news that is severely out of accord with the ways the individual believed himself to be articulated in the surrounding world" (Horowitz, 1985, p. 166). It is outside the norms of human experience.

A number of factors associated with the event of trauma are identified as influencing its outcome. Characteristics of the traumatic event itself and the severity of stressor are important (van der Kolk, 1989). Duration, potential for recurrence, and perceived control over future impact are factors that determine the magnitude of impact. Exposure to the grotesque, particularly disfiguring or mutilating disasters, tends to be more traumatic (Green, 1993). One survivor recalls a person with Kaposi's sarcoma lesions coming out of his eyes, "an image that I cannot forget."

The context in which trauma occurs, the recovery environment, and especially the availability of social support are determining factors in the degree of impact caused by a traumatic event. "Without a meaningful response from others, the victim is left isolated in the meaninglessness of trauma, and thus becomes further traumatized" (Jay, 1994, p. 31). A traumatic experience is one that overwhelms the individual (Raphael & Wilson, 1993) and is "considered injurious or harmful to the psychic apparatus" (Niederland, 1971, p. 8). Survivors experience reactions and symptoms that are typically characterized as alternating between denial and intrusion, and numbing and reexperiencing. The current diagnostic criteria incorporate these dual, simultaneous experiences.

Controllability is crucial. Efforts to control one's environment are fundamental to all species. Events and the environment must be controlled in useful ways. Thus, flexible adaptation is necessitated by changes in events and environment. The species that adapt survive, those that don't, don't. Disasters of a traumatic nature strike at the hub of this important variable. The survivor of multiple, ongoing loss is continually challenged to adapt. At some point, a threshold may be reached, and the survivor consciously or unconsciously shuts down because he or she reaches a point of ego strength depletion. A cognitive element plays a vital role in this process, and this is highly individualized. Survivors who can find meaning or a rationale for their suffering are, in effect, exerting control. "Anyone's life after trauma becomes a struggle to give meaning to the terrible truth of memory" (Jay, 1994, p. 31). This is Frankl's (1959/ 1984) ultimate position: The last of human freedoms is the ability to "choose one's attitudes to a given set of circumstances" (p. 86). Yet, Frankl spoke from a perspective after the main physical effects of his disaster had ended, a perspective that is ultimately comforting. Survivors of ongoing loss are more likely to view their situation as uncontrollable and, therefore, to generalize this state of being into other areas of their lives.

Individual responses to traumatization vary and must be understood in terms of the particular victim involved. Among Holocaust survivors, for example, studies have shown that "survivors are not a homogeneous group, and that the heterogeneity is indicative of differences in post-traumatic adjustment" (Kaminer & Lavie, 1993, p. 334). Although many survivors retain scars of various degrees, "an equally large percentage of the survivors adjusted well as individuals and became effective and contributing citizens in their new community" (pp. 334–335). In the early years of the AIDS epoch, a similar diversity of survivor response was apparent.

The individual's preexisting defense mechanisms, coping skills, personality, and resources influence the outcome of traumatic stress. In addition, the severity of stress caused by the event on a particular individual contributes to a variation in traumatization between individuals (Green, 1993; van der Kolk, 1989). Important to the process of resolution is the quantity and quality of available social support, which may either support or hinder the resolution of trauma. Variations include the existence or lack of family support (Figley, 1985b), the community-wide impact from the traumatic event (Raphael & Wilson, 1993), and the meaning assigned by the community to the victim's experience (Janoff-Bulman, 1992).

Janoff-Bulman (1992) has provided a valuable context by focusing on the meaning victims assign to trauma on the basis of disruption to their assumptive world. A traumatic event is one that "has a profound impact on their fundamental assumptions about the world" (p. 51). Not only the external world is threatened, but also the internal world, creating a "double dose of anxiety" (p. 65). Victims can no longer derive equilibrium from prior assumptions.

THE TRAUMATIC EVENT OF MULTIPLE AIDS-RELATED LOSS

Various factors influence the degree of traumatization faced by survivors of multiple AIDS-related loss. Not all of these factors are unique to AIDS-related loss. However, the clustering of so many factors in a single disaster may be unique and certainly exacerbates the potential for traumatic effect.

Quantitative Factors

A survivor of multiple loss may experience the deaths of a vast number of loved ones. It is easy to understand how quantity of loss heightens the traumatic experience. The survivor of a large number of losses loses interpersonal connections, may learn not to trust that anyone will always be there, and feels painfully isolated. Greater loss means greater traumatic impact. Quantity of death is a factor that increases the potential for traumatization. Niederland (1971), an authority on trauma, noted that "personality changes in the survivor of (traumatic) experiences are related to quantitative factors" (p. 7). The quantity of suffering and death from AIDS dwarfs most other disasters. Even if this quantity of death were distributed evenly over the general population, it would have a significant impact, but AIDS (in Western nations) has decimated subpopulations where the focus of impact is quantitatively focused.

Qualitative Factors

Various qualitative factors typical to the experience of multiple AIDS-related loss influence the event and experience of trauma.

The Disease Process of AIDS   The disease process of AIDS has three distinguishing characteristics that are recognized for increasing the potential of traumatic response in survivors:

• Trauma of a protracted nature is more likely to increase the death imprint on survivors (Lifton, 1993). The protracted nature of AIDS-related illness increases the likelihood of experiencing concurrent crises.

• Uncertainty and anxiety are heightened by the episodic nature of health problems among those living with AIDS.

• Reactions of horror, fear, and intense sadness are provoked by the physical symptoms of AIDS-related opportunistic infections, including blindness, incontinence, dementia, wasting, and death.

The experiences of two survivors of multiple AIDS-related loss illustrate the potential traumatic effect faced by those who care for people with AIDS. Eric volunteered with the Shanti Project in San Francisco. One of his clients, Billie, was a transsexual who had lived a very challenging life around Polk Street and continued to struggle with drug use despite frustrating attempts to quit. Eric endured intense anger from Billie. Still, Eric hung in there with Billie, even volunteering to clean his filthy, cockroach-covered kitchen. Eric described his last visit to Billie's.

> I called him as usual, but all I got was a busy signal. Sometimes he took his phone off the hook when he wanted to nap. I figured he was home, so I went over. He didn't answer the doorbell, but the lights were on inside, so I went in, and there was Billie, in his pearls and not much else, dead. There was shit all over the place. He'd OD'd, and panicked probably, and just shit everywhere. He had two cats. I found them in the closet, terrified. I took a deep breath and replaced the phone in its cradle. It was covered with excrement. Maybe he was trying to phone for help. I locked the apartment and went across the street and called 911. I was just barely holding it together.

Eric went on to say that the ambulance and coroner arrived quickly, and it all became very official. Amid stretched tape to cordon off the apartment and rubber gloves, Eric discovered that "suddenly my job was over because Billie wasn't there. To this day I wish that I had sat with him a little longer before going to make that call" (as cited in Garfield, 1995, pp. 117–124). Being with a dead body is an unusual experience in postindustrial nations, but it is common for those who have cared for people with AIDS.

Dan was an Alcoholics Anonymous sponsor and friend who cared for Kirk. During the last months of Kirk's life, as his dementia got worse and worse, Kirk suffered various physical ailments. Dan talked about one of the final hospitalizations.

> Kirk would not agree to go to the hospital and he fought us. Finally, I had to deceive him; I told him I was taking him to dinner. Then I drove to the ER where he was put in a wheelchair. It was a mess. I visited him every day. One day he was writhing around while a nurse changed his diaper. Do you know what it's like to watch your friend have his diaper changed and a catheter condom put over his

penis? It's awful. On my next visit Kirk was tied down to the bed by his ankles and arms. He had been pulling out his IV line. By this time he was hallucinating a lot. Still, it took him a long, long time to die.

A single personal experience like this would affect anyone. Survivors of multiple AIDS-related loss usually have many of these, and they exact a toll.

The Cumulative Toll   Psychic traumatization may involve an accumulation or a series of events at different points in time rather than a sudden single event (Schmale, 1971). More than anything else, it may be the cumulative impact of many events that makes AIDS-related multiple loss traumatic. The continual, relentless nature of the process is most devastating. One friend dies while another is hospitalized, while another is moved to a hospice, while another is currently feeling well, while memories of another are aroused, while another discloses that he has tested HIV positive. Whereas most traumatic events are defined in a specific moment of time, surviving multiple AIDS-related loss is a climate of trauma, a traumatic process more than a traumatic event.

Ongoing Traumatization   The traumatic process, in a "normal" situation, settles for most in days or weeks unless maintained or locked into high levels of response because traumatization is ongoing. Before the recognition of multiple AIDS-related loss as a traumatic process, it was speculated that an ongoing trauma would be expected to "be more disruptive . . . than a single discrete event" (Raphael & Wilson, 1993, p. 138). An example of the traumatic effect of ongoing threat occurred after the volcanic eruption of Mount St. Helens in 1980, which left survivors with an ongoing threat that complicated "the adaptive process for a prolonged period of time" (Sprang & McNeil, 1995, p. 107). In a study of Mount St. Helens' survivors, rates of anxiety, depression, and posttraumatic stress disorder were over 11 times higher than those in the control community (Shore, Tatum, & Volmer, 1986). The probability that loss will continue gives the AIDS disaster its uniquely traumatic tone; the ongoing nature of multiple AIDS-related loss makes it likely that the experience will only get worse.

Prematurity of Death   Another characteristic of AIDS-related death that provokes an intensified traumatic reaction is the prematurity of death experienced by most victims. Disasters are generally labeled disasters because of the perceived prematurity of the victims' deaths. When an elderly person dies, it is rarely labeled a disaster. There is a qualitatively different reaction to the death of someone in their younger years. Lifton (1993) noted that "the degree of anxiety associated with the death imprint has to do with . . . premature, unacceptable dying" (p. 16).

Survivors of multiple AIDS-related loss clearly experience an event that is out of accord with, and beyond, normal human experience. Quantitative and qualitative factors contribute to the uniquely traumatizing nature of the experience of survivors. Up to now, this chapter has demonstrated how characteristics of multiple AIDS-related loss affect the traumatic reaction of individuals. Now, attention is turned to the context in which AIDS-related loss occurs by analyzing its impact on community.

COMMUNITY-WIDE COLLECTIVE TRAUMATIZATION

It is impossible to comprehend the scope of impact generated by multiple AIDS-related loss without understanding collective traumatization. Quotations from Camus's *The Plague* are used throughout this book precisely because of the combined community-wide and individual effect in his story and this event.

Social Context

The social context in which AIDS occurs plays an important role in the traumatic impact multiple AIDS-related loss creates. There are two distinct ways in which the community influences traumatic effect on the individual. First, to the degree that the community itself is traumatized, the collective effect will compound trauma while decreasing the availability of support for survivors. Second, the manner in which the community responds, including the attitude it takes toward the victims and survivors, will support or hinder recovery from trauma.

Through the act of witnessing the survivor's pain, an intact and supportive community can provide relief. Support networks urge recapitulation of the catastrophe, a task important to resolution of trauma (Figley, 1985b). Communities help the survivor to find meaning in the event. Support helps a victim "reestablish psychological well being" (Janoff-Bulman, 1985, p. 27) by reconnecting the victim, in a positive way, to humanity. Over time, support networks facilitate the resolution of conflicts and ambivalence, a necessary part of recovery. "If a community denies the presence of tragedy as a part of its life . . . it only exiles those who bear its suffering" (Jay, 1994, p. 31). How the community defines the event, prescribes its response, and facilitates recovery are all factors that influence the ultimate outcome of trauma for survivors (Raphael & Wilson, 1993).

In most single-event disasters, such as a plane crash, fire, or bombing, those directly affected return to a community that has maintained its integrity and continues to have the resources necessary to provide support. The nontraumatized portion of the community responds with supportive nurturance, empathizing with the victims and survivors. A community as a whole is not typically traumatized, and the community as a whole provides support helpful for the survivor's recovery. When a community is struck by disaster, those who would have been previously relied on for support are likely to be coping with the same issues of trauma, thereby lessening their availability and ability to provide effective support. As K. T. Erikson (1976) noted, "It is difficult for people to recover from the effects of individual trauma when the community on which they have depended remains fragmented" (p. 302). Among Holocaust survivors, recovery was "made more difficult because the families and communities, through which they might have found comfort and help, no longer existed" (Harel, Kahana, & Kahana, 1993, p. 241). Indeed, this "breakdown of community structure" is an important factor in the "totality of impact" (Lifton & Olson, 1976, p. 306) identified as a characteristic of collective traumatization.

Lack of community support, or outright antipathy, magnifies traumatic stress for survivors. Survivors of the Holocaust were similarly hindered in the resolution of their trauma by a conspiracy of silence resulting from either a tendency to blame the survivors and victims or a reluctance to share or hear the experience because of its horrifying nature (Danieli, 1985). In some cases, such as that faced by Vietnam War veterans, survivors returned to a community that was not disrupted but that responded in a way that handicapped the survivor's resolution process. Because of ongoing political controversy about American involvement in Vietnam, veterans returning from the war were denied the normal moral, social, and material support expected by veterans (Figley, 1985a) and suffered the "secondary trauma of cultural rejection and hostility" (Sipprelle, 1992, p. 15), and oftentimes were confronted with stigmatization and hostility. Rage was "exacerbated by the 'unwelcome home' that many veterans received" (Scurfield, 1993, p. 883). This type of community response increases the intensity of traumatization (Janoff-Bulman, 1992) and parallels the experiences of many survivors of multiple AIDS-related loss.

Impact on the Gay Community

The impact of multiple AIDS-related loss is increased by its focus on the gay community. Because intolerance and stigmatization of gay people existed before AIDS, gay people created tightly knit communities and families of choice. Gay communities have coalesced in all of the major cities in the United States, Canada, and western Europe where gay men and lesbians can shop, eat, and socialize among gay people, in gay-owned and gay-operated businesses. Thus, AIDS devastated a community composed of people with varying levels of connection, from intimacy to acquaintance, not unlike the experience of living in a small town.

Families of origin and choice are significantly disrupted by AIDS. It has been widely acknowledged that the most emotionally devastating traumatic effects arise from catastrophes that affect the intimacy and support of families (Figley, 1985b, pp. 400–401). Further, families provide a number of functions necessary to the recognition, resolution, and recovery from trauma. As discussed in chapter 8, in the case of the AIDS catastrophe, a broadened perception of family is necessary to appreciate the devastating impact of multiple loss.

Loss from AIDS and its resulting impact on the gay community is pervasive. Already mentioned is the obliteration of social networks and the resulting fear of beginning new relationships. The gay community has also lost many of its role models, heroes, and leaders at cultural, political, and social levels. Further, there is an insidious disappearance of acquaintances and social contacts. Author Michael Bronski (1988) commented that "sometimes life feels like living under a fascist regime: People just disappear without a word" (p. 135). Among survivors, one regularly hears, "When I don't see someone I am used to seeing for a while, I just assume they've died from AIDS. That's what's so hard, people just disappear." This constant disappearance of former acquaintances has an insidious, cumulative impact. George describes life in San Francisco:

> It's a very bittersweet place, San Francisco, just because of the enormity of the loss. More so for me, maybe, because of my job. The number of people with AIDS whom I've known—friends, volunteers, clients—to catalogue all those losses is pretty incredible. People disappear here. They die, they're cremated, and they're gone. It adds a very surreal aspect to AIDS. (as cited in Garfield, 1995, p. 171)

Lessons and Comparisons to Buffalo Creek

When disaster strikes an existing community, traumatic impact is heightened. In the literature on trauma, the Buffalo Creek flood was studied for its community-wide traumatic impact on the survivors. The Buffalo Creek flood, with the experience of collective trauma and loss of community, provides a point of reference similar to the experience of survivors of multiple AIDS-related loss. The parallels will be obvious. In 1972, a flood resulted in traumatic loss to individuals and community at Buffalo Creek, West Virginia. What is important about that event, for the purpose of this analysis, is not so much that 125 people were killed, but the disaster's effect on the community. Buffalo Creek provided an opportunity to analyze the effects of trauma on individuals and community when a disaster strikes a definable and discrete community. Commenting on the collective, community-wide impact, K. T. Erikson (1976) wrote,

> By collective trauma, I mean a blow to the tissues of social life that damages the bonds linking people together and impairs the prevailing sense of communality. The collective trauma works its way slowly and even insidiously into the awareness of those who suffer from it . . . a form of shock—a gradual realization that the community no longer exists as a source of nurturance and that a part of the self has disappeared. (p. 302)

This same analysis applies to survivors of multiple AIDS-related loss. At first, the losses were separate, discrete events, sad and tragic. Over time, insidiously, the cumulative and compounding effect of multiple loss grew into a realization that the community had forever been altered. The community-wide effect provides the strongest rationale for referring to AIDS-related loss rather than to AIDS-related deaths because it is within the community-wide context that the scope and magnitude of loss is most profoundly experienced. It is important to note the impact this particular collective loss had on the sense of morale and morals. Pervasive personality changes were also observed that combined with a pervasive and consuming constellation of sadness and protest (Lifton, 1979).

FACTORS INFLUENCING THE DEGREE OF INDIVIDUAL TRAUMATIZATION

This chapter has so far reviewed the characteristics of multiple AIDS-related loss and the community-wide context that contribute to the potential for traumatization. Now, attention is directed to individual variables that influence the degree of impact on survivors. Traumatization arises out of the event of trauma. Generally, the more multiple AIDS-related loss stresses an individual's personal, social, and assumptive world, the more traumatization occurs. This information is intended to help make comprehensible the survivors' experience. It is useful as a guideline for assessing the degree of traumatization suffered by a given individual.

Severity of Stress

Severity of stress, as influenced by both quantitative and qualitative factors, correlates with the degree of traumatization. Thus, on a qualitative level, a person who loses several close friends and loved ones can be expected to experience greater traumatization than a person who loses a few friends and acquaintances. Loss of a spouse or child is most stressful. Quantitatively, the number of deaths that an individual experiences from AIDS varies considerably. The quantity of deaths can be enormous, especially for caregivers providing care and services in the midst of the AIDS crisis. Of course, the ongoing nature of this disaster means that the numbers of deaths will inevitably increase with time and will broaden the segment of the population affected.

History of Traumatization and Other Loss

A history of trauma tends to increase the degree of traumatization caused by surviving multiple AIDS-related loss. Previous experiences of trauma "create further vulnerability, especially if the trauma remains unresolved" (Raphael & Wilson, 1993, p. 108). There are a number of likely sources of prior traumatization that increase the potential for an experience of heightened traumatization in survivors. An individual who has experienced prior traumatization related to physical assault, surviving a previous disaster, or confrontation with overwhelming death or suffering is prone to having an increased reaction to AIDS. When working with survivors, it is always important to inquire about previous traumatization, including abuse. This is especially important among inner-city minorities who may have been routinely exposed to violence.

Many gay men have been traumatized by physical and verbal assault (Bridgewater, 1992). It is not uncommon for gay men to have been abandoned and rejected by their families of origin, sometimes being kicked out of their homes. The coming-out process is nearly always an ordeal, with varying levels of rejection and acceptance. Jewish survivors, for example, had a history of abuse and degradation prior to the Holocaust. Krystal (1981) concluded that the "survivors of defeat and humiliation have a multitude of unbearably painful emotions to face before the question of mastery or integration of their past can ever be possible" (p. 180).

Preexisting Personality, Defense Mechanisms, and Coping Style

An individual's preexisting personality, defense mechanisms, and coping style will influence both the degree and the outcome of traumatization (Raphael & Wilson, 1993). Each individual brings a unique background to bear on her or his experience with multiple AIDS-related loss. For example, an individual's aptitude for making new friends, the strength derived from spiritual beliefs, and the presence of a personality disorder would all influence the survivor's ability to cope with multiple AIDS-related loss. Some characteristics affecting the degree and outcome of traumatization are prevalent among survivors of multiple AIDS-related loss.

A perspective of chronic victimization is likely to produce a profound and endemic sense of helplessness. Victims of trauma often "perceive themselves as powerless and helpless in the face of forces beyond their control" (Janoff-Bulman, 1985, p. 22). Those most likely to be affected by AIDS may also be prone to attitudes consistent with victimization. Minority communities regularly feel victimized. Gay men are raised in a society where from the earliest age they are belittled, condemned, mocked, and attacked. This background can produce a culture of victimization (Bridgewater, 1992). Hemophiliacs may feel victimized from a history of "discrimination because of the public's ignorance about this rare disorder" (Brown & DeMaio, 1992, p. 93). This combination of preexisting and disaster-induced victimization can result in a chronic sense of helplessness and hopelessness. As van der Kolk (1989) noted, "If victims already have tenuous personal control, or if stress persists, they may lose the feeling that they can actively influence their personal destinies" (p. 8).

Low self-regard is another preexisting characteristic likely to be exacerbated by trauma associated with multiple AIDS-related loss. Among gay men and lesbians, internalized homophobic attitudes can contribute to problems with low self-esteem (Biller & Rice, 1990; Klein & Fletcher, 1987). AIDS can magnify these feelings through the association of a devastating and terminal illness with sexual behavior intimately associated with sexual orientation. Traumatization tends to activate negative images of one's self, and self-blame is common among survivors. As Janoff-Bulman (1985) commented, "the self-perception of deviance . . . serves to reinforce negative images of one's self as negative and weak" (p. 22). Therefore, the regular response of victims to regard themselves negatively in response to trauma is exacerbated in the experience of multiple AIDS-related loss.

Health Status of the Survivor

Physical health is a resource that may be lacking for many survivors of multiple AIDS-related loss, especially for those who have tested positive for HIV. This group is more likely to be surrounded by others dying from AIDS and thus more likely to be suffering multiple AIDS-related loss. Poor physical health and low energy interfere with the process of recovery from trauma. It takes effort and energy to do what is necessary to recover, including making new friends, seeking support, and dealing with strong emotions.

Many preexisting characteristics that contribute to the severity of trauma are likely to be present for those with HIV. Several of the variables that make an intensified traumatic reaction more likely arise in persons with HIV. Low self-esteem, with more internalized homophobia, is prevalent among persons with AIDS (Lima, Lo Presto, Sherman, & Sobelman, 1993). Personality fluctuations that arise out of dementia or high stress may push supportive people away and result in increased isolation. The HIV-positive individual may isolate and withdraw because of a reluctance to put others through the painful process of illness and death. HIV-positive individuals are more likely to feel strongly the effects of abandonment (Jue, 1994) and to have these feelings reactivated by the experience of multiple loss.

The survivor with HIV is witnessing an event, in others, that is "a threat to the physical integrity of self" (American Psychiatric Association, 1994, p. 427), a component of the definition of trauma. Each new illness and death carries with it the clear and present reminder that the same fate awaits one's self. Each time a friend experiences a painful or debilitating opportunistic infection, those with HIV think about the potential for similar suffering in themselves. These survivors report an understandable fear of waiting for the other shoe to drop.

SECONDARY TRAUMATIC STRESS

Secondary stress reactions are common in survivors of multiple AIDS-related loss, especially among caregivers, volunteers, and professionals who work with people with AIDS. "People can be traumatized without actually being physically harmed or threatened" (Figley, 1995, p. 4). There is a cost to caring. "Professionals who listen to clients' stories of fear, pain, and suffering may feel similar fear, pain, and suffering because they care" (p. 1). As a concept, secondary stress is relatively new, but there is widening respect for its effect. As a concept, vicarious traumatization (McCann & Pearlman) was first introduced in 1990. Understanding secondary stress is important to comprehend the impact on survivors. It is not only those directly touched by the death of a significant other or friend who feel the pervasive impact of AIDS-related loss.

Secondary stress response is one way that the effect of individual and community-wide disaster interrelate. Secondary stress response arises in persons not directly threatened or injured by disaster but who still respond in ways consistent to a person directly traumatized. When a disaster strikes a loved one, it is extremely stressful (Figley, 1985b). Symptoms of secondary stress parallel classic symptoms of posttraumatic stress disorder (Figley, 1995; Pearlman & Saakvitne, 1995). Survivors may experience a delayed onset of these symptoms (Beaton & Murphy, 1995, p. 59), which can "be mixed and slow to appear" (Dutton & Rubinstein, 1995, p. 92), especially when the traumatization is prolonged or likely to recur. Effects of vicarious traumatization are "cumulative and permanent" (Pearlman & Saakvitne, 1995, p. 151).

For example, war causes secondary victimization because of its community-wide effect and uncertainty regarding its end point and the scope of impact (Milgram, 1983). This effect has been noticed among crisis workers (Beaton & Murphy, 1995) and caregivers to disaster survivors.

> Death-related anxiety came to pervade the Buffalo Creek environment to the point of contagion. As in other overwhelming disasters (such as Hiroshima), such outsiders as mental health professionals and clergymen coming in actually experience some of the fear and dread described by people exposed to the disaster. (Lifton & Olson, 1976, p. 297)

Another example of this was observed after the Beverly Hills Supper Club fire, where one third of those identified as survivors were not physically present at the scene but reacted to the experience of loss of loved ones and close friends (Lindy, Green, Grace, & Titchener, 1983, p. 610). Similarly, families of the Iranian hostages in 1979 experienced more stress than did many of the hostages during their captivity (Figley, 1985b, p. 410). Traumatized children have been described as being contagious, causing traumatization among children who play with them (Eth & Pynoos, 1985).

Factors related to AIDS and characteristics of caregivers serve to heighten the likelihood of secondary stress reaction in survivors of multiple loss. Working with people with AIDS as a professional is often a commitment to a *lifestyle*, as well as an investment in a line of work. More than with most other disasters, the professional and personal selves are likely to be deeply affected.

Those therapists who earn a reputation as being helpful to survivors will see their referrals and clients increase. The poignant pleading of clients and colleagues can seem so compelling that burnout is potentiated (Cerney, 1995, p. 138). Those exposed to repetitive and cumulative crisis are prone to developing secondary stress reactions (Beaton & Murphy, 1995). Those working for years in the field of AIDS will inevitably have encountered several circumstances likely to produce secondary stress disorder. Working with survivors of trauma involves more than just exposure to the traumatic event (e.g., through the recounting of the event by the client). According to Dutton and Rubinstein (1995), "it also involves exposure to the survivor's reaction to the traumatic event (e.g. intense emotional pain, fear, rage, despair, hopelessness" (p. 91). Professionals, volunteers, and loved ones of people with AIDS usually possess a generous capacity for empathy. Although empathy helps enhance understanding of the person with AIDS's experience, it also increases the chance for traumatization. The professional whose work centers on the relief of emotional suffering in clients automatically absorbs information that is about suffering and often absorbs the suffering itself (Figley, 1995, p. 2).

Not least of the problems faced by caregivers is the "tragic transformation of hope to cynicism" (Pearlman & Saakvitne, 1995, p. 158) that can result from vicarious traumatization, a condition to which survivors of multiple, ongoing loss are particularly prone. Among this group, the burnout rate and the incidence of secondary stress is high.

SHATTERING OF ASSUMPTIONS

> How hard it must be to live only with what one knows and what one remembers, cut off from what one hopes for! . . . he realized the bleak sterility of a life without illusions. There can be no peace without hope.—Albert Camus (1946), *The Stranger*

Traumatic stress, according to one framework, is largely due to a violation of the basic assumptions that victims hold about themselves and their world and the profound impact the traumatic event has on these fundamental assumptions (Janoff-Bulman, 1992, p. 51). Certain assumptions, even when they are only implicit, guide the way people relate to themselves and their world. They establish expectations about current and future functions, goals, and developmental tasks. Meaning and purpose are derived from these basic assumptions. Throughout this book, the shattering of assumptions has been a connecting and underlying theme. Multiple AIDS-related loss strikes at many of the fundamental assumptions that define identity, relationship with the world, and future expectations. One mother who lost her son to AIDS spoke aloud to her son, saying, "I didn't consider, when I chose your name, how it would look on a tombstone." The common lament of survivors is "It was not supposed to be this way!" Bharat Lindemood (as cited in Garfield, 1995) described the kind of way it is not supposed to be:

> You walk by one room and there's a KS-lesion-covered foot hanging over the end of the bed, and in the next room someone's heaving his guts out, and in the next room you can hear a person wheezing and drowning in her own fluids, and someone else is suffering in some other way. You feel as if you've walked into a Fellini movie. It's incredible suffering, and loss upon loss upon loss—people losing their jobs, their friends, their identity as a provider, sometimes their minds. It becomes kind of hallucinogenic at moments. (p. 259)

Trauma, particularly when it results from multiple loss, severs the self "from its own history, from its grounding" (Lifton, 1993, p. 12). A person's sense of self is largely determined by connection with others and a shared history. The "individual self is interpersonal at its very core"; therefore, loss of a loved one is a "threat to one's very identity" (Uroda, 1977, p. 185). People one loves become a part of one's self (Parkes, 1972). Multiple loss strikes repeatedly at identity by severing the experience of self from its connection to meaningful others.

Previous analysis of disruption to identity arising from an experience of interpersonal loss focused on the death of one other. In this disaster, a wide spectrum of interpersonal loss occurs, from the loss of a significant other, to the loss of entire social networks, to the loss of a constellation of acquaintances, and to the loss of connection to social, political, and cultural role models. The survivor's environment is decimated in a whir of continuing devastation. One survivor said, "It seems like I am standing still while my entire environment, everything around me, changes." Discontinuity becomes the norm, as the people with whom a common history is shared are eliminated. Few historic tragedies provide a similar experience of devastation to the assumptive world through dislocation of the self as defined in relation to others.

Survivors of multiple AIDS-related loss must cope with issues not usually encountered until later in the developmental cycle, if at all. A variety of basic life expectations are undermined by AIDS besides those directly pertaining to developmental phase expectations. People expect to share a common history and grow old together with a core group of friends and loved ones. Caring for an ongoing stream of sick and dying people is not part of the expectations of any group of people, especially those in their 20s, 30s, and 40s. Parents expect that their children will outlive them but instead must bury them. No one expects to live under a constant atmosphere of death that includes the continual terror of who will sicken next and die.

Janoff-Bulman (1992) posited that invulnerability and a belief that the world is comprehensible, orderly, and sensible are assumed by most. Victims, conversely, no longer believe that what happens to them is controllable, thereby also losing the perception that they live in a safe, secure, and benign world. Survivors of multiple AIDS-related loss see these assumptions shattered continually, making comprehensible responses of extreme anxiety, anhedonia, and withdrawal.

Lifton (1993) observed a "moral dimension inherent in all conflict and suffering" (p. 18). There is a tendency to seek explanations for disasters, thereby gaining a measure of control over potential recurrence. This contributes to a tendency to blame victims, even among victims themselves, who turn blame inward in the form of guilt. This process turns the passive experience of helplessness into the active experience of placing responsibility (Lindy, 1985). When no source of blame can be determined, survivors may generalize their anxiety and "develop a life-long inability to trust" (van der Kolk, 1989, p. 11). This can create a profound disillusionment that outlasts fear and anxiety. These modes of response are all common to survivors of multiple AIDS-related loss.

THE DEATH IMPRINT

This traumatic event leaves a death imprint on survivors. The death imprint has an external, internal, and circular dynamic for survivors. Externally, the impact of multiple AIDS-related loss continually intrudes on the survivor's life. Internally, the psyche of the survivor is imprinted with self-deadening. Circularly, the survivor's death perspective is projected outward and reabsorbed. The death imprint arises in survivors as a result of the cumulative survivor experience, leaving a permanent psychological mark. Lifton (1993) noted that the death imprint can occur "gradually over time . . . [with] every death encounter reactivating earlier 'survivals'" (p. 16). This protracted nature increases the degree of anxiety associated with the death imprint. Each new death reminds survivors of earlier ones. Lifton (1979) concluded that "the degree of anxiety associated with the death imprint has to do with the impossibility of assimilating the death imprint—because of its suddenness, its extreme or protracted nature, or its association with the terror of premature, unacceptable dying" (p. 169). Although Lifton wrote these observations at a time prior to the emergence of multiple AIDS-related loss, they are predictive of the characteristics of this disaster. Surviving multiple AIDS-related loss is a cumulative experience, occurring gradually over time, leaving a permanent psychological mark.

The imprint of death seems to be on every part of the survivor's life. Each additional death reminds the survivor of previous, probably unresolved deaths. All this occurs in a context of certainty that the future holds no respite. As a result, survivors live in an environment that is permeated by death: friends calling to tell of a new illness or death, news reports reawakening anxiety, and the tangible absence of so many. Thoughts about the past recall friends who are gone, thoughts about the present involve visits to hospitals and hospices, and thoughts about the future cannot avoid a theme of hopelessness in the face of certain future loss. Defoe (1721/1969) wrote about the death imprint during the plague of 1665, noting that

> the minds of the people were agitated with other things, and a kind of sadness and horror at these things sat upon the countenances even of the common people. Death was before their eyes, and everybody began to think of their graves, not of mirth and diversions. (p. 37)

A "death spell" is cast from which there is no escape except through withdrawal and isolation.

Effects of the death imprint are observed in a fundamental change to the personality and psychic apparatus, including an entire spectrum of numbing and withdrawal responses. Survivors may come to fear, or even feel alienated from, their own emotions: "One's own emotions come to be experienced as outside the self-representation" (Krystal, 1981, p. 182). This consequence severely limits potential for successful adjustment.

Survivors regularly speak of personality changes that they observe in themselves. "My personality has changed 180 degrees," one survivor plaintively says. "I'm not the same person I used to be. I don't tell jokes, enjoy my life or look forward to anything . . . I used to laugh." Survivors of multiple loss and those closest to them notice a difference. Joy and exuberance are replaced by somber seriousness. One result observed in survivors of trauma is a "life-long inability to trust" (van der Kolk, 1989, p. 11). Survivors of the Holocaust are reported to have developed personality changes that affect their interpersonal relationships, including parenthood (Kaminer & Lavie, 1993). Especially for gay people, it is difficult to trust a connection to others when one's history is replete with abandonment.

A sense of narcissistic entitlement among survivors may arise. This tendency was observed in some Vietnam War veterans who have "pervasive egocentric, non-giving behavior" (Parson, 1993, p. 822), punctuated by frequent irrational demands and a sense of entitlement. Failure to receive sympathetic social support is shared by survivors of both Vietnam War combat and multiple AIDS-related loss. In addition, both groups have experienced an inordinate amount of suffering. The combined impact of widespread suffering and lack of support easily leads to an attitude of resentment that transfers into entitlement: "I deserve your care and I better get it!" Pervasive anger and frustration combine with a sense of having suffered enough, contributing to a justification for demanding, irritable, hard-to-please, and temperamental behavior. Although this attitudinal observation is rarely publicly admitted, caregivers working with survivors will admit it in private. This response is counterproductive because it intensifies traumatic stress; undermines the survivor's chances of attaining long-term, meaningful support; and inhibits resolution of intrapsychic conflict (Parson, 1993).

HELPLESSNESS

> This human form, his friend's lacerated by the spear-thrusts of the plague, consumed by searing superhuman fires, buffeted by all the raging winds of heaven, was foundering under his eyes in the dark flood of the pestilence, and he could do nothing to avert the wreck. He could only stand, unavailing, on the shore, empty-handed and sick at heart, unarmed and helpless yet again under the onset of calamity. And thus, when the end came, the tears that blinded [his] eyes were tears of impotence.—Albert Camus (1948), *The Plague*

Survivors of multiple AIDS-related loss are likely to feel helpless in a number of areas. They are helpless to prevent the deaths of loved ones, helpless to eliminate the pain and demise of people with AIDS, helpless to prevent collective community-wide losses, and helpless to escape a world that is saturated with AIDS. The perception of helplessness arising from incompetence and defenselessness in these tangible areas combines, in some survivors, with emotional and motivational helplessness. This manifests as helplessness to escape chronic reactive depression, helplessness to maintain emotional balance, helplessness to respond capably to ongoing loss, and helplessness to find motivation to develop and implement a vision for the future.

Learned Helplessness Theory

Learned helplessness is a relevant and useful model for understanding traumatic effect in survivors of multiple AIDS-related loss. In this section, the theory of learned helplessness is briefly outlined and applied to multiple AIDS-related loss. According to Martin Seligman (1975), helplessness is a psychological state that frequently results when events are uncontrollable. "When a person or animal has learned that the outcome is independent of responding, the expectation that responding will produce the outcome wanes; therefore response initiation diminishes" (p. 49). Later, even when the person does respond successfully in producing relief, he or she has trouble "learning, perceiving, and believing that the response worked" (p. 23). Motivation to initiate new responses is sapped, and depression and anxiety predominate.

Several studies have supported these conclusions. The most well-known involved dogs. When an experimentally naive dog is placed in a shuttle box and is electrically shocked after a signal, it frantically runs about until it accidentally scrambles over a barrier where it escapes the shock. On subsequent trials, the dog quickly becomes adept at escaping the shock and soon learns to avoid the shock altogether. At the onset of a signal for the shock, it leaps across the barrier and never gets shocked again. When a dog is given no signal before random shocks and no way to escape, it developed a strikingly different pattern.

> This dog's first reactions to shock in the shuttle box were much the same as those of a naive dog: it ran around frantically for about thirty seconds, but then it stopped moving; to our surprise, it lay down and quietly whined. After one minute of this we turned the shock off; the dog had failed to cross the barrier and had not escaped from shock. On the next trial, the dog did it again; at first it struggled a bit, and then, after a few seconds, it seemed to give up and to accept the shock passively. On all succeeding trials, the dog failed to escape. This is the paradigmatic learned helplessness finding. (Seligman, 1975, p. 22).

Not all dogs respond in the same way. One third learn to escape the shock by jumping the barrier, while the other dogs responded in the way described above. About 5% of the dogs were helpless even without prior exposure to inescapable shock. Seligman posited that these dogs had a history before they arrived at the laboratory that accounted for their helpless response.

Caution is in order when applying this theory to multiple AIDS-related loss.

Learned helplessness theories have been "overused and applied promiscuously" to situations that "misuse the concept entirely" (Peterson, Maier, & Seligman, 1993, p. 9). Three essential components must be present: contingency, cognition, and behavior. The most important contingency is uncontrollability. Learned helplessness follows "in the wake of uncontrollable events" (p. 229). Traumatic events may produce unfortunate responses, including passivity, but the other two components, which are of a learned variety, also arise in true example of learned helplessness. Cognition refers to the way in which the person perceives, explains and extrapolates the contingency. The person must apprehend the contingency (accurately or inaccurately), explain what is perceived, and use that perception to explain and form expectations about the future. "Only if the person believes events to be uncontrollable does helplessness follow in their wake" (p. 229). Behavior refers to observable consequences of contingency and the person's cognitions about it. Typically, this manifests as passivity versus activity in situations other than the one in which uncontrollability was first encountered. The person fails to initiate any actions that might allow control of a situation. In addition, other consequences follow from the individual's expectation of future helplessness, including "cognitive retardation, low self-esteem, sadness, loss of aggression, immune changes and physical illness" (p. 8).

Learned Helplessness in Survivors of Multiple AIDS-Related Loss

Uncontrollability is the main contingency provoked by surviving multiple AIDS-related loss. It does not matter what the survivor does; losses continue, and to a large extent, they occur randomly. Some who have engaged in high-risk behavior contract HIV, some do not. Some live with HIV for years, some do not. Some periods of stable health are interrupted by sudden debilitation. Some of those dying find a path of spirituality and peace, some die with bitterness and resentment. Classic learning theory states that voluntary responses that are rewarded increase; those that are punished decrease. Although there are exceptions to the typical response cycle, it still provides an implicit assumption about the way life is supposed to work. The survivor of multiple AIDS-related loss is denied this contingency. Its violation is another shattering of the survivor's assumptive world. Helplessness becomes a way of conserving energy.

Victimization, disenfranchisement, and outright discrimination are regularly the history and contemporary reality for many survivors of multiple AIDS-related loss. When an individual has developed a schema of helplessness to explain these occurrences, the survivor of later loss is likely to ignore information that contradicts it. The tendency toward helplessness is self-perpetuated (Ingram, 1986). The preexisting environment of many survivors of multiple AIDS-related loss provides fertile ground for the seed of helplessness to take root.

When the reality of helplessness to AIDS is inappropriately generalized and

applied to other situations, the cognitive element of learned helplessness is acti-
vated. "The exact nature of these cognitions is unclear" (Peterson et al., 1993, p.
229), but they are evident in attitudes and behaviors. Survivors of multiple
AIDS-related loss are devastated by their inability to control future loss. The
acute pain inherent in ongoing loss is greatly worsened by helplessness, and
this is the bridge to motivational impairment.

Two spheres of motivation are adversely affected by learned helplessness
in survivors of multiple AIDS-related loss: motivation to respond to additional
loss and motivation to proactively influence their lives. Uncontrollability over
AIDS-related loss leads some survivors to conclude that they can do nothing
about future loss. On a purely physical level, that conclusion is mainly true.
Little can be done to stop the physical deterioration and death of those already
infected. Areas in which survivors do possess control are mainly in the cognitive, emotional, and spiritual realms. These possible responses are outlined later
in the book and regularly have to do with inherently painful grief work or with
voluntarily exposing oneself to additional losses. In contrast, the main challenge
faced by many who develop learned helplessness is physical. For example, the
person who continues to live in an abusive relationship lacks the motivation to
physically escape the physical threat. In survivors of multiple AIDS-related loss,
inappropriate passivity manifests through the lack of mental action in a situation
in which effective coping is possible. Even when a successful coping response
is engaged, the survivor has "difficulty *learning* that his response has succeeded
. . . uncontrollability distorts the perception of control" (Seligman, 1975, p. 37).
Professionals who work with survivors of multiple loss will see this confounding and frustrating pattern in survivors. Apparently successful steps to treat
trauma and grief are followed by renewed helplessness. The professional, or
survivor, who is not aware of the psychodynamic rationale for this seemingly
inexplicable response is likely to become frustrated and lose motivation to continue the necessary painstaking work.

There is a second discouraging dynamic involved here. Unlike those who
can remove themselves from physical danger and immediately experience relief
from pain, the survivor of multiple loss is likely to temporarily and periodically
feel more pain. Unresolved losses need to be worked through; painful memories
need to be recapitulated. The inevitability of pain as part of an adaptive response hinders the survivor from breaking out of a pattern of learned helplessness in response to surviving multiple AIDS-related loss.

Psychological Conservatism and Motivational Disturbance

Survivors of Camus's plague were "imbued with a skepticism so thorough that
it was now a second nature; they had become allergic to hope in any form"
(Camus, 1948, p. 244). Krystal (1981) referred to a "fear of one's dreams" that
he attributed to the "posttraumatic depletion of consciously recognized spheres
of selfhood" (p. 182). Survivors become alienated from their own emotions and

hopes because of the pain associated with these emotions and hopes. One survivor of multiple AIDS-related loss said, "I am afraid to hope. It hurts too much. I know that sounds crazy but every time I allow myself to hope, I end up getting hurt by it."

Survivors frequently do not only react helplessly to AIDS but also to other areas of their lives. This has cognitive and behavioral components. Expectations that other responses to other events will be efficacious wane. A deep-seated psychological conservatism may ensue. For example, survivors of community-wide disaster at Buffalo Creek, West Virginia, developed an

> avoidance of situations that might raise the level of excitation either internally or externally. It is the defensive and ego psychological counterpart of the psychic numbing described by Lifton and Olson. We perceive psychic conservation as mental activity designed to control behavior by banking energies, surrendering ambition, reducing enthusiasm, dampening socializing and love-making, and discouraging novel experience. (Titchener & Kapp, 1976, pp. 298–299)

This adjustment hobbles the survivor, leading to existence rather than life. Many of these same characteristics are observed in survivors of multiple AIDS-related loss.

Titchener and Kapp (1976) could have been discussing survivors of multiple AIDS-related loss instead of the Buffalo Creek flood when they concluded,

> Psychological conservatism accepts survival as the only goal of existence. It is a trade-off: the individual accepts hopelessness in the present to prevent helplessness in the future, as if to say, "Better to live without hope than not to live at all." (p. 299)

This analysis of survivor response arose from a disaster with similarities to multiple AIDS-related loss, notably its community-wide effect. One crucial difference is, however, inadvertently illuminated in Titchener and Kapp's conclusion: "Psychological conservatism functions as if the disaster will recur tomorrow, thus totally distorting an individual's view of the future" (p. 299). How much more does a disaster that certainly will recur tomorrow affect the survivor's view of the future?

Emotional Disturbances: Depression and Diffuse Anger

Existing as helpless in a world of suffering leads to reactive depression. Seligman (1975) asserted that "the cause of depression is the belief that action is futile" (p. 93); "depression is not generalized pessimism, but pessimism specific to the effects of one's own skilled actions" (p. 86). Bibring (1953, p. 14) described the basic mechanism of depression as "the ego's shocking awareness of its helplessness."

Diffuse anger in survivors is partially explainable by learned helplessness.

Anyone who has witnessed someone (or one's self) hit their thumb with a hammer while trying to nail a board and then proceed to loudly curse the hammer, the nail, the board, or a coworker can understand the "transfer of helplessness" that Seligman (1975) called "shock-elicited aggression" (p. 32). "At the animal level, if a rat is shocked while another rat is nearby, the shocked rat will attack the other rat furiously" (p. 33). Humans usually have more capacity to control their aggression than rats, but anyone who has been the target of undeserved rage on the part of a survivor of multiple AIDS-related loss will notice a similarity. Helpless to rage against AIDS with any effect, survivors displace their rage. Anyone, sometimes everyone, becomes the target. Yet anger can be a very useful emotion when, instead of being diffuse, it is focused and appropriately directed. By recovering ego strength through the control of one's own emotional response, anger attacks both helplessness and depression.

Implications of the Learned Helplessness Model

Adjustment to multiple AIDS-related loss requires focused work, purposeful effort, and bolstering a sense of efficacy in the survivor. Ideally, the survivor's environment would be changed to "preclude helplessness altogether" (Peterson et al., 1993, p. 231), but that is mainly impossible for the survivor of multiple AIDS-related loss. Rather, a directive, forceful approach to combating perceptions of helplessness is necessary.

Seligman (1975) concluded that "forced exposure to the fact that responding produces reinforcement is the most effective way of breaking up learned helplessness" (p. 99). In his studies with dogs, nothing would motivate the dogs with learned helplessness to initiate a movement across the barrier and avoid shocks. The researchers tried a variety of interventions including removing the barrier, calling the dog to the other side, and offering salami to a hungry dog, but the dog just laid there.

> Finally, we showed one of our helpless dogs to James Geer, a behavior therapist, who said, "If I had a patient like that I would give him a swift kick to get him going." Geer was right: this therapy always worked on helpless dogs and rats. What it meant to us was that we should *force* the dog to respond—over and over, if necessary, and so have it come to see that changing compartments turns off shock. (p. 56)

At first the dogs had to be forcibly dragged by leash across the barrier with a great deal of effort. Gradually, the dogs began to become more and more receptive to crossing the barrier, even when it was raised, to avoid shock. Eventually, all began to respond on their own. Once the "correct response had occurred repeatedly" each dog "initiated its own response, and thereafter never failed to escape" (p. 57).

A perception of control may be extraordinarily difficult to muster. However, if survivors of multiple AIDS-related loss are going to positively adjust, they must believe that control is possible. Michael Callen survived many friends, lived with AIDS for 12 years, and wrote a book called *Surviving and Thriving with AIDS*. He wrote, "I have railed against, and cursed, and challenged hopelessness wherever I have encountered it" (Callen, 1988, pp. 34–35). Later chapters of this book focus on survivors' recovery and offer suggestions for proactive responses where control is possible. This challenge can be met on a variety of levels, including purposeful engagement in grief work, involvement in positive response to AIDS, increasing support, personal growth through a search for meaning, choosing a balance of engagement and detachment, creating rituals, and seeking a definition of one's spirituality.

ALTERNATING EXPERIENCES OF NUMBING AND INTRUSIONS

Traumatic symptoms typically include avoidance of thoughts and feelings related to the traumatic event along with emotional numbing and withdrawal from activities, relationships, and future planning. Intrusions arise frequently in survivors of trauma and include nightmares, flashbacks, and intrusive and distressing recollections. Survivors of trauma do not experience one cluster of these symptoms to the exclusion of the other cluster of symptoms; both can occur in alternating patterns. The survivor of multiple AIDS-related loss experiences these classic symptoms of trauma.

Numbing and Withdrawal

Psychic numbing is referred to as the most universal response to disaster (Lifton & Olson, 1976, p. 299). It is the "diminished capacity to feel" (Lifton, 1993, p. 18) and is observed in survivors of multiple AIDS-related loss. Charles Garfield, who pioneered the Shanti Project in San Francisco and wrote a book about AIDS caregivers, titled his book *Sometimes My Heart Goes Numb*. Survivors frequently report being unable to cry anymore, even as they attend memorial services and witness the ravaging effects of illness on their closest friends. Some are shocked by how numb they do feel, critically describing themselves as cold and unfeeling. One survivor complained that "my best friend died over a year ago and I haven't cried yet. Can you believe that? My best friend died and I don't shed one tear!"

Diminished capacity to feel, characteristic of psychic numbing, manifests in a number of ways. Caregivers find that the "end effect of numbing is burn out" (Garfield, 1995, p. 263). The caregiver may demonstrate cynicism, insensitivity, or a dehumanized response to the one being cared for. The survivor of multiple AIDS-related loss sometimes seems to be stuck in a very narrow range of emotions. Answers to the question "How do you feel?" are met with simplified responses such as "good" or "bad." Sometimes even this simplified range is abandoned in favor of monoaffective expressions. For example, the survivor reports only feeling angry. Krystal (1981) concluded that "the survivor has to maintain intrapsychic barriers against the ambivalence, doubts, guilt, and rage. A widespread constriction of fantasy results" (p. 185). Feelings of happiness, joy, and spontaneity are also muted. A survivor in Shrader's (1992) study said that he "had become a great deal more serious and less fun-loving and spontaneous" (p. 102).

Withdrawal from various forms of living, particularly withdrawal from social settings and events, frequently occurs. Fear of future abandonment is realistic given the ongoing nature of the AIDS catastrophe. The only way to avoid the pain of future loss is to avoid contact with those who might die. Adjustment requires a certain amount of recapitulating the traumatic experience, but survivors may seek to avoid the feelings that naturally emerge. Unfortunately, efforts to overcome trauma by avoiding traumatic content are ineffective (Kaminer & Lavie, 1993).

Withdrawal also occurs in connection with a pulling back from life. Some survivors lose motivation. Nothing seems to matter anymore; what's the point? One survivor who lost his lifetime partner and all his meaningful friends said, "I expected to die before them all. Now, I don't know what to do." Sadly, he sits alone most days in a dark basement apartment, waiting to die, existing only in a physical sense.

Krystal (1979, 1981) has offered an interesting perspective on alexithymia in survivors of trauma that has relevance to multiple AIDS-related loss. Alexithymia has affective and cognitive components. Emotions are undifferentiated, poorly verbalized, and often somaticized. Thinking is operative, dominated by noninterpretive, chronological, banal facts. Survivors with alexithymia are often aware of their deficiency, but like color-blind people still experience a narrowed range of qualitative experience. Another characteristic of these survivors is their tendency to have a

> sudden outburst of what are assumed to be strong emotions: for instance rages which cease as abruptly as they start. The subject is not quite sure whether he really feels what he seems to be expressing . . . they tend to behave as if they suddenly switched to another personality. (Krystal, 1979, p. 18)

These survivors "show a marked impairment in their capacity for creativity, especially in regard to drive gratification fantasy" (Krystal, 1979, p. 19). Alexithymia is especially prevalent in survivors with a history of substance abuse and personality disorders.

Intrusive Thoughts and Reexperiencing of Trauma

Intrusive symptoms are wide ranging and typically include preoccupation, "labile or 'explosive' entry into intensely emotional and under modulated states of mind," and "repetitive thoughts, images, emotions, and behaviors" (Horowitz, 1985, p. 162). The long-term, ongoing nature of multiple AIDS-related loss affects the manner in which intrusive symptoms manifest in survivors. The trauma of AIDS-related losses are not typically associated with a specific, limited moment of horror, like many other trauma-inducing disasters. Therefore, symptoms of intrusion and reexperiencing are often generalized and related to manifestations of the death imprint.

Explosive Emotional Response   When capable of emotional expression, the survivor of multiple AIDS-related loss may tend to express labile and explosive emotions. Outbursts of anger and rage are common (Houseman & Pheifer, 1988). Although anger is an appropriate response in the face of AIDS, these outbursts are often generalized against people, events, and situations unrelated to AIDS, similar to observations made by Horowitz (1985) regarding psychological response to stress. "This rage is especially difficult to contemplate because it may be a diffuse theme, aimed at anybody, having therefore an irrational quality because the linkage in terms of causation is not clear to the subject" (Horowitz, 1985, p. 162). Frequently, rage and diffuse anger are directed against caregivers (Lloyd, 1992), especially those closest, and therefore "safest," for the survivor. This behavior may be self-defeating, especially when it makes it difficult for people to be supportive and hinders the establishment of new support.

Repetitive Thoughts   Repetitive thoughts of AIDS-related losses occur among survivors, a common symptom associated with traumatic stress response. These have a different flavor than the flashbacks experienced by Vietnam War veterans, who sometimes relived battle tragedies. Survivors of multiple AIDS-related loss are more likely to speak of intrusive thoughts and memories that well up from within them. A dissociative flavor permeates their descriptions of drifting away into memories or confusion. Anniversary reactions provoke a recurrence of feelings. The world of survivors of multiple AIDS-related loss is full of reminders about loss from AIDS. In the gay community, for example, triggers to repetitive memories abound in social settings such as bars, events such as gay pride celebrations, and ongoing memorial services.

Repetitive thoughts are frequent at times when sleep is sought. One regularly hears survivors report dreams that sometimes include horrifying exaggerations of the actual illness ordeals of dead loved ones. Russ Berst, a survivor of two partners, described some of his dreams as horrible flashbacks. When survivors lay down to sleep, their quieting minds may be bombarded with both memories and worries of loss. Sleep disturbances are common among survivors of the Holocaust (Kaminer & Lavie, 1993) and other disasters. Increased sedative use documented among survivors of multiple AIDS-related loss is necessitated by sleep disturbance (Martin, 1988).

Voluntary Reexposure to Trauma

Voluntary reexposure to trauma is a phenomenon noted among some survivors of traumatic events (Horowitz, 1976a; van der Kolk, 1989). The ongoing nature of AIDS allows the phenomenon to be actualized repeatedly. Survivors of multiple AIDS-related loss frequently engage in volunteer efforts and caregiving capacities related to AIDS. Lesbians and gay men who have suffered more loss from AIDS tend to be more involved in gay-related support efforts, increasing their reexposure to AIDS-related loss. Perhaps voluntary reexposure to AIDS-related loss provides the survivor a degree of control inasmuch as feelings can be anticipated. There may be a similarity to the common human tendency to touch an aching tooth.

Volunteer efforts in response to AIDS have been impressive. It is difficult, and perhaps unnecessary, to separate compassionate response to an ongoing crisis from voluntary, repetitive, almost masochistic reexposure to traumatization. Volunteer work, caregiving, and social involvement connected directly to AIDS serve a number of functions for the survivor. These include the creation of meaning from tragedy, a modicum of control in an environment of powerlessness, social connection to fellow survivors, and human empathic response. Whatever the reason, many survivors devote much of their lives to efforts guaranteed to reexpose themselves to trauma.

IMPLICATIONS OF A TRAUMATIC PERSPECTIVE

Assessment and treatment of traumatic stress response resulting from multiple AIDS-related loss is complicated by two factors. First, chronic passivity, frequently seen in survivors of trauma (van der Kolk, 1989, p. 14), combines with tendencies to isolate. "The experience of any trauma makes one a stranger in one's world; one is pushed into an exile where connection between people is impossible, where memories are not shared" (Jay, 1994, p. 34) This prevents victims of trauma from being identified and, therefore, treated. Constriction of emotional affect and psychic numbing may mute the ability of survivors to express their experience of traumatization. Treatment for trauma entails a degree of reexperiencing the painful event and inherently involves pain and anxiety. There is, therefore, a tendency to avoid the work required for recovery from surviving multiple AIDS-related loss related to the conservation of energy principle. Survivors commonly avoid the necessary, painful work that involves reactivating painful feelings. Krystal (1981) observed that

> although it may be painful and difficult for an individual who has endured serious psychic traumatization to achieve intrapsychic integration, this is what the survivor needs most of all. One of the most devastating aftereffects of trauma is the widespread use of repression, denial, and psychic splitting. (pp. 181–182)

Only when the accumulation of unresolved grief and trauma becomes more unbearable than reexposure to the memories required for trauma and grief work do many willingly engage this difficult and painful process.

Another difficulty faced by clinicians assessing and treating survivors of multiple AIDS-related loss is the possibility that traumatic response is masked by more obvious symptoms such as chemical dependency, self-destructive behaviors, intimacy impairment, emotional numbing, or personality disorders. As van der Kolk (1989) noted,

> People who become fixated at a level of helplessness and loss of control are likely to end up in the mental health system, where they will receive a variety of psychiatric diagnosis, depending on the particular presentation during any particular admission. (p. 22)

A survivor of trauma who presents with diffuse rage, inappropriate anger, or narcissistic entitlement may be diagnosed with a personality disorder. Lindy (1985) observed that "clinicians tend to presume the presence of long-standing chronic mental disorder" (p. 155).

Even when psychotherapeutic work is engaged, it is often ineffective. Krystal (1975) attributed this ineffectiveness to the survivors' impairment of affect tolerance due to their fear of emotions, which are experienced as heralds of trauma. Beyond this difficulty, survivors who cannot recognize their own emotions because of problems related to alexithymia suffer "a severe impairment to utilizing dynamic psychotherapy" (Krystal, 1979, p. 29). These survivors may complain more of physical than emotional symptoms.

Some common survivor responses can be traced to reactions to both trauma and grief, such as survivor's guilt, depression, helplessness, emotional shutdown, and diffuse anger. Therefore, it is essential that both problem paradigms be assessed and treated. Also essential is a realization that a history of trauma and grief will exacerbate the impact of multiple AIDS-related loss. Assessment, and treatment, may need to include previous losses and traumatization.

Diagnosis Difficulties

Current diagnostic criteria are wholly inadequate and may also hinder assessment of trauma associated with multiple AIDS-related loss, especially by clinicians unfamiliar with this unique phenomenon of trauma and grief. Acute stress disorder, one possible diagnosis that incorporates traumatization, is inappropriate for survivors of multiple AIDS-related loss because it excludes disturbances lasting more than 4 weeks (American Psychiatric Association, 1994, p. 432). Secondary traumatization is inadequately addressed in the diagnosis and in posttraumatic stress disorder. Most events and experiences of traumatization are diagnosed as posttraumatic stress disorder. However, this diagnosis presumes an event that is "post"; one that is historic, not ongoing. Figley (1995) concluded that "PTSD should stand for primary traumatic stress disorder, rather than post-traumatic stress disorder, since every stress reactions [sic] is 'post' by definition" (p. 9). Although Figley's recent book on compassion fatigue is groundbreaking and useful, it fails to account for ongoing traumatization that occurs with multiple AIDS-related loss. Lack of appreciation for secondary stress reactions in survivors includes an inability to assess and diagnose symptomatology. Beaton and Murphy (1995) concluded that a barrier to coworkers and family members is their lack of ability to "detect secondary post-trauma symptoms as most post-trauma symptoms are subjective in nature." Family and friends may find the trauma symptoms difficult to understand since "they [the crisis workers] must have known what they were getting into" (p. 75). This is precisely the situation of many survivors of multiple AIDS-related loss.

Clinicians who are outside the group of people most affected by multiple AIDS-related loss or who are unfamiliar with the analysis presented in this chapter are unlikely to recognize the effects of trauma among survivors, thereby making effective treatment unlikely. It is time to recognize the traumatic effect of multiple AIDS-related loss and begin the process of developing effective intervention strategies.

Given the fact that survivors of multiple AIDS-related loss face a unique form of trauma and grief with significant symptoms of distress for which no adequate diagnostic label is available, justification exists for naming a new syndrome. An approach to naming a cluster of symptoms that characterize a condition of trauma has precedent. Buffalo Creek syndrome (Titchener & Kapp, 1976) was identified in realization that the flood event produced unique characteristics arising from its impact on a community and individuals. Rape trauma syndrome (Burgess & Holmstrom, 1974; Seligman, 1994) has similarly been identified. Survivors syndrome has been identified by Lifton and Olson (1976) and Niederland (1971). Similarly, *multiple AIDS-related loss syndrome* is justified by the unique characteristics of this event and experience.

CONCLUSION

Survivors of multiple AIDS-related loss contend with more than a traumatic event, they live amid the reality of an ongoing traumatic process. That reality influences both the event and the experience of trauma and has serious implications for treatment of survivors. The first priority in traditional trauma recovery efforts is to terminate the external traumatic event or remove the person from contact with it (Horowitz, 1976a). Neither is a feasible option with survivors of multiple AIDS-related loss. Rather, survivors of AIDS-related loss face a situation conceptually similar to leaving abuse victims with the abuser, telling them that there is nothing that can be done and to expect more abuse. The abuse victim might, however, at least garner widespread public sympathy.

Although divided for the sake of clarity and organization, factors contributing to traumatic stress reactions, preexisting characteristics making traumatic reaction more severe, and consequences of trauma all interrelate. Understanding this interconnection is essential to any effort to appreciate the magnitude of this disaster. The overlapping processes of grief and traumatization significantly affect the experience of surviving multiple AIDS-related loss and the process of recovery. Lifton (1993) noted that "many of the symptoms in the traumatic syndrome have precisely to do with impaired mourning" (p. 17). As discussed in chapter 6 on grieving and bereavement, survivors of multiple AIDS-related loss regularly exhibit symptoms of unresolved grief and complicated bereavement. Grief may never be resolved. Consequent symptoms of depression, guilt, isolation, despair, emotional shutdown, and anxiety arise as a result of a response to both grief and trauma.

Theories about the prioritization of either grief or trauma work conflict. On one side, grief work may only proceed "after issues regarding helplessness and traumatic overload" (Lindy, 1985, p. 160). Unresolved trauma may hinder the resolution of grief (Raphael & Wilson, 1993; Lindy, Green, Grace, & Titchener, 1983). Yet unresolved grief hinders the resolution of trauma because symptoms of unresolved grief such as isolation, emotional shutdown, despair, and guilt all hinder the process of recovery from trauma. Thus, survivors of multiple loss face the bind of having their grief response hinder traumatic resolution while their trauma response hinders resolution of grief.

The community-wide impact of multiple AIDS-related loss increases the severity of individual response to trauma and handicaps the recovery process. In addition, traumatic response in individuals serves to hinder establishment of social support. The process is two-directional: The community is less available to support the individual, and the individual is less able to solicit support because of anxiety associated with future loss and behaviors that push away potential support. Because of the crucial role support plays in the resolution of trauma, the implications for recovery are significant.

Survivors of multiple AIDS-related loss experience a traumatic event and respond in ways characteristic of traumatization. Recognition of this fact makes comprehensible the sometimes chronic and severe cluster of symptoms observed in survivors of multiple AIDS-related loss. Understanding multiple AIDS-related loss within the framework of traumatization may assist in strategies for resolution and treatment.

Chapter 8

Familes of Origin
and Families of Choice

Experience is a brutal teacher, but it hurt, it hurts.—C. S. Lewis in Attenborough & Eastman (1993), *Shadowlands*

AIDS kills families. Families of origin and families of choice are disrupted when the functions and roles of family members are affected by multiple AIDS-related loss. The term *dying family* was coined to refer "not only to families experiencing multiple deaths, but to the dissolution of the family through incarceration, addiction, illness, abandonment or court removal of children, hospitalization, sibling separation, or homelessness" (Dubik-Unruh, 1989, p. 11). Although this particular definition of dying family was clearly written with families of origin in mind, this book, and particularly this chapter, demonstrates that families of choice are also dying families.

This chapter is meant to increase awareness of two issues that have been relatively ignored. First, families of choice serve valuable functions; this is highlighted by the impact of multiple AIDS-related loss on these families. The importance of families of choice is underlined by the disruption many such families have faced and the crucial roles these families have fulfilled in response to AIDS. Second, the impact of multiple AIDS-related loss on families of origin has been neglected in favor of focusing on what has been assumed to be an almost exclusive impact of AIDS on nontraditional families.

Debra, whose case was presented in the first chapter, is the mother of two sons, both of whom have hemophilia and HIV. Her only sister had two sons who were both hemophiliac, contracted HIV, and died of AIDS. Debra is involved with many other hemophiliac families and friends. Over the past several years, she has witnessed the deaths of many people she has loved. She finds it difficult to make others understand the depth of her ongoing grief and the fear she holds for a future that will undoubtedly hold more suffering and death. Debra keeps a scrapbook of photos and mementos to commemorate her losses.

Greg is a gay man who has little contact with his family of origin, and his family of choice has been decimated by AIDS. He has had HIV for over a decade. In that time, he has lost two partners to AIDS. All of his close friends died a few years ago. Courageously, he made new friends and established a new family of choice. Now, they have all died too. Greg cannot bring himself to make new friends for fear of being hurt and abandoned again. He is prone to episodes of rage and irritability, and so people tend to avoid him.

Nick lost his partner, Morgan, to AIDS. He has been no stranger to multiple AIDS-related loss in both personal and professional capacities. Everyone associated with Nick and Morgan lavished praise on Nick's care for Morgan, especially during the final months. During those last months, some of Morgan's family of origin were especially supportive and helpful. At Morgan's memorial service Nick said, "When I used to hear about family values it sounded to me like fingernails on a chalkboard, but no more. Now I know what family values mean. It's like I've gained a couple of brothers and a new nephew."

These three families have been overwhelmed by the effects of multiple AIDS-related loss. They are representative of three different family scenarios: the heterosexual family of origin, the gay family of choice, and the interface of both types of family.

A variety of trends prophesy an increasing impact on families of origin. The family, in the context of AIDS, has been neglected (Bor, Elford, Hart, & Sherr, 1993). An analysis of the effect of multiple AIDS-related loss on families has not previously been offered. Recent trends indicate that women, Blacks and Hispanics, and persons with heterosexually acquired HIV infections account for the highest growth in the future (CDC, 1995). Adolescents are increasingly affected by AIDS (Atwood, 1993); one in four new HIV infections are in persons under 20 years of age (Neergaard, 1996). A "second wave of infection is underway" (Ramos, 1995, p. 29). Therefore, the impact of AIDS on traditional families and society will continue to increase into the foreseeable future.

FAMILIES DEFINED

At least one family is affected by every person infected with HIV. Even if one narrows understanding of the familial impact of AIDS to the traditionally defined, nuclear family, the impact is vast. However, many of those most affected by multiple AIDS-related loss belong to nontraditional families of choice. Thus, families may include the traditional nuclear family, extended family and relatives, friends, lovers, sexual partners, and drug-related connections. To fully understand the scope of impact of multiple AIDS-related loss on families, it is imperative to consider the consequences on both families of origin and families of choice (Nord, 1996b).

Traditional Families

Many traditional families—composed of relatives connected by blood, marriage, or adoption—suffer multiple AIDS-related loss. Although there are no measures of incidence, it is not uncommon for a traditional family to have suffered multiple AIDS-related loss. This occurs in a variety of ways related to the etiology of HIV transmission. For example, families with hemophilia often cope with multiple loss. A family may have more than one member who is gay or an IVDU. In a family where one of the partners or spouses tests HIV positive, the other partner may become infected. For example, more than 10% of hemophiliacs' wives were infected. One hemophiliac who was married in 1986 wrote that he never realized the danger he was putting his wife in (Goss, 1994).

Children may be conceived and born before knowledge of HIV infection. The CDC predicts that between 93,000 and 112,000 children will be born to mothers who will die of AIDS between 1992 and 2000; these women will give birth to between 32,000–38,000 children infected with HIV (Levine, 1992). Also, some partners may choose to take risks with an HIV-infected partner, which can result in either their own infection or the birth of an infected child. Therefore, it is not uncommon for families to experience the death of both parents, more than one child, or a combination of these deaths (Chachkes & Jennings, 1992). Finally, a strong case can be made that any individual family death involves multiple losses.

Traditional families may face the simultaneous impact of acknowledging a member's HIV status, news about sexual orientation, sexual partners, or drug use. Families have a double adjustment to undergo when coping with a son who has AIDS in "those unfortunate cases where two facts are forced into awareness at the same time" (Shearer & McKusick, 1986, p. 163). The level of denial in such families is probably high to begin with if the family was "unaware" of the son's homosexuality.

Lifestyle choices may have been unknown or ignored. News of HIV infection may include news of marital infidelity, bisexuality, rape, parental drug use, and subsequent risk to other family members, notably the spouse through sexual contact. The family may react with shock, disapproval, disappointment, resentment, and anger. Adolescents with hemophilia and HIV find it awkward to talk with their parents or other adults about HIV. "After all, it is no secret that talking about HIV infection includes talking about sex, and talking about sex is often not easy" (Steinhart, 1990, p. 1). Natural fears about the HIV threat may be displaced into feelings that divide the family rather than bring it together.

Many families have both children and adults who are infected with HIV. The majority of infected children are born to mothers who are themselves infected (Dubik-Unruh, 1989). Children will make the connection between their own illness and the death of parents or siblings. One boy's experience highlights the painful poignancy of this possibility.

> Jimmy had a sore on his foot which was being treated some months after the death of his mother. During the process the toddler observed: "Mommy sick. Mommy die. Jimmy die too?" This fall, Jimmy's disease progressed. . . . In all probability, Jimmy will die too. . . . Jimmy has lost his home, his mother, his father, two sisters, two brothers, maternal and paternal grandparents, aunts, uncles and cousins, staff members to whom he was attached, and, progressively, his health. Some of his family was lost to death, some just don't come to visit anymore. (as cited in Dubik-Unruh, 1989, p. 10)

Between 25% and 33% of infants with AIDS will not be cared for by their biological parents (Tourse & Gunderson, 1988). Although Jimmy lost his family before he became sick with AIDS, in many families, the first sign of HIV infection in the parents is observed in a sick child. The child is discovered to have AIDS-related illness, then the parents are tested. Intense feelings of parental guilt often accompany this double blow.

Nontraditional Families

In the movie "Torch Song Trilogy" (Gottfried & Boggart, 1988), Arnold, who is gay, stands in a cemetery over his lover's grave saying kaddish while his mother says kaddish for her husband in the background. When she notices what Arnold is doing she confronts him.

> Arnold: "Momma, you know who this is, it's my lover!"
> Mother: "Wait. Wait. Wait! You're going to compare my marriage to you and Alan? You dare to compare yourself to that?"
> Arnold: "I'm talking about my loss."
> Mother: "What loss did you have? You fooled around with some boy. . ."
> Arnold: "Momma, I lost someone I loved very much."

Arnold's mother persists in her disgust and yells at her son. A time for ritual healing is destroyed. Later, Arnold despairs, "Queers don't love and those that do deserve what they get." A similar scene occurs regularly for survivors of multiple AIDS-related loss.

The impact of AIDS, especially multiple AIDS-related loss, has highlighted the importance, value, and function of families of choice. By decimating families of choice, multiple AIDS-related loss instructs about the vitality of these families. In part, one can recognize what existed in its absence.

Available vocabulary about families of choice is not only limiting, it is disturbingly devaluing.

> We have terms or labels that signify most types of grievers. Wives and husbands become widows and widowers; children become orphans; brothers and sisters are said to experience sibling loss; but there is no term to describe those who grieve friends. Titles give rise to identity. (Deck & Folta, 1989, pp. 82–83)

Relationships between lovers, for example, whether heterosexual or homosexual, are seen as purely sexual and mainly flippant. Fudin and Devore (1981) wrote about another type of nontraditional relationship, concluding that

> Not all functional relationships receive societal sanction. Minimal support is given the long-term, extramarital relationship entered into by a husband who remains with his wife and family. Perhaps the external relationship satisfies unmet needs of the husband and wife and helps to maintain the marriage. If so, the extramarital relationship may be functional, although it receives no sanction. (p. 134)

The phrase *family of choice* is used with purpose in this book because choice is the key to appreciating the importance of these social arrangements. Family members are chosen because of characteristics not always present in families of origin: shared values, interests, trust, loyalty, and support. As time passes, the importance of family members deepens. Deck and Folta (1989) asserted that "throughout the life cycle, peers are often more significant in importance than kin . . . friends often provide the most meaningful and psychologically close relationships" (p. 78).

Families of choice exist for heterosexuals and homosexuals. Almost everyone is a member of both. Yet, nowhere is the value of family of choice seen more clearly than in the families created by gay men and lesbians. Gays and lesbians have often been forced by necessity to create families of choice because their family of origin is nonsupportive, rejecting, or hostile. One gay man said, "My family rejected me because I was gay. When I was young I left home and rarely have contact with them. I found a new family, but now I am losing it too." It is not uncommon for those with AIDS to have been rejected by their families of origin (Macklin, 1988). To the extent that a family structure provides essential functions, the lack of its availability for many gay men and lesbians in their family of origin has created a vacuum of family function that has been filled by family of choice.

The main functions of family are "rarely fully achieved" (Bozett & Sussman, 1990, p. 1) for gay or lesbian family members by their families of origin, especially in regard to coping with the many stresses brought about by AIDS. A study by Britton, Zarski, and Hobfoll (1993) determined that "family support did not surface as a powerful resource under any conditions" (p. 52). Instead of providing support and nurturance, stressful family-of-origin relationships are the norm for gays dealing with AIDS (Christ & Weiner, 1985).

Families of choice take on the roles that are "usually performed by biological family members in the heterosexual culture" (Britton et al., 1993, p. 46). Gay couples—living together, supporting a household, supporting each other materially and financially, coping together with difficulties, planning vacations, marking rites of passage, sharing holidays, sharing intimacy, and committing to each other—fulfill the functions of family. Gay couples are very similar, in almost every respect, to heterosexual, married couples. There are no significant differences between them (Mendola, 1980).

Extended families of choice are especially important in the gay community. For gay men, especially those dealing with AIDS, friends provide the functions of relatives (Hays et al., 1990). Most gay men and lesbians insist that family members are the people who are really there for them, the people they can count on emotionally and materially (Weston, 1991). Many gays expect, rely on, and receive more support from their family of choice than from their family of origin. There can be no denying the importance of family of choice. To ignore this nontraditional form of family is to play with semantics, denying function for form.

Among IVDUs, both types of families may be directly affected by multiple AIDS-related loss. A traditional, heterosexual family may be devastated if one or both spouses are infected with HIV or children are born infected. Little is known about the family relationships and friendship networks of IVDUs, but it has been demonstrated that social networks and friends appear "more important than biological family in providing support especially for those dealing with HIV" (Stowe et al., 1993, pp. 31–32). Whether it is biological or affiliation, family is the most important social system for IVDUs (Bor, Miller, & Goldman, 1992).

It is clear that many of those dealing with AIDS will find at least as much, if not more, support in their family of choice than in their family of origin. Unfortunately, closeness is usually attributed only to blood relations rather than functional ones. In today's mobile society, blood relations may have only infrequent contact (Fudin & Devore, 1981). Indeed, close affiliation with family of choice makes multiple AIDS-related loss more likely because of the link between family of choice and the etiology of HIV transmission. Gays and IVDUs are simultaneously more likely to have formed families of choice and to have been infected with HIV.

Nontraditional family arrangements may include commitments to monogamy that are as meaningful as similar commitments in traditional families. Misconceptions about sexual and relationship instability still exist. Therefore, it should not be surprising that similar feelings about betrayal arise in homosexual and heterosexual couples. Choices about ongoing sexuality need to be addressed directly.

Society has not recognized the importance of families of choice. Deck and Folta (1989) observed that

> social protocol still assumes that kin are the most important relationships even when the members are isolated or estranged from each other. There appears to be a

cultural lag between the social definition of rights and responsibilities of family members, and the reality of social relationships. (p. 81)

The AIDS epoch has helped improve understanding for, and appreciation of, families of choice. In the early years, friends and lovers were routinely excluded from hospital rooms. By shining a light on the value of these relationships, AIDS has served a valuable function by marking the salience of these relationships.

Interface of Two Families

The process of illness from AIDS, or the planning and event of the memorial service, may be the first time the family of origin and the family of choice must associate with each other. Many people with AIDS have compartmentalized their families and friends, especially in the gay and IVDU communities. Families of origin may be separate from family of choice who are separate from heterosexual, non–drug-using friends.

Parents may blame the dying person's family of choice for contributing to the lifestyle that "caused" AIDS or use the family of choice as a scapegoat (Dworkin & Pincu, 1993). When the family of origin does not acknowledge the viability of their son's sexuality or the rights and grief of his partner, "conflict can result" (Shearer & McKusick, 1986, pp. 164–165). Anyone who has worked extensively with people with AIDS will recall many tragic examples of hostility between the family of origin and the family of choice. The partner of the person with AIDS is sometimes the target of wrath. Parents may force the person with AIDS to choose between them and the family of choice. Intolerant religious views make matters worse. A lifetime partner to a man with AIDS had the following experience

> Phillip had an impossible choice to make. But—I was there for him, day and night, month after month. Then his parents came and cried and told him how much they loved him and wanted to take him home, if he would repudiate evil and evil-doing [being gay]. Finally he said that he repented his sins and would turn his back on evil. They swooped him up and he was gone, without a word. (as cited in Fuller, Geis, & Rush, 1989, p. 35)

The cruelty of these stories is truly heartbreaking, yet most survivors will have endured the reality of them directly or indirectly, sometimes repeatedly. The lifetime partner cannot prove legal rights to property or control the loved one's remains.

> Frequently, biological family members appear during the last few weeks of the patient's life. While he is alive, they many not be able to force the patient to reject his lover and life-style, but immediately following the death, they often take over and assert their legal prerogative to make decisions. (Fuller et al., 1989, pp. 36–37)

Obviously, the interface between the families of choice and origin can be a source of tremendous and lasting stress and pain. Families of choice and origin may find themselves in "love triangles, bitter struggles over who will assume responsibility for the patient's medical management, financial management, emotional support and physical care" (Lovejoy, 1990, p. 303). A rivalry may develop between the lover of the person with AIDS at the same time parents are having trouble adjusting to having a homosexual son.

One area where conflict can negatively affect the coping of survivors is in connection with memorial services. Sometimes the family of origin will co-opt all planning and arrangements. Friends and family of choice are entirely excluded or the remains are taken far away. One gay man recounts his experience with his partner's family of origin.

> Greg and I talked over everything. In those last months he'd really gotten into Zen meditation. We planned a simple service with some poetry and chants and everything. We were going to put his ashes under the willow tree in our back yard. But that last week his parents swooped in and took over. Greg tried to stop them but he was too weak. I tried to stop them, but I didn't count. . . . They decided everything, the words and music. Everything. They had the service in a funeral home. Of course they didn't want me to sit with the family. They really didn't even want me to come. Greg would have hated the whole thing, that was the hardest part. . . . Then they got a court order and took everything they thought was Greg's out of the house. . . . They acted as if they deserved it for all the pain Greg and I had caused them. . . . They left me with nothing to remember him by. (as cited in Fuller et al., 1989, p. 37)

Unfortunately, it is not uncommon for the family of origin to exclude or minimize the family of choice at the memorial service. Friends and the family of choice are sometimes shunned or ignored. This creates bitterness at a time intended for healing.

The importance of memorial services, or funerals, to the grieving can hardly be overstated because they serve a number of important functions for healthy grieving (see Rando, 1984, pp. 173–196). A common predeterminant to the development of pathological mourning is that the memorial service did not go well for the bereaved (Volkan, 1975, p. 338). Families of choice are frequently ignored or minimized in the planning and execution of these services. The family of origin may control everything. They may decide to hold no service, hold only a private service, or hold a service in the deceased's home town, far away from the family of choice.

The author once attended a traditional religious service completely organized by the deceased's family of origin. The service focused on Lou's childhood and hopes for his eternal soul and included several religious prayers, most of them in Hebrew. Although his lifetime partner and many friends attended, not one mention was made of Lou's family of choice or his active life in the gay community. Near the end of the service, one of the deceased's friends who could contain himself no longer burst into an angry tirade, pointing out the presence of Lou's partner and friends. Instead of providing a ritual where feelings of grief could be validated and supported, the service produced bitterness, resentment, and rage.

However, memorial services are frequently times when the family of origin and family of choice come together for the first time. Both learn about the "other life" of the deceased. The family of origin is gratified to see the number and quality of friends. The family of choice appreciates learning more about the history of their loved one. The optimal situation for healing occurs when both families support each other. Therefore, given the importance of family of choice and family of origin in understanding the impact of multiple AIDS-related loss, and the similarity in functions provided by both types of families, this chapter refers to both types of families whenever it speaks of families, unless specifically noted.

IMPACT ON FAMILY FUNCTIONS, ROLES, AND MEANING

Multiple AIDS-related loss unavoidably alters a family. It moves its members into an environment of profound change, turmoil, confusion, and anxiety and may call into question the very meaning of issues fundamental to what it means to be a family. Almost no area of family life is left unaffected when a family members has AIDS (Lovejoy, 1990). When multiple AIDS-related loss affects a family, the impact is enormous, permeating every aspect of family life. Because it is impossible to completely separate the effect of multiple loss on the individual from its effect on the family, many of the struggles confronted by individual members affect the family as a whole.

Family Roles and Tasks

Having even a single family member sick with AIDS shuffles the roles and functions of family members. Loss of a spouse requires rearrangement and restructuring of the survivor's life and "typically produces a crisis" (Nichols & Everett, 1986, p. 172) in the family. The death of a family member interrupts a family's ongoing process and initiates a crisis and rebuilding of family identity both in managing family roles or functions and in managing intense shared emotions. Shapiro (1995) reasoned that

> Our deepest emotional experiences, our attachments to beloved family members, are lived out within the mundane work of day-to-day family living. The death of a family member disrupts the work of the family, which must reorganize the ways it fulfills family work roles as well as family emotional functions. (pp. 170–171)

When more than one family member is living with AIDS, or there are serial cases of AIDS, the impact is overwhelming. Children may have to take care of parents. Parents, who thought they were finished caring for the physical needs of children, often find themselves caring again for their children. Often this care involves tasks that were never expected and are particularly difficult. A family member may have to change diapers or clean up after incontinence. Many must learn to work with catheters and IV lines on a daily basis. Medicines must be administered while keeping track of dosage and frequency. Family members with AIDS may lose their sight or be unable to walk or clothe themselves.

Multiple loss from AIDS often strikes the same family or peer group. It is not uncommon for a family to experience the death of both parents or children. Under these conditions, it is exceedingly difficult for parents to adequately plan for the future care of their children, thus the children's losses may continue through multiple foster home placements (Chachkes & Jennings, 1992). Mothers who are ill themselves watch in despair as their children die. The father and mother are in the conflicting roles of needing care and needing to provide care.

Some of the infections that regularly occur in people with AIDS cause tremendous disruption to family roles and tasks. For example, coping with the effects of dementia can be particularly frustrating on various levels. The personality of the person suffering dementia may seem completely changed; family members observe that the person with AIDS is "not the same person" they used to know. Not uncommonly, the person with dementia can become extremely irritable and difficult to be around. Dangerous situations can arise when the family member with dementia forgets to turn off a stove or lights a cigarette and leaves it burning in an unsafe manner.

Families assign roles to various members. The diversity of ways families divide responsibilities is matched only by the number of families affected. What is consistent is the ensuing disruption brought about by the impact of AIDS, especially when a family is shaken by multiple AIDS-related loss. Families in which one member is especially dominant in terms of decision making, earning power, or influence are particularly susceptible to role reversals that result in profound instability and anxiety. The formerly dominant family member may become extraordinarily dependent.

Children

Illness and death within a family draw attention and energy away from the needs of the children. The scenario described by Kastenbaum (1977) has regularly occurred in hemophiliac families.

> When one parent dies, for example, the surviving parent's grief can interfere with the ability to care for the emotional or even the physical needs of the children. . . . Sometimes it is the sibling who dies. In this situation the parents may be so involved in the plight of the dying child that other children are neglected. (p. 257)

Children are prone to face two extreme sources of instability and stress. First, they are deprived of normal familial support while another's is prioritized. Second, they must deal with their own bereavement and adjustment process.

Children who lose their parents inherently face multiple losses including the loss of home, parents, safety, and security. Children who lose a parent are at increased risk for physiological and psychological problems if the loss is accompanied by disruption in environmental routines, such as moving to a new location or changes in caregivers. Fortunate children who are raised by their grandparents still face some challenges. The family itself has lost a generation; the children are raised by people who may be twice as old as their parents. There are probably both positive and negative implications in this occurrence.

A common fear in these children is the loss of the remaining parent (Osterweiss, Solomon, & Green, 1984). The death of a parent is a psychological, social, and spiritual crisis for a child. Orphans from AIDS often face a future of multiple personal loss arising from developmental and behavioral problems resulting from a lack of consistency in their lives, including difficulty trusting and bonding with adults (Doka, 1992). Children and adolescents who grow up in an environment of death and AIDS are "likely to worry about their existence. They may assume that the world is not a safe place" (Dane, 1992, p. 24). This may have long-term implications for the child's developmental process.

Children who are dying of AIDS themselves are often moved "from one chaotic system to another" when others in the family are also infected (Dubik-Unruh, 1989, p. 10). The death of the family may precede physical deaths as problems arising from HIV are coupled with addiction, illness, incarceration, abandonment, court removal of children, hospitalization, sibling separation, and homelessness (Dubik-Unruh, 1989).

Certain tasks may intrude on the family that were previously ignored. Families who will continue to lose more members need to prepare. Decisions have to be made about medical care and life support. Routine aspects of bereavement—including plans for memorial services, disposition of the body, and payment for services—will be necessary. This planning may pale in comparison to even bigger decisions about placement of children, housing, and financial provisions. Family members may be actively involved in a rational suicide strategy. "Many simply want their loved one's misery to end, with action taken, at a predetermined stage of illness, to terminate prolonged agony" (Lippmann et al., 1993, p. 75).

Shifts that occur in family roles and functions are certainly not all injurious. Members of families of origin and choice regularly respond with impressive care and growth. Even when the family of origin begins with rejection, very often they come around and allow both the person dying and the survivors to work toward a place of peace. Unfinished business is finished. Things that were left unsaid are said. The response of families of choice has been heroic from the first days of the AIDS epoch. When most of society feared and attacked people with AIDS, families of choice were often the only ones who cared. As the years have gone by, their consistent commitment and dedication to helping over the long haul has been awe inspiring.

Emotional Adjustment

The family will inevitably face a variety of strong emotions that will require adjustment on the part of all members. Relative stability of emotions that may have existed before AIDS will be severely disrupted. Suddenly, or gradually over time, emotions of grief, shock, anger, sadness, anxiety, and helplessness emerge. "Surprising emotional reactions may be forthcoming," which cause other family members to be "shocked and upset by the emotional reactions that erupt" (Nichols & Everett, 1986, p. 173). These may be particularly destabilizing for children who see their parents falling apart and provoke fears of abandonment that couple with the very real threat of abandonment through death. Dependence and vulnerability, pain with inadequate comfort, separation and subsequent depression, changes in routine due to frequent hospitalization, and erratic care taking are all a part of what these families must endure. Disappointment cannot be avoided and may provoke relational divisions; anger frequently results. If subsequent anger either is not expressed or is expressed inappropriately, the resulting harm to both those with AIDS and those surviving is immense.

When children die before their parents, it provokes an especially intense grief response (Rando, 1984). Compounding the age inappropriateness of AIDS-related death is the confounding of expectations that normally occurs. Children are expected to outlive their parents. Parents face multiple losses each time a child dies; they experience the loss of the child, loss of family, loss of continuity, loss of future plans, loss of normal expectations, and loss of future grandchildren.

Family members may wish that those with AIDS would die. These feelings and thoughts are usually not expressed.

> Such yearnings are more prominent when HIV is an embarrassment or if they feel ostracized from support networks. Families may wish for such a death to diminish their own anguish or to stop an over-extended commitment to a sick and/or dependent AIDS relative. (Lippmann et al., 1993, p. 75)

When these thoughts and feelings are not expressed, they nearly inevitably lead to internal dissonance that is troubling for the survivor. Worse yet, they may contribute to survivor's guilt after death.

Concurrent Stressors

A significant number of children orphaned by AIDS come from "socially disorganized and poorly functioning families" (Chachkes & Jennings, 1992, p. 80).

Families dealing with concurrent stressors have a particularly difficult time coping with the stress of family members living with and dying of AIDS. Nowhere is this more apparent than in impoverished, inner-city families in which various coexisting stressors such as financial strains, poor housing, inadequate health care, drug abuse, mental illness, discrimination, and the stress of inner-city life may strain life, even without AIDS. An example of this was presented by Shapiro (1995), who observed that "many children in Latino families grow up exposed to systematic risks such as poverty, community violence, deficient urban schools, limited access to health and mental health care, and racism" (p. 162). Coping with multiple AIDS-related loss is much more difficult for people dealing with socioeconomic stress because it interacts with the mourning process, making it more difficult to mourn (Johnson-Moore & Phillips, 1994).

A family member who faces the concurrent stress of being HIV positive is prone to a number of factors leading to increased distress as a result of multiple AIDS-related loss. Fears related to stigmatization, including fear of rejection, often serve to encourage family members to seek support outside their traditional network. Feelings of abandonment may be severe, especially if the person has been abandoned by his or her family of origin. As the person who is HIV positive watches family and friends sicken and die, it is natural to dread his or her own future and experience intense anxiety.

The emergence of AIDS in a family will inevitably alter its structure and functions and raise a number of issues likely to create anxiety or conflict. AIDS, or even disclosure of HIV status, may result in lost employment, lost insurance, exclusion from religious associations, dismissal from school, or threats to housing. Even when these threats do not materialize, the risk of such threats undermines the stability of the family and provokes stress and anxiety. Those with AIDS may be blamed. After death, the family is never the same, and some form of adjustment is inevitable.

Values in the family, and the meaning ascribed to the illness, may provoke bitter struggles. Fears may go unspoken and fester as anxiety. Family members of known gay men are observed to experience more anxiety, through all phases of the AIDS trajectory, than do the gay men with AIDS (Church, Kocsis, & Green, 1988) as they worry about the prognosis, pain, and death of their family member. Issues related to the dying person's family of choice, including a significant other, may provoke anxiety. Normal grief reactions may reignite previous feelings of unresolved loss and conflicts within the family.

Many of the issues discussed earlier in this book will prove especially stressful for families. Stigmatization may provoke a wide range of stressors. Decisions about who to inform and who not to inform may create rancor and resentment. Conflicting needs for support and protection may arise. If fear of stigmatization initiates a cycle of withdrawal and isolation, the family's emotional instability will be seated within the family. Little opportunity will exist to disperse and discharge tensions, fears, anxieties, and frustrations.

172   THEORETICAL PERSPECTIVES

Cultural Considerations

Cultural beliefs and traditions play an important role in the way families are affected by AIDS. A variety of cultures within the United States are severely affected. The year 1994 was the first when Blacks and Hispanics together accounted for the majority (53%) of all AIDS cases reported among men. Among women, the majority of AIDS cases has been among this group for some time (CDC, 1995). Shapiro (1995) asserted that the "death of a family member exposes our culture's social arrangement, since the bereaved are forced to recognize the social losses precipitated by the loss of a pivotal member" (p. 171). Surviving multiple AIDS-related loss is even more likely to expose and confront cultural social assumptions.

Black families "frequently include nonrelated individuals as family members or legitimate parts of the system" (Fudin & Devore, 1981, p. 134). Certain factors related to AIDS and culture influence the ability of many African Americans to receive support from their families. The "mode of transmission seems to be important in determining how significant others in the black community respond to a person with AIDS" (Johnson-Moore & Phillips, 1994, p. 104). There may also be a reluctance to ask for support or go to support groups because of fear of racism and discrimination. Homophobia, in ways that are salient in this community (Dalton, 1989), may prevent disclosure of AIDS-related loss. Some African Americans believe AIDS is "a tool to promote hatred of racial and minority groups" (Dworkin & Pincu, 1993, p. 278) and that AIDS is "a form of genocide against blacks" (Rosin, 1995, p. 23). Churches frequently play a significant role in the belief systems and support available for survivors of multiple loss. Although the church has been a stabilizing force in the family and community since slavery (Johnson-Moore & Phillips, 1994), it may also promote judgmental beliefs about the victims of AIDS that hinder disclosure (Rosin, 1995).

Hispanics account for 8.2% of the U.S. population but suffer 17% of total AIDS cases and 24% of pediatric cases (Chachkes & Jennings, 1992), although the CDC believes that Hispanic AIDS cases are understated by at least 30% (Bardach, 1995). The family has special significance for most Hispanics. Disclosure of AIDS-related loss is hindered by the shame it might bring to the family (Chachkes & Jennings, 1992). Intimate matters are usually not discussed outside the family, especially issues related to sexuality. To seek support outside the family may be viewed as compromising the family's pride and dignity (Dillard, 1983).

Hispanic families tend to have an especially difficult time cooperating with a member's family of choice. Strong cultural traditions related to machismo serve to cast homosexuality in a highly negative light. Families are frequently structured in a patriarchal arrangement, with the husband and father holding authority and acting as the decision maker. Illness from AIDS can bring a reversal of this role, resulting in severe stress and anxiety.

Familial Support Handicapped

The family is likely to be the individual's most important support system, whether it is the family of origin or the family of choice. Yet, multiple AIDS-related loss decimates the family, from whom support would be most useful. Multiple AIDS-related loss is a compounded disaster in that it simultaneously destroys families, producing the need for support, while destroying the best available source of support. The very people most able to give meaningful support are the ones eliminated.

Realizing the importance of extended families of choice is crucial in the context of multiple AIDS-related loss. Even when disaster strikes a family, other members of the extended family are traditionally available for support. This backup source of support is often unavailable for survivors of multiple AIDS-related loss for a variety of reasons. Especially in the gay community, the extended family is likely to be decimated by ongoing death and illness. Even when an extended family is physically available, when they are not themselves sick or dead, they may be unable to provide meaningful support because they are already overburdened, overwhelmed, and stressed by a multitude of ongoing loss. The deleterious impact of community-wide stress is profound. For the gay community, although the need for support is tremendous, many survivors report simply being unable to provide any more.

IMPLICATIONS FOR FAMILY THERAPISTS

Multiple AIDS-related loss presents a uniquely challenging set of problems for survivors and those who provide them services. Special considerations must be given this growing population. Survivors of multiple AIDS-related loss are increasingly likely to seek the services of family therapists as a result of the demographic shift in the incidence of AIDS into traditional family structures. Therapists may have to confront a variety of issues that range from emotional to physical.

Trends in Professional Understanding
of Families of Choice

For a variety of reasons, family therapists and other professionals have previously been unprepared to effectively help families deal with issues related to multiple AIDS-related loss. A lack of appreciation for issues of multiple loss is understandable given the relative recency of this phenomenon in connection with AIDS and the fact that it is, only now, becoming recognized as an historically unique form of traumatization and grief.

Until now, a lack of awareness of these special issues has handicapped the capacity of family therapists to be effective in this area. Professional family therapy journals "have been curiously silent" (Green & Bobele, 1994, p. 349) about AIDS, with many of these journals publishing nothing about AIDS for several years. Therefore, an awareness of the special issues raised by multiple AIDS-related loss is the first, and most important, step a clinician can take in an effort to be helpful and useful to survivors. Green and Bobele (1994) concluded that

> The significant correlation between knowledge and attitudes gives credence to the importance of knowledge in enhancing the quality of therapy for [people with AIDS] and their families. Training which expands the knowledge base of therapists working with this population is essential. (p. 362)

Another area in which family therapists working with survivors of multiple AIDS-related loss may need additional information and exposure is in the area of minority concerns. Unfortunately, family therapists "often lack the necessary knowledge and understanding of the minority client's cultural and community experience to provide effective care" (Green & Bobele, 1994, p. 352).

Recognition of, and information about, families of choice remains scarce. Most psychotherapists remain "remarkably uninformed about the issues pertaining to this diverse population" (Carl, 1990, p. xiii). Because of outdated and disproved notions, such as the stereotype that gays lack the ability to sustain long-term relationships, many psychotherapists fail to understand and work with the variety of issues encountered by gay men and lesbians (Stein, 1988). This reality is particularly alarming given the important role the family plays in coping with AIDS (Lovejoy, 1990). It is impossible to fully comprehend the impact of multiple AIDS-related loss on families without an understanding of the family forms affected. This book was written to contribute to that understanding.

Several forces have combined recently to improve professional understanding of issues related to family of choice (Stein, 1988). The 1973 decision by the American Psychiatric Association to depathologize homosexuality contributed to a shift in professional understanding of gay lifestyles. Social trends that allow a greater appreciation of nontraditional family arrangements help, as do changes in traditional gender role arrangements. Legitimization of gay social and political identities, along with scholarly interest in gay individuals and social structures, have contributed to an expanded understanding of social arrangements that include families of choice. Finally, the emergence of AIDS itself has increased awareness of gay lifestyle and support systems, and has for many people put a human face on homosexuality. The response of gays to AIDS has fostered an appreciation for the cohesiveness and generosity of the gay community.

Issues for Family Therapy

Therapists who already have a reputation for competence and compassion in the working with homosexuals will probably see more survivors. Green and Bobele

(1994) demonstrated a connection between the amount of knowledge and contact family therapists have with persons with AIDS and therapists' attitudes. More knowledge and contact correlates with more positive attitudes and, presumably, more effectiveness. Those clinicians who regularly see populations most affected by AIDS should be aware of the unique phenomenon of multiple AIDS-related loss in order to avoid casting the issues faced by survivors as simply grief related. Family therapists are in an ideal position to help families cope with the uniquely devastating consequences of multiple AIDS-related loss, a phenomenon that will increasingly affect families of both origin and choice. Understanding the consequences of multiple AIDS-related loss and realizing that this disaster requires a modification of traditional grief and trauma therapy will help family therapy be effective.

Psychoeducational efforts are important throughout the process. Fears of contagion should be addressed directly. Some family members may not raise the issue even when fears about it are pronounced. Those who have sexual relationships with each other need appropriate sexual safety information. Families will need to directly address issues related to sexuality and fears of contagion. Families may lack competency in dealing with HIV/AIDS-related issues; therefore, an ability and willingness to engage in a frank, clear, and rational discussion of HIV risks and prognosis are useful. Explicit discussion about which sexual acts will continue and which will be modified often needs to be facilitated by the therapist. The therapist who is unwilling or uncomfortable promoting a discussion of these issues is not well qualified to work with these families and should not.

Other family members will find reassurance in education about the safety of normal household contact. Almost always there exists a need to educate families and individuals about the need to do grief work together. Two tendencies conspire to promote an avoidance of this process: the intense pain commonly associated with it and the misdirected desire to avoid causing pain in a loved one.

Therapists are regularly called on to help with practical planning concerns. Encouraging the family to purposefully preplan medical care options and make decisions about whether to continue life support measures through the use of durable powers of attorney and living wills prevents greater upset at a later time when stress will be higher. Most especially, families of origin must be encouraged to plan for the eventualities of death. Although this is normally not the role of the therapist, in this case this intervention can prevent massive pain and serve to facilitate a positive response. Therapists who deny their role in this process might remember the story of John's partner.

> What happened after he died was unbelievable. His parents appeared and came rampaging through our house and just packed up everything except my clothes. They came in like vultures and took everything, saying that it had been John's and was now theirs. They were his heirs. They looked at me as if I were dirt. I talked

with an attorney. I don't have any rights. Spouses have rights. Children have rights. But legally, I don't exist. (as cited in Fuller et al., 1989, p. 38)

Family members may need support and referrals for dealing with financial concerns, the placement of children, and other issues. Children who will be left without a parent "should be informed about the process at a level commensurate with their maturity" (Lippmann et al., 1993, p. 74). Custody or guardianship issues need to be discussed up front and directly. Children should not be left in the dark about the forthcoming deaths of parents, siblings, or members of the extended family. This task is obviously difficult and is helped along with the skilled and caring facilitation of a therapist.

Children may need special attention whether they have HIV or not. Children will make a connection between the deaths of parents and siblings, and possibly, themselves. "Questions raised by them require honesty and support" (Dubik-Unruh, 1989, p. 14).

The therapist dealing with a family experiencing multiple AIDS-related loss must be prepared to deal with issues related to the stigmatization surrounding this disease. It should be assumed that these issues are present even when they are not verbally expressed. AIDS-related anxiety can take a variety of forms, from fear of personal infection to issues related to the illness process; therefore, a therapist knowledgeable in these matters will be more helpful. Families may find that their religious leader or congregation is unwilling to provide support, and may possibly present a negative attitude. This can be especially troubling for families and can create additional schisms within the family itself. Guilt can manifest itself in a number of ways in connection with surviving multiple AIDS-related loss, so a therapist must be on the lookout for implicit signs of survivor's guilt, including statements that are self-condemning.

Family therapists with a grounding in systemic family therapy will have a useful perspective on the impact of multiple AIDS-related loss on the symbiotic relationship of families and how it is disrupted. Families may present with problems not attributed to multiple AIDS-related loss but that have everything to do with a shift in the reciprocal relationships of family members. As Kerr and Bowen (1988) noted,

A family usually comes to therapy with a fairly narrow perspective on the nature of the problem. It is the therapist's responsibility not to get pulled into the emotional whirlpool of the family and into this narrow perspective, but to be able to back up, achieve a reasonably broad perspective, and make decisions accordingly. (p. xii)

Rather than compartmentalizing problems, family systems theory is an excellent model for addressing the shift in roles, functions, and relationships instigated by this tragedy. Allow the survivor to discuss the loss, find a context for the loss, and recount a history. Having family members make a list of their losses, a technique sometimes used with elderly persons who have experienced multiple loss (Freeman, 1984), is helpful, especially when it is combined with use of ritual to commemorate the loss. Rituals are an important tool in adjustment and are covered in chapter 9.

Therapists should be prepared to mediate conflicts, competitions, and jealousy between families of origin and choice. This task is complicated when either side perceives that sides are being taken by the therapist. It is not uncommon for the family of choice to assume that they are right and that any competent clinician would "obviously" take their side. In such cases, the therapist must intervene with care to avoid seeing the family of origin flee and reentrench itself in a stance of intense judgmentalism and hostility against the family of choice. Negotiation may sometimes carry a businesslike tone in the midst of anguish and fears. A mother may resent the lover's time with her son when they both know that time is short. A plan to divide time alone with the person may be a workable compromise.

CONCLUSION

Multiple AIDS-related loss and the family inevitably bring many issues to the surface that may previously have been ignored. These are the most difficult times that a family will ever face. Issues that family rules previously prohibited need to be discussed. Physical and emotional issues must be dealt with forthrightly. Severe disruption to family roles, functions, and expectations is inevitable. Whether the family is one of origin or choice, these issues are a challenge for everyone involved.

Part Three

Healing and Surviving Multiple AIDS-Related Loss

This part shifts the book's attention from describing the problem of multiple loss to offering some perspectives for healing. Chapter 9 begins by pointing out how profoundly AIDS affects the survivor's identity. This chapter offers a philosophical perspective on this experience, arguing that embracing the despair inherent in the fate of surviving multiple loss is the first step to recovery. Chapters 10 and 11 offer constructive suggestions for coping with, and healing, the suffering of survivors. Professional issues are addressed in chapter 12. Conclusions, which arise out of this historic phenomenon, are explored in the final chapter.

Chapter 9

Existential Issues and Self-Identity

Life is more alive, more zestful, when we are aware of death; and death has significance only because there is life.—Rollo May (1981, p. 66)

A survivor's sense of self is forever altered by multiple AIDS-related loss. Identity is challenged by an experience that disrupts interpersonal connections and sometimes alters personality. Normal developmental stage issues and tasks are scrambled.

It is not uncommon to think of AIDS as provoking social, political, and psychological issues, but it also provokes philosophical issues. AIDS provokes existential issues, including questions of being versus nonbeing, desire for relationship versus ultimate isolation, of responsibility and choice, and of meaning in the face of apparent meaninglessness. Spiritual concerns are nearly always an important part of the individual's adjustment to multiple, ongoing loss. This chapter discusses how these three areas are affected by this extreme experience. In so doing, it shifts the focus of the book from an exposition of the circumstances and problems of surviving multiple AIDS-related loss to a look at how survivors adjust to this overwhelming reality. Implied throughout this discussion are suggestions for making "sense" of this disaster. Survivors are regularly challenged to live purposefully and deliberately.

SENSE OF IDENTITY

The individual survivor's identity is affected by multiple AIDS-related loss. The survivor experiences three levels of disruption to his or her pre-AIDS self. First, perspective of self is altered by identification with HIV status, impact on sexuality, one's projected future self, personality changes, questioning of value systems, and developmental stage disruptions. Second, self-identity is interrelated with other persons. When multiple, ongoing loss steadily disrupts these connections, the survivor's sense of self is thrown off balance. Third, self as connected to the world as a whole is disrupted. Basic assumptions about the universe are challenged. For many, exposure through the nakedness of grief or forced "coming out" amends their relationships to the world. These three areas are divided solely for the sake of organization and clarity; they interrelate and overlap.

Individual Sense of Self

Below are reviewed a number of ways of seeing one's self in the context of surviving multiple AIDS-related loss.

HIV as Self   One of the most startling ramifications of this disease is the tendency of those most likely to be affected by HIV to assume the identifying label of HIV status, to use a variation of the verb *to be* to describe themselves. One regularly hears gay and hemophiliac men say, "I am HIV positive" or "I am HIV negative." These labels are simply not applied to most other diseases. It would sound crazy to say "I am cancer" or "I am diabetes."

Diseases are normally something people have, not something people are. Possibly one of the reasons that those most affected by HIV readily assume a disease identity is that it is "easy" to be a disease; it provides an identity. Odets (1995) asserted that "AIDS has given gay men a disease that, in all its horror, can provide an easier identity than being homosexual" (p. 106). Even the labels *positive* and *negative* connote a judgment about self. "I am positive" equals "I am dying of a horrible disease." "I am negative" equals "health."

Those who do not know their HIV status refer to themselves as "HIV indeterminate." What message does that give people about their identity? "I am not one thing or another; I am indeterminate." Taking on a disease identity has profound implications. For example, Odets (1995), who subtitled his book *Being HIV Negative in the Age of AIDS*, wrote that "Being gay and uninfected in America today is an identity" (p. 99).

The ease with which this disease was assumed as identity is telling. The only other diseases that popularly carry the verb *to be* to describe their sufferers are alcoholism and drug addiction. All carry severe stigmatization. Punitive judgment is prevalent in connection to all three. These are the diseases of blame, carrying a presumed culpability even more condemning than the diseases of smokers.

Assuming an identity based on disease status is rampant and pervasive in the AIDS epoch. There is an HIV-positive community and an HIV-negative community. From the beginning of AIDS, there has been a committed effort to divide people by their AIDS status. People had AIDS-related complex or full-blown AIDS or were Class I, II, III, or IV. Relationships with others and communities are affected. Those with HIV do not have AIDS *yet*. Each group has reason to feel disadvantaged and marginalized.

For the most part, only those with the most advanced and shockingly debilitated symptoms of AIDS have been permitted the liberty to openly discuss their feelings. The same scenario is encountered regularly in groups where persons with various HIV progression meet: Those with less advanced AIDS, and especially those without HIV, are shy, almost ashamed, to express themselves. The attitude that one's issues are not as important as another's alters one's perspective of self. "I am not as important as you. My needs don't count as much." This meshes smoothly with underlying shame prevalent in communities affected by AIDS, and this shame becomes "a state of being" taking "over one's whole identity" (Bradshaw, 1988, p. vii).

Krystal (1981) offered an interesting analysis about survivors of the Holocaust that may have relevance to the internal psychodynamics behind the assumption by so many gay men of an HIV identity.

> The survivor of the genocidal Holocaust stands the risk of polarizing the object and self-representations into victim and perpetrators [propelling] the survivor to continue to experience his- or herself as the victim, and with this comes the longing to change places with the oppressor. But the identification with the aggressor must remain unconscious or else it will flood the self-representation with psychotic rage. (p. 180)

Instead of unconsciously identifying with the object of a prison guard, the survivor of multiple AIDS-related loss identifies with the object of HIV. Some of those with HIV regularly refer to themselves or others as the virus ("I am HIV" or "he is HIV").

These distinctions are more than semantic, they influence the individual survivor's concept of him- or herself. After a lifetime of living as and being treated as an outsider, the gay man who still tests HIV negative is an outsider again. As those without HIV gain a voice nearly two decades into the AIDS epoch, it is no longer uncommon and hardly shocking to hear envious and bitter talk about the sometimes generous services available to those with HIV.

Surprisingly little or no attention has been paid to this peculiar tendency to identify oneself as the disease. This is explainable in part because people are used to, and therefore comfortable with, this labeling. Yet, those who are made aware of this identification with HIV are usually shocked by their previous blindness in regard to this matter. It is important to use correct language. This disease has exposed a number of issues related to language that affect the survivor's experience. Throughout this book, people are not identified as disease or lack of disease. People are infected or not infected with HIV.

Sexuality   AIDS has certainly affected sexual identity. The physical threat of illness and death casts a pall over sexual expression. Psychological threat of annihilation is inherent in certain sexual acts that had previously been routine.

For many gay men, sexuality was identity. This was especially true in the years before AIDS. After AIDS became a threat, they wondered how could they be gay if they couldn't do the things they used to? (Acevedo, 1986).

> Most men—gay or heterosexual—do not develop their self-definition solely on the basis of sexual orientation. Sexuality and sexual expression are only part of one's total experience and development of sense of self. For some gay men, however, sexual expression is a critical aspect of identity. When sexual expression results in an incurable and fatal infection, both identity and self-esteem may be threatened. (Lloyd, 1992, p. 96)

Sexual rituals, specialized practices, exotic locations, and active fantasy lives formed the identity of many gay men. The majority of their lives revolved around ghettos of men who devoted their lives to particular sexual practices and customs. AIDS undercuts much of that. Where caution failed to mandate change, accumulated deaths effected profound change in sexuality. Sexual spontaneity and desire have decreased. Back-room bars became scarce or nonexistent; bath houses were closed. One study of gay male sexual behavior demonstrated that more than 86% had decreased or eliminated various sexual practices (Stulberg & Smith, 1988).

An advantage that many, many gay men recognize in the aftermath of AIDS is a change to more balanced modes of relational interaction. Rather than primarily viewing other gay men as sexual objects to take and use for a limited time and depth of interaction, gay men have had the opportunity to deepen relationships beyond the purely physical. There is less promiscuous sexuality, and monogamous relationships have increased.

Personality Alterations   Survivors sometimes report significant distress about self-perceptions that their personalities have changed. Grief is a narcissistic injury that Freud identified as damaging the self-esteem of the aggrieved. This outcome is more likely given the specific characteristics of this disaster. Many personality changes were noted in the chapter on trauma, notably a decreased capacity for fun and playfulness. This distress often expresses itself in fears about going crazy. It is not the norm for persons in the their late 20s to early 40s to experience a change in who they are. Confused thoughts and fluctuating emotions often resemble adolescence.

Survivors also note positive changes in their personalities. They see themselves as more open to diversity, more compassionate, and more in touch with themselves. A mother who lost her son to AIDS, who had been exposed to more human diversity through her experience than she ever expected, noticed many positive changes in herself. "I learned about people, that they were people, you know? I'd never want to go back to that little, little, narrow person."

Future Self   A normal part of identity formation is the projection of one's self into the future. What relationships will be important? What career goals will be pursued? What will be priorities for spending time? All of these future projections of self involve other people. Yet survivors of multiple AIDS-related loss are likely to distrust any plan for the future when so many of their previous plans have been undermined. Many gay men assume that they will become infected with HIV and so neglect future planning. The only question is when infection will occur.

The future holds uncertainty and mistrust. The survivor's assumptions and expectations, formed over years, are shaken. Outliving one's parents seems less sure; saving for retirement, less important. Pursuing career objectives is evaluated in a different light. Dramatic shifts in values, even when ultimately positive, are destabilizing. Perspective and planning for the future are transformed.

Developmental Stage Disruptions and Recapitulation   One of the most striking features about surviving multiple AIDS-related loss is the potential, in survivors, for normal developmental stage progression to be confused or replayed. Erik Erikson's (1959/1980) conceptualization of development offers a valuable framework for understanding this aspect of the survivor's experience.

Erikson (1959/1980) called basic trust the first component and cornerstone of a healthy personality, not only in terms of its chronological development but also in terms of its importance for all of the remaining stages. The survivor of multiple AIDS-related loss is sadly likely to reexperience issues related to fundamental trust. "Is the world a safe place? Am I able to count on anything?" In adults whose basic trust is impaired, Erikson observed "withdrawal into themselves" (p. 58); this is frequently observed in survivors.

Autonomy develops, as opposed to shame and doubt, after trust is established. Erikson (1959/1980) asserted that shame is characterized by feeling "completely exposed and conscious of being looked at—in a word, self-conscious" (p. 71). Bereavement overload results in the sense of being inappropriately and regularly exposed in public. Survivors often report crying in public and feeling ashamed. One survivor said, "It's like I am always walking around buck naked. People can see right inside of me. I have no privacy."

Survivor's guilt may contribute to lack of initiative in survivors or the redirection of initiative into self-destructive avenues (see chapter 6). Survivors who believe, through the "logic" of guilt, that their survival is blamable may renounce or stymie normal developmental tasks. Friedman (1985) used the example of the child who avoids autonomy and individuation because of guilt that he or she would harm the parent. Similarly, the survivor of multiple loss may avoid forming intimate relationships for fear of betraying the deceased. Symptoms of alexithymia (see chapter 6) have a self-evident connection to the developmental process (Krystal, 1979, p. 24). Severe anhedonia, lack of future orientation, and excessive rumination are all symptoms of a breakdown in initiative.

Identity formation, characteristic of adolescence, is often recycled in the survivor of multiple AIDS-related loss. Fundamental issues related to one's choices about relationships, spirituality, belief systems, and careers may be rethought and affect the survivor's ego identity. Saying "I am a totally different person" is so common among survivors as to seem clichéd. Erikson (1959/1980) noted that ego identity "develops out of a gradual integration of all identifications" (p. 94) and confidence in one's ability "to maintain inner sameness and continuity" (p. 95). Might ego identity "undevelop" in the face of disintegration?

An opportunity is also present here. The survivor has the chance to choose an identity that may be more in keeping with the values and insights brought about by his or her survivor's experience. Previous problems with overidentification or faulty identification can be corrected, and a more satisfying authentic identity may develop.

The adult developmental stages of intimacy versus self-absorption and generativity versus stagnation are obviously affected by surviving multiple AIDS-related loss. These issues are outlined in detail in chapters 6 and 7 in terms of problems that survivors have with anhedonia and forming new relationships. The final developmental stage of life, integrity versus despair, because it is so vital to the survivor's experience, is analyzed in some detail next. Survivors yearn to move on to a place beyond the survivor in Camus's *The Plague* who is characterized by being "hostile to the past, impatient to the present, and cheated of the future" (Camus, 1948, p. 68).

Survivors seem to exist firmly on one side or the other of the integrity versus despair dichotomy. They are almost always catapulted into this stage, which Erikson (1959/1980) proposed as the final life stage, before an age-appropriate time. The survivor of multiple loss who has HIV is especially prone to the challenges presented by this stage. Erikson's description of despair sounds like the description of many survivors of multiple AIDS-related loss. It is characterized by the lack or loss of "accrued ego integration" (p. 104). The "one and only life cycle is not accepted," and despair is "often hidden behind a show of disgust, a misanthropy, or a chronic contemptuous displeasure" (p. 104). As is asserted later in this chapter, all survivors of multiple AIDS-related loss must pass through the attitudes described here.

Fortunate survivors are able to move past despair to a place of integrity about their experience in life, specifically as it has been irrevocably altered by multiple AIDS-related loss. The next section of this chapter discusses in some detail the survivor's opportunities to develop a meaningful sense of integrity about this extreme experience. Erikson (1959/1980) observed that "only he who in some way . . . has adapted himself to the triumphs and disappointments of being . . . may gradually grow the fruit of the seven stages. I know no better word for it than *integrity*." The survivor must accept "one's own and only life cycle," a life that "permitted no substitutions" (p. 104). One's own life is viewed as one's own. Erikson (1950) described the integrity to which many survivors strive:

> The possessor of integrity is ready to defend the dignity of his own life style against all physical and economic threats. For he knows that an individual life is the accidental coincidence of but one life cycle and but one segment of history, and that for him all human integrity stands or falls with the one style of integrity of which he partakes. (p. 232)

What Erikson describes here are the fundamental existential issues of meaning and the dilemma between destiny and responsibility that inevitably arise in the survivor of multiple AIDS-related loss. Establishing an individual integrity about the experience is the essence of adjustment and the "very goal and essence of all psychoanalytic psychotherapy" (Krystal, 1981, p. 177).

Positive Gay Identity Formation   The process of forming a positive gay identity had been well studied before the AIDS epoch, with developmental stages proposed for the process (Cass, 1979, 1984; Troiden, 1989). The impact of the AIDS epoch on this process has not yet been studied. However, some impact can be assumed. Dworkin and Kaufer (1995) concluded that grief "reactivates emotions related to the developmental experiences involved in establishing one's gay or lesbian identity. In experiencing such loss, one's identity, self-esteem and body image are challenged" (p. 47).

Because of the perceived connection between homosexuality and AIDS, the person who is in the process of forming a gay identity will necessarily need to include issues related to AIDS. Social interaction is a crucial part of forming a positive gay identity, but AIDS may promote isolation. Coming to terms with a positive HIV status is a second coming out. The same stage development process may need to be replayed in connection to HIV status. In the case of forming a positive gay identity, much time is typically required (Troiden & Goode, 1980); the same assumption is true for survivors who must incorporate the realities of AIDS into their identities.

Self as Connected to Others

In Buber's (1970) classic book, *I and Thou,* he concluded "Man becomes an I through a You" (p. 80). Although this book underlines the various types of losses emanating as a result of AIDS, the primary losses that affect one's identity in connection to others are multiple deaths. These result in a physical disconnection from others. One inevitably evokes the I whenever another is acknowledged. "When one says You, the I of the word pair I-You is said too"

(Buber, 1970, p. 54). Every self exists only because it connects to others. Even the hermit is defined by his or her connection to others.

This section focuses on the individual survivor's connection to others as individuals; the next section focuses on connection to others at a community-wide level. The longing for connection to others is primary, even at the earliest human consciousness. "The development of the child's soul is connected indissolubly with his craving for the You, with the fulfillments and disappointments of this craving" (Buber, 1970, p. 79). The survivor of multiple AIDS-related loss continually copes with the disappointment of this visceral craving.

Image of Self as Reflected in Others Buber (1970) concluded, "I require a You to become; becoming I, I say You" (p. 62). He repeated that relation is reciprocity. People derive a large part of their definition of self from their reflection in others. Writing about survivors of a community-wide disaster, Erikson (1976) concluded,

> People normally learn who they are and where they are by taking sounding from their fellows. As if employing a subtle form of radar, we probe other people in our immediate environment with looks, gestures, and words, hoping to learn something about ourselves from the signals we get in return. But when there are no reliable objects off of whom to bounce those exploratory probes, people have a hard time calculating where they stand in relation to the rest of the world. In a very real sense, they come to feel that they are not whole persons, not entirely human, because they do not know how to position themselves in a larger communal setting. (p. 304)

To a large extent, humans perceive themselves the way others perceive them. It is reasonable to assume that when others are not available for this identity-forming reflection, sense of identity is shaken.

John Donne wrote that "any man's death diminishes me" (cited in Bartlett, 1968, p. 308). The self is less whole when a part of one's living relationship to an other is severed. People also define themselves by their roles in connection with others. For example, the hemophiliac family survivor may have been a mother, wife, and family provider. When death eliminates the male members of her family, she is no longer a mother, wife, or family provider. Friends, too, foster a sense of identity. "From friendship we derive a sense of self-confirmation, a sense of who we are, of self-worth and self-esteem" (Deck & Folta, 1989, p. 79). "Their death creates a loss of our identity and a threat to our self-esteem, and it renders our role as friend meaningless" (p. 86). This source of identity is severely challenged in most survivors of multiple AIDS-related loss. Caregivers to people with AIDS often note that their identities as caregivers are eliminated when someone dies. This loss of identity is especially difficult when the caregivers give up the role entirely, ceasing to be AIDS caregivers.

Others reflect self-identity through memory. Shrader (1992) concluded that "for subjects who had suffered massive losses (i.e. fifty or more), there was a sense of losing not only their history, but a large part of their sense of self" (p. 110). One survivor interviewed by him said

> And then when you lose them you lose a lot of yourself. . . . What it is is the reflection of you in them dies. Their shared aspect of you, their memories of you and their image of you dies . . . the other half of you that is in them. (p. 90)

The reader must remember that these principles may be true for any death, but are multiplied for survivors of this disaster. This is the sense conveyed by the survivor who said, "If my life is a book, no one knows more than one chapter of it."

Self as Member of a Social System   Survivors of multiple AIDS-related loss, by definition, always confront disruption to their view of self as part of a social system. Parkes (1972) recognized that even the death of one close person had an effect on individual sense of identity.

> If I have relied on another person to predict and act in many ways as an extension of my self then the loss of that person can be expected to have the same effect upon my view of the world and my view of myself as if I had lost a part of myself. (pp. 96–97)

The only way this reality can be theoretically avoided is to have experienced the loss of no one important, but this is never the experience of the survivor of multiple AIDS-related loss. As a member of a social system that has been decimated by multiple loss, the survivor's identity is inherently altered.

> It may be that accepting the death of a friend is even more difficult than accepting the idea of one's own death. The death of peers destroys the social network in which the individual is a member. Most friendship groups are dyads. Therefore the death of one means the demise of the group. (Deck & Folta, 1989, p. 84)

The self as part of a group no longer exists. Memories may persist, but the survivor is no longer a friend of his or her friend. Todd, a survivor of multiple loss, said, "I don't have any friends anymore, I have acquaintances." The survivor may treasure previous membership in a peer or social group, but he or she can no longer be personally identified as part of that group. This disconnection is particularly potent in the gay community where tightly established groups of friends viewed themselves as part of a group. For example, it was common on the East Coast for groups of gay men to have a yearly tradition of gathering at Fire Island or other beachfront locations. Over and over, survivors note the disappearance of these traditional gatherings, and therefore their membership and identity as a part of them. Uroda (1977) observed,

The individual self is interpersonal at its core, arising out of and continuing to be dependent on the other. In other words, we establish our self-image and identity in terms of our relationships to significant persons. (p. 185)

Of course, the most devastating loss of connection is to those the survivor loves. This connection is mainly severed at death. Loss of a loved one is a "threat to one's very identity" (Uroda, 1977, p. 185). Love exists because of connection. "Love is responsibility of an I for a You" (Buber, 1970, p. 66). Love is the ultimate risk, and its disruption by death is the focal point of loss from AIDS. Love "binds us to things"; the beloved "is part of ourselves" (Ortega y Gasset, 1961, p. 33). People "we love seem to become a part of our self" (Parkes, 1987, p. 97). When the survivor loses loved ones, they lose a part of their self. Maslow (1968) observed that "not only does love perceive potentialities but it also actualizes them" (p. 98). That being true, the survivor of multiple loss inevitably suffers the loss of potentialities.

Unstable Future Relationships   Brad was a client in psychotherapy whose main concern was his disconnection "from everyone." He reported trouble holding a job, severe anhedonia, no future direction, and increased substance abuse but connected none of it to the fact that would come out in later psychotherapy sessions: Every one of his close friends had died from AIDS. When that reality finally sunk home, Brad gasped as he said, "I expected to grow old with my friends. We joked about having the first gay retirement home. What am I going to do? I have no one to grow old together with!"

The reality that so many gay men are disconnected first from their families of origin and then from their families of choice has no historic parallel. Intimacy has been identified as a particular challenge for many lesbians and gay men. Fear of loss and challenges to trust, inevitable in this crisis, heighten the difficulty of forming future intimate relationships. One trusts in the context of expectations about the future. The survivor has some of her or his most fundamental areas of trust undermined repeatedly by a future that is untrustworthy.

Self as Connected to World

This section explores how the survivor's perception of self in relation to the world at large is affected, both negatively and positively, by multiple AIDS-related loss. Parkes (1972) concluded that "my view of myself is inextricably bound up with my view of the world" (p. 96). Survivors' identities are shaken by disruption of their world, and they are very often cut off from their world, their community. Their landscape, their environment, has changed. They are literally left separated and isolated. May (1983) asserted that the chief source of modern Western man's anxiety and despair is the combination of loss of being and loss of world. Yet, the experience of multiple AIDS-related loss also frequently has the salutary effect of promoting greater connection to community and an increased sense of belonging.

Self and Safety in the World   This disaster strikes at core assumptions and expectations about how the world is "supposed to be" akin to other shocking events that undermine perceptions of relative social security. The Oklahoma City bombing, the Holocaust, Jonestown's mass suicide, and Susan Smith's drowning of her children all affect the self through an affront to security that far outweighs actual quantitative risk or personal threat. Yalom (1980) explained why such events so strongly affect the individual who is not directly involved.

> They also stun us because they inform us that nothing is as we have always thought it to be, that contingency reigns, that everything could be otherwise than it is; that everything we consider fixed, precious, good can suddenly vanish; that there is no solid ground; that we are "not-at-home" here or there or anywhere in the world. (p. 361)

The individual feels threatened, and isolated, because the world is not safe, nothing is secure, foundations crumble. Realization of threat, lack of stability, increased vulnerability, and disappearance of a social safety net all contribute to existential isolation. The survivor of multiple, ongoing loss feels less protected and more alone and powerless.

Besides the disruption to identity related to the survivor's world view and fundamental expectations, the survivor who is coping with secondary stress reactions also faces a different challenge to self-identity. Those who suffer secondary traumatization may experience "the loss of a familiar sense of identity" because of a disruption to the way they "understand the world, including causality, life philosophy, and moral principles" (Pearlman & Saakvitne, 1995, p. 160).

One way in which the survivor's sense of identity and safety in the world can be significantly affected is through the forced coming out that many gay men experience as a result of enduring multiple loss. Exposure of homosexual identity is mandated by various factors. This experience "flushes out an identity that might have remained hidden from neighbors, jobmates, family, friends" (Sontag, 1989, p. 25). Lesbians and gay men "were forced out of the closet by the circumstances of caring for sick and dying friends" (Mancoske & Lindhorst, 1995, p. 28). Kayal (1994) observed that

> AIDS has created a third period and politic in gay history. Because of AIDS-homophobia, coming out is no longer a private or arbitrary choice. It is a social, personal, and political necessity, demanded by the need and desire to survive both individually and collectively. (p. 42)

It is simply impossible to bear the amount of pain inevitable with the survivor's experience without almost everyone in the survivor's life being made aware of it. When the reason for that pain is publicly acknowledged, people may assume that the survivor must be gay. Survivors call this a second coming out. All the adverse consequences of stigmatization related to homosexuality and AIDS may affect the survivor's sense of security in the world.

It was a sad reality for many survivors of multiple AIDS-related loss that the act of seeking much-needed support also resulted in exposing an identity that opened them to judgment and condemnation. Martin and Dean (1993a) observed

> More than any other disease, AIDS can be deeply stigmatizing, for both the person who is sick and for those close to him. For many gay men AIDS forces into the open one's identity as a homosexual to previously uninformed family members, friends, and co-workers, as well as a cadre of strangers encountered in the course of obtaining necessary health care. Not only is this "forced coming out" stressful to the individual with AIDS, but it also frequently strains individuals and relationships in the social network. (p. 322)

In the long run, however, many survivors report that the problems initially confronted in this second coming-out phase of their lives had benefits. Although it was difficult to face the challenge of exposing one's gay identity at a time of personal vulnerability, the ultimate impact was positive. The many benefits of leading a congruent life, without the need to carefully guard private matters, were realized.

Self in Community   Membership in community as a defining characteristic of self has been greatly affected by experience of surviving multiple AIDS-related loss. Although identity disruption certainly occurs, the survivor has, in many cases, experienced an enhancement of positive identity. Early neglect and hostility toward those with AIDS promoted a coming together of those most affected. This was especially true in the gay community. A study by Stulberg and Smith (1988) noted that "many members of the gay community have responded to the physical, emotional, and psychological assault of the AIDS epidemic by pulling together and taking care of their own. The result is an unprecedented level of political involvement and voluntarism" (p. 277). Besides organized community relationships, respondents reported increased interest in becoming closer to their families and friends. Nearly half of those in relationships "believed that AIDS actually had improved their relationships" (p. 280). Although these community-based improvements in self-identity have yet to be quantified, their impact is significant. A regular topic among those affected by multiple AIDS-related loss is the enhanced value they place on relationships. "I feel better about myself now that I have meaningful friends, not just casual buddies," one survivor reported.

Volunteer work in response to AIDS has done much to help the condition of both people with AIDS and survivors of multiple AIDS-related loss. In many cases, voluntary involvement has provided survivors a new community. It is not uncommon for volunteer organizations to provide support services for their volunteers, typically including support groups or regular training follow-up. These bring caregivers together as a group and provide a sense of camaraderie and mutual support. Many survivors now report, nearly two decades into the AIDS epoch, that they met some of their best friends through volunteer involvement, and they frequently note that the overall quality of their friendships is improved.

EXISTENTIAL ISSUES AND PSYCHODYNAMICS

Anxieties that are normal and healthy and that potentiate personal growth arise in response to this existential crisis, but so too do anxieties that are neurotic and unhelpful. The survivor is faced with choices about which issues to engage. This section is organized by focusing individually on the four classic existential issues: being versus nonbeing; responsibility, choice, and fate; isolation versus desire for connection; and meaning versus meaninglessness. Finally, conclusions are offered that may be used to challenge survivors to a higher level response in the face of this overwhelming and unique catastrophe.

Being Versus Nonbeing

Survivors of multiple deaths receive a potential gift: the opportunity to face life head on because they are forced to face death head on. Consideration of death enriches rather than impoverishes those willing to think deeply and feel meaningfully. Yalom (1985, p. 30) said it best: "Although the physicality of death destroys man, the idea of death saves him." Fear of death is always the beginning of wisdom (de Unamuno, 1921/1954). Facing death is an important part of the paradoxical benefit acknowledged by many survivors. Many survivors assert too, the need to face away from death, toward life.

Those with HIV certainly confront the reality of their own physical death and choices about their psychological life each time they watch AIDS destroy a loved one's body. Survivors who test positive or negative are surrounded by death symbols, death anxiety, death meditations, and death itself. Each loss experience confronts survivors with their own mortality. The continual drum of threat to being is the existential anxiety that Tillich (1952/1980) defined as "the state in which a being is aware of its possible non-being" (p. 35). Anxiety arising from confrontation with nonbeing is far more tremulous than simple fear of death. This anxiety is related to ceasing to be, obliteration, annihilation, and the inevitable sense that one's existence never mattered. This dread is often present in survivors of multiple AIDS-related loss and partially underlies the anxiety provoked when a survivor forgets the names and faces or various experiences with loved ones. "If they are forgettable, so am I!"

This basic anxiety provokes an anxiety of guilt. The threat of death always awakens and increases "consciousness of guilt" (Tillich, 1952/1980, p. 53). Condemnation of the self centers on failing to live up to one's destiny, failing to meet expectations, for not being as good as loved ones who have died. Frankl's (1959/1984) assertion that the good ones all died is similar to the lament heard from many survivors of multiple AIDS-related loss. This is especially likely in survivors with active issues of survivor's guilt. This is a despair that cannot be avoided, even by suicide, for even the survivor's inevitable lack of being taunts him or her. Facing this despair is essential to coping with multiple AIDS-related loss; those who never experience it are unlikely to engage in meaningful choice.

Kierkegaard (1849/1989) understood that despair is a defect and merit. The possibility of despair is "man's advantage over the beast, and it is an advantage that characterizes him" (pp. 44–45). In the face of this despair and continual confrontation with issues of being and nonbeing, survivors may respond with the courage of despair. In the face of ultimate uncertainty, all are simultaneously given the fortuitous opportunity to intentionally decide how to live and what to live for. This despair can be the basis of a vigorous life. The "greatest heroes, perhaps the greatest of all, have been men of despair and that by despair they have accomplished their mighty works" (de Unamuno, 1921/1954, p. 130). One can react with the courage of despair, the courage to take that despair upon oneself, and can resist the radical threat of nonbeing by the courage to be as oneself.

Heidegger (1962) distinguished between two modes of existence: an "inauthentic" life characterized by forgetfulness of being and an authentic life characterized by mindfulness of being and self-awareness. This distinction is remarkably clear in survivors of multiple AIDS-related loss in whom this attitudinal and intentional difference is, at times, stunning. Those who move from the "normal" world into contact with survivors of multiple loss regularly observe something in caregivers of people with AIDS similar to a man who began volunteering in AIDS services in the early 1990s.

> At first I was shocked. You all talk so casually about death! But there is something more that is hard to put my finger on. You all live so honestly, so directly, so authentically. You don't tolerate any bullshit. Someday, I hope that I can be more like you.

After a few months working with people with AIDS, assisting four clients who died, and meeting regularly with other survivors, he underwent a noticeable shift in consciousness. For some time this was destabilizing and provoked more anxiety than comfort because the process takes times and requires thoughtful internal contemplation and interpersonal support. The extreme nature of multiple AIDS-related loss again provides a generalizable lesson: The process of inner growth rarely occurs in isolation. It requires contact with others, either through support of those living or through the deaths of loved ones. Heidegger realized that one does not move from forgetfulness to enlightenment only through effort or contemplation. Certain urgent experiences are necessary, experiences that are unalterable and irremediable. Living through extreme and constant confrontation with death, the survivor of multiple AIDS-related loss is overtly placed within the struggle, which Karl Jaspers (as cited in Barrett, 1958/1962) described as a struggle to awaken in the individual the possibilities of an authentic and genuine life, in the face of modern drift toward a standardized mass society.

Jaspers (as cited in Barrett, 1958/1962) referred to these experiences as border or boundary situations. One permutation of this kind of border or boundary experience arises regularly in survivors of multiple AIDS-related loss. Survivors regularly observe that the line between life and death is blurred, indistinct, unclear. Physically, the distinction between life and death is diffuse, existing along a continuum:

> HIV infection—Asymptomatic—Early infections—AIDS diagnosis—Major opportunistic infections—Final stage—Coma—Bodily death—Memorial service—Memories —Bearing witness

The episodic course of AIDS makes the distinctions between life and death even more diffuse. Bodies wither away or quickly deteriorate; people with AIDS seem near the edge of death, then recover strength again. This lack of distinction is important to the existential experience of survivors. First, it largely removes the denial of death so common in postindustrial nations. Second, it sets survivors of multiple AIDS-related loss apart from those around them who blithely ignore implications of being and nonbeing. Third, it has practical consequences in terms of choice and responsibility, both of which become more purposeful in the preponderance of survivors. Not only physically but psychologically, "life and death merge into one another" (Yalom, 1980, p. 30). Gerry, a survivor of multiple loss with HIV, asked, "Are we all living or are we all dying?" It is a serious question with implications deeper than the physical.

Raleigh, a survivor, talked about experiencing the presence of ghosts, the shadows of people whom he used to physically encounter. Garfield (1995) quoted a caregiver, George, as saying that "in San Francisco there are all these ethereal people floating around" (p. 171). Garfield asked, are these ghosts a destructive fantasy? Psychopathology? "Not at all; in fact such glimpses are a common experience for caregivers, especially for those who have experienced the deaths of many clients and friends and lovers, and whose losses number in the dozens or even hundreds" (p. 171).

Russ Berst, who has lost two partners, speaks matter of factly about visits from them. "They visit me in my dreams; sometimes we talk. It isn't scary. I think they just want to help me." Although these assertions may strike some as dubious or odd, they are such a regular feature of the survivor's experience. Attempts to rationalize them away as simply characteristic of grief-related searching are inadequate.

Not all responses to this overt confrontation with death are noble and self-enhancing. Fear of death may overwhelm zest for life. Some survivors take on a stance of survival and mere existence instead of living. Anxiety of nonbeing is anxiety without object and can express itself in loss of direction and lack of intentionality (Tillich, 1952/1980). Others may develop a hedonistic attitude summarized in the outlook "Party now, for tomorrow we die."

Although it seems contradictory, fear of death emanating from continual death exposure leads many to suicide. With suicide, anxiety about death threats is permanently eased. Besides overt suicide, however, the variety of subintentional suicidal behaviors becomes more comprehensible given this perspective. Frankl was noted for asking some clients, "Why do you not commit suicide?" (as cited in Allport, 1959, p. 9). That question allows the survivor an opportunity through confrontation with nonbeing and moves the discussion to the next existential issue, responsibility and choice.

Responsibility, Choice, and Fate

It is not a coincidence that so much of the world's genius has struggled with suffering, especially illness and dying. It's reported that Beethoven said, "I will take fate by the throat," and he did. Fate and destiny are essential to the survivor's experience and crucial to healthy coping with multiple, ongoing loss. Ortega y Gasset (1961) asserted, "I am myself plus my circumstances" (p. 45). Railing against the unfairness of this tragedy will profit the survivor nothing except a pat on the shoulder. The hard and bitter fact is that destiny has prescribed, for the survivor, the experience of surviving multiple AIDS-related loss. The lot is cast, but it is a fate complemented by freedom. Choice is most apparent in decisions whether to engage the pain inevitable in this personal crisis and use it to one's advantage. Maslow (1968) observed that "growth forward is in spite of these losses and therefore requires courage, will, choice, and strength in the individual. . . . Growth has not only rewards and pleasures but also many intrinsic pains and always will have" (p. 204).

Buber (1970) asserted that "fate is no bell that has been jammed down over man; nobody encounters it, except those who started out from freedom" (p. 106); "nothing can doom men but the belief in doom" (p. 107). At some point, every survivor who wants to live as something more than a victim must do what Frankl reported doing in the concentration camp. Survivors of the Holocaust had to realize "that *it did not really matter what we expected from life, but rather what life expected from us*" (Frankl, 1959/1984, p. 98). This inevitably leads to choices, including responsibility for responding to one's destiny.

> We needed to stop asking about the meaning of life, and instead to think of ourselves as those who were being questioned by life—daily and hourly. Our answer must consist, not in talk and meditation, but in right action and in right conduct. Life ultimately means taking the responsibility to find the right answer to its problems and to fulfill the tasks which it constantly sets for each individual. (p. 98)

Choice is mandated by the extreme nature of continual loss. This is the self-affirming courage to live "in spite of."

At the point of despair, the utter certainty that suffering will continue and that one's destiny involves ongoing loss, the survivor has the opportunity to give up false hope. May (1981) said it best:

> *Authentic despair is that emotion which forces one to come to terms with one's destiny.* It is the great enemy of pretense, the foe of playing ostrich. It is a demand to face the reality of one's life. . . . Despair is the smelting furnace which melts out the impurities in the ore. Despair is not freedom itself, but is a necessary preparation for freedom. (p. 235)

The survivor of multiple AIDS-related loss is usually comforted when directly confronting this very real despair. The beginning of relief is felt when survivors acknowledge that their experiences are indeed extreme, that their suffering is profound. It is perfectly understandable that they feel and behave the way they do. At this spot, survivors can support each other and professionals can join with survivors to commence the healing process.

The survivor who withdraws, shutting down to avoid painful emotions, simultaneously experiences a restricted spectrum of emotions. Conversely, the survivor who can embrace healthy despair can experience wider, deeper, and more intense emotions, including joy and pleasure. This is the point Jean-Paul Sartre made in *The Flies* when Orestes argues with Zeus, asserting that "human life begins on the far side of despair!" (Sartre, 1947, p. 123). It is also the point made in the 1993 movie *Shadowlands* by C. S. Lewis's wife, Joy, when she encourages her husband to face her inevitable death and asks him to accompany her through the pain. "The pain then is part of the happiness now."

At this point, fortunate survivors begin to test life's most basic assumptions and values. In a study of survivors of multiple loss, Carmack (1992) noted that "previous goals, values and priorities were simultaneously and interactively appraised and reappraised" (p. 12). The concept of freedom takes on new and expanded meaning. Many survivors concur with Frankl's assertion that the last of human freedoms is to choose one's attitude. Freedom is less a negative stance (a freedom to not) and more a positive stance (a freedom to). It becomes less a freedom to do as a freedom to be. The survivor is free to decide values, explore new avenues of personal power, and, very often, establish relationships that are deeper and more meaningful. Many existential writers have made the point that people avoid the threat of nonbeing by avoiding being. Otto Rank (1945) described a neurotic as one "who refused the loan [of life] in order to avoid the payment of the debt [death]" (p. 126).

May (1981) noted that freedom of this sort is "the mother of all values" (p. 6). Survivors testify that they were given a second chance at living. Buber (1970) noted, "Fate and freedom are promised to each other. Fate is encountered only by him that actualizes freedom" (p. 102). This is the challenge and opportunity for the survivor of multiple AIDS-related loss. Some compare their experiences to the near-death experiences of others, especially as they provoke a shift in life priorities. A smothering of trivialities (Yalom, 1980) becomes the norm as choices are made with purpose. Honesty and integrity permeate life. Living an authentic life is vitally important to many survivors. "I simply will not tolerate lack of genuine feelings, thoughts or intentions from myself or anyone else." Survivors report choosing to do only what they want. Even when they are helping others, there is a perception that these choices are their own.

One of the hardest choices survivors make is to go on living and pursuing personal pleasures. Survivors often must shift their outlook, moving from comparing their deceased loved ones' inability to seek pleasures to their worthiness to "deserve" good things. A past-centered focus with retrospective thoughts can foreclose future goal setting. This change in outlook inherently involves a shift to a focus on the here and now and creating a vision for the future. One perspective that helps survivors, and is frequently observed in the AIDS epoch, is the perception that people die the way they lived. The survivor is well-served who heeds Friedrich Nietzsche's insight:

> I have known noble ones who lost their highest hope. And then they disparaged all high hopes. . . . But by my love and hope I conjure thee: cast not away the hero in thy soul! Maintain holy thy highest hope! (p. 44)

Isolation Versus Desire for Connection

All humans are confronted with "an unbridgeable gulf between oneself and any other being" and a fundamental "separation between the individual and the world" (Yalom, 1980, p. 355). For the survivor of multiple AIDS-related loss, the sense of isolation is reinforced by tangible realities (e.g., the deaths and disappearances of loved ones and disconnection from community). A history of abandonment may contribute to a sense of aloneness. Finally, the realities of stigmatization and disenfranchised grief may provoke perceptions of aloneness. The belief that no one understands, that no one else is experiencing this same suffering, leaves the survivor psychologically isolated.

Although aloneness and loneliness are certainly not the same thing, many survivors of multiple, ongoing loss promote their own aloneness and loneliness. Schizoid traits of detachment, separation, lack of affect, and depersonalization are frequently witnessed. On top of loved ones literally disappearing, survivors who isolate or withdraw exacerbate their sense of aloneness. Those relationships that are maintained may be marked by distance rather than intimacy. In the wake of the AIDS epoch, all sorts of distance-keeping scenarios arise. Among some gay men, even anonymous sexual encounters took on a greater distance. Physical contact at bath houses was replaced by strict prohibitions against physical contact at "jack-off clubs" that only allowed individual masturbation. In the gay and heterosexual worlds, phone- and computer-linked sex contact flourished, promoted for its safety. Intimate physical contact is discouraged because it is dangerous. These caricatures of relationship exacerbate, however, the survivor's basic aloneness.

The survivor of multiple, ongoing loss is challenged with choices about relationships: whether or not to have them, how deep to allow intimacy to grow, and how much to invest in the other. After losing love so regularly, the survivor must assume the challenge of loving again. Frankl (1959/1984) discovered the power of love while a concentration camp prisoner.

> A thought transfixed me: for the first time in my life I saw the truth as it is set into song by so many poets, proclaimed as the final wisdom by so many thinkers. The truth—that love is the ultimate and highest goal to which man can aspire. . . . *The salvation of man is through love and in love.* (p. 57)

Frankl went on to explain the importance of love to the quest for meaning. Love "finds its deepest meaning in his spiritual being, his inner self" (p. 57). Those fortunate survivors who discover this truth are well-served. The love of today permits a perspective that does not dwell on the past and, in changing perspective, soothes the pain of yesterday's hurt.

Yalom (1980) asserted that existential isolation is "the major developmental task" (p. 362). It is "the facing of aloneness that ultimately allows one to engage another deeply and meaningfully" (p. 362). May (1981) quoted Maslow as writing, "Death and its ever present possibility makes love, passionate love, more possible. I wonder if we could love passionately, if ecstasy would be possible at all, if we knew we'd never die" (p. 105). Survivors observe in themselves the fact that relationships are based on intent. They may still maintain several acquaintances, but friendships are carefully chosen and nurtured. Family of choice takes on heightened meaning. Stulberg and Smith (1988) surveyed gay men to assess the psychosocial impact of AIDS. Among survivors, almost half of the respondents in relationships believed that AIDS had improved their relationship. Another significant finding was "substantially increased interest in spending time with friends and family" (Stulberg & Smith, p. 280). The survivor's existential sense of aloneness typically promotes inquiry into issues of self, relation to the world, assumptions about the universe, and questions of identity.

The hard reality of isolation made palpable by multiple AIDS-related loss prompts many survivors to look, for the first time, at issues of attachment versus detachment, enmeshment versus individuation. Separation from relationships in which one has been enmeshed is invariably a difficult and painful process, but in the long run, this separation can lead to personal growth through differentiation. Many people want to be individuals, but not everyone is willing to give up the togetherness required to achieve more individuality, according to Kerr and Bowen (1988). The experience of surviving multiple loss can force this giving up of togetherness. "Basic differentiation is functioning that *is not dependent on the relationship process* [emphasis added]" (Kerr & Bowen, p. 98). The well-differentiated individual "does not have a 'need' for others that can impair functioning" (Kerr & Bowen, p. 107). Maslow (1968) observed that the self-actualized person "showed a surprising amount of detachment from people in general" (p. 182) and a need for privacy. They have a "self-governing character" with a "tendency to look within for the guiding values and rules to live by" (Maslow, p. 182). The opportunity for personal growth in these areas is another one of the potential paradoxical benefits available to the survivor of multiple, ongoing loss. Forced to go it alone, survivors may discover within themselves resources and strengths of which they were previously unaware. Viewing the experience of loss as an opportunity, survivors may build individual capacities.

Meaning Versus Meaninglessness

Adjusting to multiple AIDS-related loss mandates a look at issues of meaning. A perception of the world as meaningless is almost inevitable unless this breed of suffering is faced as an issue of meaning. Without an individually discovered and personal sense of meaning, the survivor continues to live in a despair of meaninglessness. Without a sense of personal meaning, the other three existential dilemmas cannot be approached in a way that enhances the survivor's existence.

What meaning can be made of this disaster, this suffering, this life? "How does a being who needs meaning find meaning in a universe that has no meaning?" (Yalom, 1980, p. 423). Unresolved grief, so common in survivors, has implications for an individual's sense of purpose. "The consequences of blocked expressions of grief can be devastating and result in a life that lacks meaning and purpose" (Martocchio, 1985, p. 337). Not surprisingly, Shrader (1992) discovered in his study of gay survivors of multiple loss that questions of meaning predominated. These questions arise in connection to suffering; "disaster tends to engage our search for meaning" (Kastenbaum, 1977, p. 111). Basic assumptions about predictability and security are crushed. The survivor will often be heard declaring, "It is not fair!" or "There is no meaning to this." These are cries for meaning.

Similar to the paradoxical benefit of despair described earlier, this pure encounter with meaninglessness is essential to the survivor of multiple AIDS-related loss. The question of meaning cannot be shirked without effect. Yet, a rational and objective search for meaning is likely to frustrate. A survivor, David, discussed his search for meaning:

> For the first few years of AIDS, I was relentless in trying to make meaning from the cyclone of suffering and death around me. Then, after many frustrations, I concluded that there was *no* meaning to AIDS. There was no way to make sense of it. That is just the way it is! It does not matter one bit whether or not I like it. Asking these questions is worse than pointless. So now, I don't torment myself with seeking meaning but I seem to find it when I don't look for it.

Frankl (1959/1984) noted a similar outlook in Holocaust survivors.

> Long ago we had passed the stage of asking what was the meaning of life, a naive query which understands life as the attaining of some aim through the active creation of something of value. For us, the meaning of life embraced the wider cycles of life and death, of suffering and of dying. (p. 99)

Most existential thinkers have concluded that meaning is not a destination, but a process. Meaning is not caused, it is created. Kierkegaard (1849/1989) observed that "for it to be true that someone is not in despair, he must be annihilating that possibility every instant" (p. 45). Meaning is necessarily an individual creation. Survivors of multiple AIDS-related loss must have an ongoing quest for meaning that matches the ongoing suffering around them.

A few paths allow survivors to pursue this quest. Each individual's experience with multiple loss is unique. No one else has the same experience. "What you have experienced, no power on earth can take from you" (Frankl, 1959/1984, p. 104). And that same experience profits the survivor through the development of inner strength. Nietzsche's famous dictum, "That which does not kill me, makes me stronger," holds particularly true here: Over and over, caregivers to people with AIDS report that they could not do before AIDS what they routinely do since AIDS. Survivors note an increased capacity of strength and ability to care, to ask for support, and to love. Survivors also find meaning in a tangible response to AIDS. Volunteering is a choice example of this approach.

Some survivors embrace suffering. Rather than viewing their pain as pathological, they are able to appreciate the existential dilemma and opportunity for growth it portends. Suffering screams for an answer. Humans appear unique in their ability to project and predict their own deaths. This capacity increases the potential to suffer by anticipating suffering. Humans also strive to assign meaning to suffering. Frankl asserted that suffering may be a human achievement. This is one area where individual psychotherapy is particularly important for the survivor of multiple, ongoing loss. The survivor will need to be comforted, supported, and piloted through the "existential crisis of growth and development" (Frankl, 1959/1984, p. 125). Trying to avoid the suffering of multiple AIDS-related loss is pointless; therefore, the wise survivor accepts the destiny of suffering and continually creates an evolving meaning. This process of purposefully seeking meaning assists survivors by providing a restorative process (Williams, 1983).

Spirituality   Spirituality provides many benefits to the survivor of multiple AIDS-related loss, not the least of which is a path toward meaning. Long before trained psychotherapists and traumatologists theorized about psychic numbing, complicated bereavement, and treatment strategies, humans found healing power in their spiritual beliefs. The survivor who faces this disaster, like so many before, is greatly benefited by the strength, perspective, and wisdom available through spirituality. Faced with so much suffering, survivors regularly enhance their spiritual lives.

Gay survivors of multiple loss often have a history with religion that has alienated them (Booth, 1995; Clark, Brown, & Hochstein, 1989). As a result, mainstream religion may not serve to buffer death concerns as it does for traditional heterosexual populations (Neimeyer & Van Brunt, 1995). Despite a poor history with religion, the impact of AIDS has motivated many gay men to reevaluate the importance of religion and spirituality in their lives. In Stulberg and Smith's (1988) study of gay men, more than one quarter of the respondents indicated an increased interest in religious-spiritual ideas. The age group of 31–40 was more likely than any other age group to express increased interest in spiritual concerns. Gay men who adhere to a spiritual belief system that is not affiliated with formal religious structures have been found to have lower death anxiety (Franks, Templer, Cappelletty, & Kauffman, 1990).

Miguel de Unamuno (1921/1954), a Spanish philosopher, wrote *The Tragic Sense of Life*. Although he had no idea that multiple AIDS-related loss would arise in later years, de Unamuno's insights into spirituality in the face of tragedy are remarkably fresh and challenging while providing a useful perspective on reconciling spirituality with this disaster. Connected to the futility of determining meaning through rational inquiry, "we may say that everything vital is anti-rational, not merely irrational" (p. 34).

> There is simply this human feeling, just as underlying the enquiry into the "why," the cause, there is simply the search for the "wherefore," the end. All the rest is either to deceive oneself or to wish to deceive others; and to wish to deceive others in order to deceive oneself. And this personal and affective starting-point of all philosophy and all religion is the tragic sense of life. (de Unamuno, 1921/1954, p. 37)

Faith, he asserted, is "simply a matter of will, not of reason, that to believe is to wish to believe" (p. 114). So, the survivor's attempt to find meaning through spirituality is necessarily a task of faith. Acceptance of fate is an act of faith. It provides considerable relief to many when they realize that the meaning of life or the answer to spiritual matters does not come solely through hard work and rationality. Tennyson described it well in *The Ancient Sage*:

> For nothing worth proving can be proven,
> Nor yet disproven: wherefore thou be wise,
> Cleave ever to the sunnier side of doubt,
> Cling to Faith beyond the forms of Faith!
> (as cited in de Unamuno, 1921/1954, p. 34)

Spirituality must be a part of adjustment to multiple AIDS-related loss for most survivors. Every participant in Shrader's (1992) study of survivors had "struggled with their spirituality," and for most "the result has been a feeling that their spirituality is a more integrated part of their daily existence" (p. 104). The individual must engage this work on a deeply personal level, and part of the work is inherently private. However, psychotherapists working with survivors should be willing to engage these issues. It is impossible to survive multiple, ongoing loss without addressing fundamental questions related to spirituality. Spirituality will not eliminate suffering, but it will help provide a way to cope with suffering and personally grow from it. Spirituality is, importantly, within the survivor's control, unlike so much else. "It is this spiritual freedom—which cannot be taken away—that makes life meaningful and purposeful" (Frankl, 1959/1984, p. 87).

CONCLUSION

The experience of surviving multiple AIDS-related loss is not a problem to be solved, but a challenge to be confronted and a catalyst for personal and community growth. Judy, a caregiver to people with AIDS, wrote,

> Even towards the end of life, when you have trouble finding your friend in those blankets. . . . And you are still standing at the ready trying to do the things he needs, take care of the small stuff, and every once in a while, through the veil of pharmaceuticals or the anger that surfaces, you see your old friend. The one you used to know before. . . . And in that one small moment, you realize that you wouldn't trade your place right now with anyone else on earth. That as hard as it is to be where you are, it is the best, holiest place on this earth and you are in awe that you are privileged to be here. (Gough, 1996, p. 11)

Judy's experience and perspective is not rare. She has been given a glimpse into a world beneath superficial appearances. The survivor whose true desire is recovery and growth will find many opportunities in this crisis. Maslow (1968) observed that "the person who hasn't conquered, withstood and overcome continues to feel doubtful that he *could* [emphasis added]" (p. 4). AIDS gives the survivor the opportunity to prove to him- or herself that he or she can.

The immediacy of concerns surrounding AIDS helps promote a here-and-now focus. A survivor is not well served by dwelling on future worries, as real as they are and as persistently as they present themselves. A constant meditation on the "what-ifs" inherent in this crisis will only serve to paralyze and terrorize the survivor. This is seen in the tendency not to postpone things that really matter. It also involves the deepening appreciation for the "elemental facts of life" (Yalom, 1980, p. 35), including flowers, trees, and seasons of nature. Heidegger (1962) said it brilliantly: "Being-in-the-world *is* itself in every case its 'there'" (p. 171).

Those survivors who have not yet arrived at a place where healing can occur need the support of other survivors and professionals knowledgeable in this field. Counselors should not be shy about engaging survivors in existential issues or reluctant to talk openly about spirituality. These issues will be on the survivors' minds and must be a part of their recovery. Ochberg (1993), an authority on treating trauma survivors, wrote about the importance of therapeutic involvement in the search for meaning.

> The therapist, however, should have the aptitude to guide a search for meaning, to recognize existential despair, to confront self-pity, to reinforce recognition of one's responsibility for one's life. A final phase . . . includes articulation of the meaning of life in terms that are specific to the individual, not general or abstract. (p. 781)

At any time, all survivors have the capacity and freedom to change their perspective toward multiple AIDS-related loss. Nietzsche's maxim applies well here: "He who has a why to live can bear with almost any how" (as cited in Frankl 1959/1984, p. 97). The dilemma between freedom and destiny is profound, and this is exactly the point at which psychotherapy is useful. May (1981) asserted, "I propose that *the purpose of psychotherapy is to set people free*" (p. 19);

> Our old way of thinking—that problems are to be gotten rid of as soon as possible—overlooks the most important thing of all; that problems are a normal aspect of living and are basic to human creativity. This is true whether one is constructing things or reconstructing oneself. *Problems are the outward signs of unused inner possibility.* (p. 20)

This spot of personal power is an excellent avenue into the treatment of learned helplessness in survivors of multiple AIDS-related loss. Once they realize that they are not simply being done to, they can begin to help themselves. "If others can survive and thrive in this experience, so can I!" The ability to take control of one's own spiritual, mental, and attitudinal life counteracts helplessness and hopelessness. The critical question for survivors of multiple AIDS-related loss is the one posed by May (1983): "What am I pointing toward and what will I be in the future" (p. 97).

Survivors of multiple AIDS-related loss are given the glorious opportunity to live in a way described by de Unamuno (1921/1954):

> Above all, I shall have lived. In a word, be it with reason or without reason or against reason, I am resolved not to die. And if, when at last I die out, I die out altogether, then I shall not have died out of myself—that is, I shall not have yielded myself to death, but my human destiny will have killed me. Unless I come to lose my head, or rather my heart, I will not abdicate from life, life will be wrested from me. (p. 130)

Chapter 10

Helping the Survivor
of Multiple AIDS-Related Loss

> If people bring so much courage to this world the world has to kill them to break them, so of course it kills them. The world breaks every one and afterward many are strong at the broken places.—Ernest Hemingway (1929), *A Farewell to Arms*

This chapter is written for both survivors and the professionals who help them. Because this phenomenon is new, little attention has even been devoted to explaining the issues that arise for survivors. Nearly no attempts have been made to offer suggestions for the treatment and recovery efforts of survivors facing this disaster. Because many of the characteristics of this event are historically unique, there are few preexisting models to which either the survivor or the professional can refer. More study of survivors who seem to develop optimal coping strategies is needed (Dworkin & Kaufer, 1995). Responding to this challenge will require pioneering work that involves trying approaches that seem like they should help. As years go by, a body of anecdotal accounts and, one hopes, research will document the relative efficacy of the approaches presented here. Future editions of this book, it is also hoped, will include feedback and suggestions offered by readers who are either survivors or professionals working in this challenging field.

Every survivor needs an individually meaningful approach to recovering from multiple AIDS-related loss. There is no right way to respond to this disaster, and there is no cookie-cutter approach to treating the effects of surviving this disaster. Survivors will respond to the crisis in a wide variety of ways, from drug abuse to spiritual enlightenment, from social withdrawal to volunteering to facilitate support groups. Much of a survivor's response will be related to grief. Manifestations of grief are highly variable and individual (Martocchio, 1985).

A number of variables affect the survivor's response to multiple AIDS-related loss. First, survivors' experiences vary widely. The hemophiliac mother, urban gay man, and inner-city Hispanic woman are affected in dramatically different ways even though all may experience multiple loss. Second, different survivors use different resources. Some benefit greatly from support groups, and others never attend one. Some are greatly assisted with the help of a trained professional, such as a psychotherapist, and others will not use one or believe they cannot afford one. Third, survivors vary greatly in terms of what they find supportive and nonsupportive. Whereas one person might want to be listened to empathetically, another prefers direct advice. Whereas ritual may be important to one survivor, another will find it meaningless. Finally, an issue that greatly influences the recovery efforts of survivors is their interpersonal skills. Survivors who isolate themselves, withdraw, or are prone to diffuse, inappropriately expressed rage have greater difficulty. Survivors who are outgoing, willing to ask for support, and volunteer in an AIDS service organization fare much better.

The phrase *recovery from multiple AIDS-related loss* needs some explanation. Complete recovery from this disaster is impossible, especially while it is ongoing. If, one day, the communities suffering multiple loss from AIDS no longer must face an accumulating impact, the disaster will certainly live on in their memories, outlook, and identity. There will be no getting over this experience, ever. Survivors are indelibly imprinted with an accumulation of grief, a shattering of assumptions, and a distrust for the future that will continue long after AIDS is no more. An overriding reality of this experience is the constantly changing nature of loss and its impact. The cumulative toll will mount, fresh losses will change the survivors' perspectives, and coping will shift within people "depending on their appraisal and reappraisal of an event or situation" (Carmack, 1992, p. 10).

The foundation of all recovery efforts must be the recognition that fate has cast this experience into survivors' lives. Survivors' responses must not include any attempt to make it go away. It will not. Survivors must, instead, find a way to incorporate this experience into their lives, using it to maximum advantage as a tool that fosters insight and growth.

This chapter is divided into three sections. The first deals with the question of seeking help and explains the value in working with others. Following this, special issues that arise for survivors of multiple, ongoing loss are addressed, with suggestions for working on them. The next section focuses on the unique issues related to grieving that arise from multiple AIDS-related loss and how to treat them. Attention is paid to recovery from traumatic stress.

SEEKING HELP

Without the help of others, the magnitude of impact generated by surviving multiple AIDS-related loss cannot be adjusted to with positive outcome. Survivors who attempt to cope with multiple, ongoing loss alone only contribute to a destructive cycle of isolation prompted in the first place by AIDS. Survivors in Shrader's (1992) study were "adamant that multiple losses cannot be successfully resolved on one's own, and that survivors must utilize support wherever the survivor may find it" (p. 140).

The extent to which the survivor's preexisting support network has been decimated by AIDS is of consequence to the recovery effort. The urban gay man is most likely to face the elimination of the same people who would have been expected to provide support. However, the professional caregiver who has experienced countless losses from AIDS may return to a support network relatively intact and functional. Whether to seek professional counseling help is the individual decision of each survivor.

Social Support

Nothing is more important to the recovery effort than social support, and nothing so distinctly divides survivors who fare well from survivors who fare poorly than their level of social support. "It is a remarkable fact of life in the cerebral cortex that simply sharing an experience makes it meaningful" (Odets, 1995, p. 267). First and foremost, survivors who associate with other survivors quickly discover that they are not alone. Others have endured similar pain, and others have developed helpful coping skills. This is often the first breakthrough toward healing that survivors experience: the realization that they are not isolated, that others exist to help, that there is hope. Those who work with survivors notice the palpable insight of survivors who realize that they are not alone. "Others understand!"

Support is crucial, especially for those who are traumatized, but lacking for most survivors of multiple AIDS-related loss. A trained professional can help by legitimizing the mourner's status. "Whatever social validation and acceptance of the loss can be secured from others in the environment should be promoted" (Rando, 1993, p. 499).

The Jewish community has developed traditions that serve both to validate and to commemorate its survivors. Judaism views major traumas such as the Holocaust as the community's legacy and "obligates the community to respond—both immediately and over time—to the person's suffering" (Jay, 1994, p. 31). Something on that order is needed in response to multiple AIDS-related loss.

Individual psychotherapy may help the individual to the extent that he or she is able to heal the self, but it will never be wholly successful in treating the effects of this disaster. Ramifications are too deep and involve tears in the community fabric that can only be healed by community. In the gay community, there has been some early attempt to mark this disaster through such events as a yearly candlelight vigil in San Francisco, an AIDS Memorial Vigil in Seattle, and the Names Quilt. Even in the gay community, however, recent years have seen an increase of intracommunity bickering and allegations that AIDS has gotten too much attention.

Those survivors who can rely on a social system of friends and family are fortunate. "Close relationships provide ongoing support, comfort, and a sense of security and stability in a life filled with ambiguity" (Jue, 1994, p. 325). A study of gay men who had lost friends or lovers during the early years of the AIDS epoch demonstrated that "perceived adequacy of instrumental and emotional support reduced the impact of bereavement on subsequent grief reaction symptoms" (Lennon, Martin, & Dean, 1990, p. 482). Survivors of multiple loss who are also living with HIV are particularly well served by social support (Hays et al., 1990; Jue, 1994). Families of origin are often a tremendous source of nurturance for survivors. Unfortunately, fears about a family's potential reaction keep many from seeking this valuable source of support.

There is a downside to social involvement, especially when it centers on others who are connected to AIDS. In an Australian study on the psychosocial impact of AIDS, it was determined that although social support networks "provided invaluable physical, psychological, and spiritual support, they also provided the means through which community members were confronted with more deaths of people with whom they had become emotionally involved" (Viney, Henry, Walker, & Crooks, 1992, pp. 153–154). This is a very real risk and is sometimes the reason given when volunteers quit their commitment or when friends decide that they need to spend time with other people.

In a study meant to measure the influence of social support on the grief reactions of gay men, Lennon et al. (1990) determined that social support was a crucial variable in the level of distress experienced by survivors. Those who felt that they had received adequate support reported less adverse grief reactions than those who felt that their support had been inadequate. Lennon et al. concluded that "although the presence of support systems may ease the burden of death and grief, they also may have the effect of bringing the losses into sharper focus" (p. 478). Lennon et al. gave the Names Project as an example of this, because it is designed to emphasize the catastrophic impact of AIDS.

Giving Help

There is a paradoxical benefit of personally receiving help from efforts to help others. "I have gotten far more out of my volunteer work than I have given." No other single act seems to help survivors more than volunteering in AIDS-related service. Recent research on "social support suggests that providing support to others may actually be more stress-buffering than receiving support" (Hays et al., 1990, p. 381). Gay and bisexual men involved with AIDS service have significantly lower levels of death concerns, including less fear of premature deaths (Bivens, Neimeyer, Kirchberg, & Moore, 1994).

Steve, a survivor who volunteers, said, "I do so much volunteer work because it gives me some sense of control when I'm surrounded by feelings of helplessness." Volunteering in an AIDS service organization is not the only effective type of volunteer work for survivors. However, such work is a direct response to AIDS and offers the survivor a sense that she or he is doing something tangible to counteract the negative consequences of AIDS. This feeling of efficacy is important in the AIDS epoch because survivors so easily feel powerless. Volunteering counters these perceptions. In a study designed to assess the psychosocial impact of AIDS on gay men, Stulberg and Smith concluded that "one of the most helpful methods of coping with AIDS-related psychological stress is to volunteer for an AIDS organization" (Stulberg & Smith, 1988, p. 280) Volunteer work "provides an individual with some sense of efficacy by allowing him to contribute, with other gay men, to the fight against a common foe" (p. 280). Gays who volunteer in response to AIDS make a statement about self-acceptance by undermining homophobic attitudes and empowering the gay community through "the communalization of AIDS" (Kayal, 1994, p. 33). Those persons who engage in AIDS service work experience self-fulfillment by supporting others and feel that they make a positive difference for others.

The wonderful thing about volunteering is that the volunteer can select what type of work to do and what level of commitment to offer. Work can range from walking the pet of a person with AIDS to delivering meals, from driving clients to doctor appointments to emotional support, from doing weekly chore service to providing hospice care in the final days of life. Volunteer work does not have to be for persons with AIDS. Benefit is also derived from helping those who help people with AIDS. Facilitating emotional support groups for caregivers, families, and survivors or helping in the emerging area of caregiver support networks all prove helpful.

Volunteering truly does make a difference. Because there is so much need, a volunteer's work may not get done without his or her effort. There is a peril inherent in this reality. Nearly every person who volunteers or gives care faces the dilemma of deciding when to say no. It is vital that volunteers learn to balance engagement and detachment (Carmack, 1992). People need to protect themselves against overinvolvement so that their efforts maintain a perception of choice.

For survivors with HIV, volunteer work can be especially important. Volunteer work in the AIDS field helps "to objectify and externalize the illness. Other benefits from AIDS work include feeling positive about contributing to society and giving to others. This may help foster a sense of pride in their identity" (Dworkin & Pincu, 1993, p. 277). Working with other people with AIDS in a reciprocal setting allows survivors to break out of the role of always being the one helped and receiving services.

> For the person with AIDS, the opportunity to reciprocate support and assistance— as opposed to constantly being in a dependent, "victim" role—may promote a valuable sense of self-esteem that one is still capable of being an active, contributing member of one's social world. (Hays, Chauncey, & Tobey, 1990, p. 381)

Learned helplessness and depression are particularly well treated by tangible, physical efforts to assist others. Seligman (1975) asserted that

> exposure to the fact that responding produces reinforcement is the most effective way of breaking up learned helplessness. . . . In summary, I suggest that what produces self-esteem and a sense of competence, and protects against depression, is not only the absolute quality of experience, but the perception that one's own actions controlled the experience. To the degree that uncontrollable events occur, either traumatic or positive, depression will be predisposed and ego strength undermined. To the degree that controllable events occur, a sense of mastery and resistance to depression will result. (p. 99)

Volunteering naturally leads to distraction from one's own problems. Patty, a survivor of multiple loss who gives car rides to people with AIDS every Thursday, said,

> A lot of times I go to my volunteer work upset and worried about this or that in my life. You know, my husband didn't take out the garbage, can we afford a vacation this summer, my boss is a real ass. Let me tell you, all that disappears the second my first client gets into the car. Last week, for example, the first man was on the way to the doctor for a brain biopsy; they think he has PML [progressive multifocal leukoencaphalopathy]. The next women was going to the Social Services offices to straighten out her Medicaid spend down and find out what happened to her food stamps this month. The next client was going to the public clinic to have half his teeth pulled. My so-called problems seemed petty in comparison, and it may sound terrible, but I felt a lot of gratitude when I finished my shift that day.

The act of volunteering shifts one's thoughts from the self, distracting survivors from their own problems.

Problems with self-esteem underlie problems with depression and learned helplessness, so it should be no surprise that the action of helping others also benefits the survivors' sense of self-esteem. Maslow (1968) observed that "if we do something honest or fine or good, it 'registers' to our credit" (p. 5). The net result ultimately is that "we respect and accept ourselves" (p. 5). Work as a volunteer is likely to be seen in such light, to the benefit of survivors.

SPECIAL ISSUES ARISING WITH MULTIPLE AIDS-RELATED LOSS

Survivors face problems coping with multiple AIDS-related loss; these have been reviewed earlier in the book, especially in chapters 6 and 7 on grieving and traumatization. The following discussion is meant to offer suggestions for survivors dealing with diffuse rage, survivor's guilt, self-destructive behaviors, anxiety, stigmatization, and ongoing loss.

Diffuse Rage

To those around the survivor, there may be no doubt that he or she is suffering from inappropriate outbursts of anger. The survivor, however, may think it is perfectly appropriate to yell at the deli clerk who put too much mayonnaise on a sandwich. The significant other who is frustrated at the survivor's short temper, mood swings, and outbursts about a puppy may not be able to comprehend the survivor's response to a confrontation about kicking the dog. "The stupid dog should have known I was going to walk that way and gotten out of my way!" Those in the survivor's life may feel perplexed and frustrated, but soon they usually become hurt and resentful. Many relationships break up or suffer terribly.

Usually, survivors can see that their behavior is sometimes inappropriate. They have some insight that they are always on edge, sometimes inappropriately attacking others, and are viewed as volatile by those around them. A trusted friend, or a professional, is sometimes needed, however, to connect the pieces of their behaviors and attitudes with the responses of those around them. "Maybe you have lost your friends because you are behaving unfriendly."

Once survivors who struggle with inappropriate anger gain insight into their attitude and behavior, specific steps can be taken to address the problem. However, survivors must be willing to acknowledge the problem and address it; some are not willing to do either. A psychotherapist can be useful in this process. Validating the profound anger that is simmering beneath the surface and allowing survivors to vent that anger appropriately can greatly help. Survivors have good reason to feel extraordinarily upset, and this reality needs to be legitimized. Self-defeating behavior, however, needs to be seen as such, helping neither those around the survivor nor the survivor.

Anger is an emotion that men are more likely to express because of social conditioning that relatively encourages it in men and discourages it in women. Because anger may be a relatively easy emotion to express, some survivors may ignore intermediary emotions such as fear, anxiety, sadness, grief, frustration, and helplessness. Instead of jumping immediately to a stance of anger, survivors are better served by exploring other valid emotions and learning to express them. Again, the professional counselor can help. Rando (1986a) noted that too often the physical effects of emotions are overlooked by caregivers who fail to capitalize on this important dimension of intervention. Offering physical outlets, such as pounding a pillow, playing a sport, smashing old dishes or glasses in a safe area, punching a punching bag, kicking an empty and open paper bag, and so forth, will provide avenues for the siphoning off of emotions that, lacking other means of release, may prompt emotional and physical acting out in inappropriately aggressive ways. (p. 110)

Anger is a frequently acknowledged component of grief, but the extreme and protracted nature of multiple AIDS-related loss magnifies its potential impact on survivors and those in relationships with them. Addressing anger directly is an important part of improving coping skills for many.

Anger can be used to benefit survivors. Appropriately expressed anger gives survivors a sense of mastery, an opportunity to have their concerns heard and appreciated. Anger can motivate constructive action. A mother who lost a son to AIDS and continued to feel angry volunteered to help other mothers. "That's my way to get even at whatever took my son away." Another mother who volunteers said, "Anger is what keeps me active and I hope I never lose my anger." Seligman (1975) discussed the value of anger in treating depression that arises in response to learned helplessness.

Stigmatization

Part of the rage that many survivors feel stems directly from perceptions of indifference fostered by stigmatization. Survivors are left without the socially recognized right, role, or capacity to grieve publicly. Because survivors are likely to be denied the normal sources of support available to the victims of other disasters, special provisions must be made to find or invent alternatives.

Survivors have every right to decide to whom disclosures of AIDS losses are made. The stigmatizer and the stigmatized carry out prescribed roles in the process of stigmatization (Goffman, 1963). By "interrupting the transaction and refusing to assume the role of either perspective" (Dworkin & Kaufer, 1995, p. 50), survivors can gain a sense of control. This option addresses only overt stigmatization that is hostile and blaming; more subtle effects of stigmatization that serve to minimize the survivors' experiences must be addressed differently.

To counter the impact of society-wide stigmatization requires the active involvement of outside sources such as support groups, professionals, friends, and family who have education and insight about issues related to AIDS. Especially helpful is the support of others who are coping with the same issues related to stigmatization and grief. Sprang and McNeil (1995), who wrote a book on stigmatized grief, concluded that "these authors propose that individual therapy, in combination with other supportive or therapeutic services, is indicated in the majority of the cases due to the alienation and stigma associated with the loss" (p. 173).

Expression of affect is likely to be severely restricted because stigmatization makes emotional expression feel unsafe to survivors. Therefore, safe places and people must be found where this necessary emotional discharge can safely occur. Stigmatized AIDS-related grief is likely to have a cognitive component. A surviving parent, for example, may have guilty perceptions that he or she is somehow responsible for the deceased's death from AIDS. A common erroneous cognitive assumption is the extent of stigmatization that still exists regarding AIDS. Survivors are likely to perceive disclosure of their losses as more dangerous than it actually is.

> Cognitive interventions should focus on reframing irrational and self-destructive thoughts. Clients may verbalize thoughts such as . . . "If I had been a better parent my child would not have been gay, and therefore, would not have gotten AIDS." Counselors can detect irrational or inaccurate thought processes and assist clients in replacing them with more healthy cognitions. (Sprang & McNeil, 1995, pp. 172–173)

Therapy with survivors should not focus only on the effects of stigmatization but on the fact of stigmatization itself. Psychoeducational efforts to explain the realities of stigmatization and its impact on survivors' experiences should be explicit. This process helps to normalize the abnormal situation faced by survivors and provides some relief based on the contextual perspective it permits.

Anxiety

Many survivors report symptoms consistent with generalized anxiety disorder (American Psychiatric Association, 1994, pp. 435–436).

> A. Excessive anxiety and worry (apprehensive expectation), occurring more days than not for at least 6 months, about a number of events or activities.
> B. The person finds it difficult to control the worry.
> C. The anxiety and worry are associated with three (or more) of the following six symptoms. . . .
>   1. restlessness or feeling keyed up or on edge
>   2. being easily fatigued
>   3. difficulty concentrating or mind going blank
>   4. irritability
>   5. muscle tension
>   6. sleep disturbance

It is not difficult to understand the source of anxiety in survivors, especially those who are continuing to experience the infection, sickness, and death of friends. Yet, understanding the source of anxiety does little to mediate its effects.

Survivors are often helped when given the opportunity to talk about the source of their anxiety. It helps them to feel validated and understood. Another of the benefits of normalizing the abnormal event of multiple, ongoing loss is that survivors feel less anxious about feeling anxious. It helps when a professional can assist survivors to "break down the anxiety into its component parts" (Rando, 1986b, p. 113). Worries about John's wasting away should be separated from worries that Mike may be secretly infected, which should be separated from worries that Miguel has dementia, which should be separated from worries that Jackson is still shooting drugs.

> In this fashion, specific fears and concerns are delineated and each one can be addressed and problem-solved individually. It is always easier to cope with well-defined, explicit fears than to attempt to grapple with more global, undifferentiated, and thus more terrifying anxiety. (Rando, 1986b, p. 113)

Self-Destructive Behaviors and Attitudes

Self-destructive behaviors and attitudes create problems for some survivors of multiple AIDS-related loss. Among these behaviors are suicidal risk, abuse of alcohol and drugs, withdrawal and isolation, chronic patterns of risky sexual practices, and explosive episodes of rage. Self-destructive attitudinal problems include intense resentment, bitterness, and emotional shutdown. Severe anhedonia, unresponsive depression, and diffuse anger may have both behavioral and attitudinal components.

Attitudes and stances toward the world that inhibit healing are self-destructive. Krystal (1981) made an interesting point about survivors of the Holocaust and patterns of self-destructive attitudes that has relevance here.

> The issue of moral and ethical judgment is often substituted for self-healing. It seems virtuous to "feed" righteous indignation and treasonous to stop the rage. In this respect, it is useful to consider that hate, anger, guilt, and depression are forms of pain. It is a masochistic perversion for survivors to promote the continuation of these pains within themselves. Rather, to the extent possible, they should soothe themselves and gain peace through self-acceptance. (p. 182)

The stance of bitterness, rage, blame, hate, and attack is sometimes overriding in survivors of multiple AIDS-related loss. These attitudes are corrosive for the individual holding them and inevitably drive others away.

Once survivors gain sufficient insight to enable them to view certain behaviors and attitudes as self-destructive, these problems can be treated through behavioral and cognitive approaches that may require hard work. For example, a problem with alcohol or drug use that has taken on addictive characteristics may require outpatient, or even inpatient, treatment. Anhedonia that has become behavioral may require behavioral therapy wherein survivors obtain rewards for marginally increasing involvement in formerly pleasurable activities. Like so much of the grief work that must occur in survivors of multiple, ongoing loss, education about the need to view this process as hard work, requiring diligence and effort, is crucial. Underlying any treatment should be a process of uncovering the issues that stand behind self-destructive behaviors and attitudes. These are apparent in the many issues faced by survivors of multiple AIDS-related loss, but they may also include issues related to survivor's guilt, early trust development, and abandonment concerns.

Survivor's guilt contributes heavily to self-destructive behaviors for reasons described in chapter 6 on grief. Survivor's guilt is usually based on irrational beliefs and faulty assumptions that are amenable to psychotherapy. Cognitive work can go a long way to address these concerns, especially in cases of gross cognitive distortions. However, many of the issues underlying the development of survivor's guilt have long-standing and deep-seated roots. Odets (1995) observed that

> The psychotherapeutic approach to men suffering with survivor guilt is straightforward, and, indeed, much "ordinary" psychotherapy is about survivor guilt in the broadest sense of the idea. All psychotherapists work with problems about separation from family, ambivalence about success, and relationship difficulties. Such issues routinely involve survivor's guilt, even when working with those not living in an epidemic. (p. 284)

Current feelings of guilt about surviving are often related to earlier issues of perceived abandonment, shame, undifferentiated family connections, and, for gay men, deep-seated internalized homophobia and heterosexism. The crisis of surviving multiple AIDS-related loss may make overt issues that simmered hidden beneath the surface for some time. Odets (1995) explained the hope for survivors:

> When it is understood that guilt about surviving those who are lost to HIV is irrational and unrealistic and that it is compelling because it connects so powerfully to earlier feelings of guilt, the psychotherapy patient may then begin to feel that he has a right to have the best life he can—at any rate a decent one—and that trying to do so is not violence against, betrayal of, or abandonment of those less fortunate. (p. 285)

As issues with guilt are uncovered, an opportunity to uncover and treat other problems may arise.

Survivor's guilt seems to respond well to volunteer work. In a study of gay male survivors of AIDS-related loss who experienced guilt, "there was a high correlation between involvement in gay and/or AIDS organizations and relief from survivor guilt feelings" (Boykin, 1991, p. 256). This correlation makes sense to the "logic" of survivor's guilt. The logic of guilt supposes failed behavior and responsibility for negative outcomes. Volunteer work nearly inevitably leads to self-gratification, pride, and responsibility for positive outcomes. Self-condemnation is replaced with self-affirmation.

GRIEVING AND RECOVERY

The fact that survivors of multiple AIDS-related loss need to grieve is self-evident. What is presented here are the unique issues that arise from this phenomenon. These may also apply to other types of multiple, ongoing loss that occur at both an individual and a collective level. Because of the many complicating issues involved with AIDS and multiple loss, grief work must be approached in a way unique to this experience. Biller and Rice (1990) concluded

> The complexity of AIDS as a social phenomenon, including the stigma, the variety of forms that the disease process may take, and the fear of contagion, all point to the need for specific practice interventions addressing the unique phenomenon of grieving for people who have died from AIDS. (p. 288)

Four overriding considerations distinguish this experience from that of the normal grief experience: the cumulative impact of multiple loss, the ongoing nature of the tragedy, the global scope of loss, and the concurrent traumatization that is so often a part of this experience. This look at the issues of grieving multiple AIDS-related loss begins with some issues that are fundamental to understanding multiple loss and recovering from it.

A Perspective on Grieving Multiple Loss

"What use is grief to a horse?" asks the psychiatrist in Peter Shaffer's (1988/ 1973, p. 17) play *Equus.* To a gay man who has lost all of his close friends and his lifetime partner or to a mother who has lost her children and husband, one might readily ask, What use is grief? Perhaps it is not that a survivor grieves in response to painful loss so much as in response to love. This is the point Tolstoy made when he said that "only people who are capable of loving strongly can also suffer great sorrow" (as cited in Worden, 1991, p. xi). If a horse has no use for grief, it is because a horse has no use for love. Survivors of multiple AIDS-related loss suffer because they loved. To never hurt would require never loving. So, the pain of survivors can also be the comfort of survivors: "At least I am capable of loving." Shearer and McKusick (1986) noted that "there is a hidden asset in this psychologically painful epidemic. These men have experienced many of the necessary ingredients of love: devotion, putting the other person first, seeing the best of oneself in the other" (p. 168).

This is part of the foundation that must be established for survivors of multiple AIDS-related loss: They hurt because they loved, but that same love heals them. This framework provides relief and hope.

Grief is the Process and Work of Adjusting to Irrevocably Lost Objects, Relationships, and Dreams   This is the definition presented in chapter 5; it has particular relevance here. Survivors of multiple loss experience an irrevocable change to their world resulting from irrevocable loss. This realization is difficult for most bereaved persons, but survivors of multiple loss are particularly challenged to accept so many irrevocable losses. There is no way to replace these losses. Grief work must begin at acknowledgment of this hard reality. Sometimes survivors of multiple, ongoing loss will feel overwhelmed and try to believe that it cannot possibly be true. All manner of bargaining-type defenses are used. Survivors are helped most, however, by direct confrontation with reality.

The Pain of Grief Work

Grief work is painful. A lot of loss means a lot of pain. Parkes (1972) concluded that anything that avoids or suppresses the pain prolongs the grief. Survivors of multiple loss are going to have difficulty working through their grief for a variety of reasons. Many survivors are experiencing bereavement overload, the accumulation of so much unresolved grief that knowing where to starts seems impossible. If these reasons were not sufficient to dissuade survivors from engaging in grief work, the added burden of dealing with stigmatization and the cruel judgments that surround AIDS create even more anxiety.

The threat of ongoing loss may tempt survivors to ignore past losses. Emotional shutdown may seem more comforting than the painful memories provoked by the work of grief, but emotional shutdown is denial and persisting in denial means remaining stuck in a very early stage of the grief process.

Pain is essential to the healing and growth process. It is unavoidable, if any degree of recovery is going to occur. Maslow (1968) asserted, "If grief and pain are sometimes necessary for growth of the person, then we must learn not to protect people from them automatically as if they were always bad" (p. 8). The professional who works with survivors of multiple AIDS-related loss must be willing and able to push pain. Survivors must be willing to lean into the pain.

Survivors must see the recovery process as work, as a job that needs to be done. A pioneer in grief, Erich Lindemann (1944), noted that "the duration of grief reaction seems to depend upon the success with which a person does the *grief work*" (p. 143), and nothing has changed about the need for grief work since he wrote that. If grief is work for the aggrieved of a single death, how much more work is it for survivors of multiple and ongoing loss? The professional who works with those affected by multiple AIDS-related loss should strive to educate survivors that there are tasks of mourning (Worden, 1991, p. 10).

Counselors need to use evocative language that is clear and unambiguous. Loved ones are dead; they are irrevocably lost and will never return. The world has forever changed; things will never be the same. Those outside the immediate scope of impact from this disaster most need to be reminded of these fundamental truths of grief counseling. It is refreshing to observe how groups of multiple-loss survivors will naturally turn to direct, specific, and poignant language.

"When Will I Get Better?"

When the survivor is willing to do the difficult work required to recover from this disaster, he or she will inevitably ask, "When do I get better? How will I know when I am improving?" These are difficult questions. First, the culmination of recovery "will not be to a pre-grief state" (Worden, 1991, p. 18). Survivors must realize that they will be permanently marked and changed by this experience. Neimeyer (as cited in Marino, 1996, p. 13) said it well: "Loss is never something we are done with. We relate to our losses differently throughout our lives." A mother who volunteered on a phone line for mothers told one mother who had just found that her son had AIDS, "It's never going to go away. It's going to change."

For perspective, it may help to describe the survivor who is certainly not healing, the survivor who is overwhelmed by loss, despair, and hopelessness. This survivor is always looking backward to the past, to a history that is no more. Ask about life today, and you will hear about yesterday. A passivity of mind and resignation marked by doom distinguish this survivor's attitude. In *The Expression of Emotions in Man and Animals*, Charles Darwin (as cited in Mogenson, 1992) noted that "he who remains passive when overwhelmed with grief loses his best chance of recovering elasticity of the mind" (p. 58). Self-defeating behaviors and attitudes may be present, including subintentional suicide risks, mood-altering chemical abuse, extreme isolation, and diffuse rage. Worden (1991) asserted that the best description of the survivor who has not recovered from grief enough to move on with life is "not loving." The survivor's adjustment to loss is "hindered by holding on to the past attachment rather than going on and forming new ones" (Worden, p. 17). One might characterize this survivor as hard, even brittle.

The attitude and focus of the survivor who is recovering from multiple AIDS-related loss is more future oriented and flexible. The survivor is able to "reinvest his or her emotions back into life and in the living" (Worden, 1991, p. 18). This survivor's outlook will accept the terrible and painful reality of this disaster with a sense that fate has prescribed an experience that would not have been chosen, but that exists. There is no attempt to deny the pain of loss or avoid the fact of future loss, but there is an attempt to move on with life. Those who have died are still cared about and missed, but thoughts of them do not paralyze the recovering survivor. "We will always miss those we loved and lost, but when our mourning is successfully completed, we are not only healed, but strengthened by our sorrow as we step into the world again" (Oda, 1992). This survivor has an elasticity of mind that allows for change. More than anything else, survivors who are recovering from multiple AIDS-related loss will present a here-and-now and future-based focus. Life is lived in the present, plans are made for the future, and enjoyment is permitted.

This shift in survivor outlook cannot be forced and does not arise by pure exertion of effort. It is a gradual evolution. The trend of recovery begins before it is observed. In a number of little ways, survivors will begin to reinvest in life. Survivors may notice themselves laughing during dinner with friends. Plans to date may be arranged. A class might be taken. There is a reconnecting to life and a re-creating of life.

Cumulative Loss

Survivors face a range of accumulated loss. As discussed in chapter 3, "Understanding Multiple AIDS-Related Loss," quantitative and qualitative factors affect survivors' experiences. The hemophiliac mother presented in chapter 2, who has two sons dying and has already had her nephews die and whose involvement with other hemophiliacs has exposed her to additional loss, will have a different experience than the urban gay man who has HIV and has lost two partners and most of his friends. What these two survivors will share, along with most survivors of multiple loss, is the experience of unresolved, accumulated loss. Some of the grief may have been worked through, but most likely a large portion remains unresolved and contributes to symptoms of complicated bereavement.

Survivors may feel the full force of bereavement overload, express thoughts and feelings of being overwhelmed, and say that they have no idea where to start. The prospect of being completely overwhelmed once grieving begins is terrorizing to many survivors. Survivors, who are about to enter the challenging work of resolving accumulated loss, need a counselor or other survivors to educate them about the normalcy of their thoughts and feelings. "It is necessary to normalize the person's grief because unrealistic expectations or negative feelings about essentially normal reactions cause the majority of problems with grief" (Rando, 1984, pp. 96–97). The clinician can help to structure and focus the client as he or she sorts out issues that can be dealt with one at a time. Regardless of the number of losses, each individual loss will need to be acknowledged and grieved independently.

Overshadowing Death

Sometimes survivors will have an overshadowing death that dominates others. In Shrader's (1992) study of gay survivors of multiple loss he noted that

> in most cases, one significant death seemed to overshadow all the other losses the survivors experienced. This single death was usually the same death that had had the biggest impact upon the survivor; a lover, a close friend and/or the first AIDS-related loss. (p. 87)

This is very typical. For gay men, the overshadowing death is usually the first partner or best friend who died. In families of origin, it is usually the first child who died. The grief from these is surprisingly fresh; one gets the sense that the loss was recent when in fact it may have occurred years ago. Of course, for many survivors there was never any time to fully mourn this first significant loss before others occurred. A common sign that one loss is overshadowing and unresolved is the inability of survivors to hold ambivalent thoughts and emotions about the deceased. Typically, the deceased is all good, never did a thing wrong, and left this earth in a state of sainthood.

Another type of overshadowing death involves the death of someone with whom the survivor had an ambivalent or conflicted relationship. Mourning is complicated when ambivalence is present because "mourners are often reluctant to acknowledge that negative emotions—particularly anger—play a part in a relationship" (Rando, 1993, p. 469). In families of origin, it is common for a gay son or IVDU to die while the family has unfinished business. The person with AIDS may wait until the very end of her or his life to inform the family of origin about the AIDS diagnosis, leaving little time for reconciliation or adjustment. These deaths become overshadowing primarily because of the unresolved issues left for the survivor to process after the death of the person with AIDS. Guilt and intrafamilial conflict can stymie attempts at recovery. Professional counseling and peer support groups are well suited to help these survivors.

An overshadowing death can interfere with work on all other losses in a way that is damaging to the process of recovery from multiple AIDS-related loss. Biller and Rice (1990) discussed the interrelation between an overshadowing death and the ability of a survivor to grieve a contemporary death.

> Interestingly, after each new loss, survivors seemed to further grieve the loss they had identified as most significant. They then began to deal with that loss as if it were the only one, which had a further impact on the intensity of that loss. Furthermore, the most recent loss did not get the attention it needed for its resolution to begin. Recent losses were minimized and the grief wounds for the most significant loss never healed. The pattern makes it impossible for people to smoothly transfer from one phase of grief to another. (p. 288)

This tendency to be rigidly transfixed by the impact of a single loss that remains unresolved is common. Neither the overshadowing loss nor the subsequent losses are addressed appropriately.

The overshadowing death always needs to be addressed first even though it is the most difficult. Any other grief work will become stuck in comparison to the dominating and blocking loss. This loss will take much time because many of the problems characteristic of unresolved grief and complicated bereavement will center around it.

Profound pain often accompanies the first significant death and complications, such as debilitating survivor's guilt, may be present.

Working through Cumulative Grief

Survivors of multiple AIDS-related loss face the daunting task of needing to methodically work through years of accumulated unresolved grief. There is no exact parallel for it. Typically, survivors will have responded, early in the AIDS epoch, like almost anyone would respond to two or three deaths occurring in succession. They will have been shocked, gone to memorial services, been supported by friends and family, and then tried to move on with their lives. At some point, survivors usually felt overwhelmed by the crush of loss. During this phase, survivors concluded that they could not take anymore. Often this demoralization translated into behaviors that contributed to an accumulation of unresolved grief such as refusing to mourn. In many cases, this was a conscious decision typified by refusal to attend any more memorial services.

After any overshadowing death is processed to a point of reasonable completion, survivors who wish to recover must move on to more long-term grief work. Survivors who fare best are the ones who see this process as a long-term one and who are committed to sticking it out. A commitment to psychotherapy or a support group is beneficial. One necessary part of grief work that takes considerable time is uncovering the meaning of each loss. Parkes (1972) observed that "in any bereavement, it is seldom clear exactly what is lost" (p. 7). This is especially true for losses that are not specifically tied to a death event such as community-wide losses. However, even deaths of individuals require survivors to uncover the various meanings the deceased person played in their lives. "The survivor usually is not aware of all the roles played by the deceased for some time after the loss occurs" (Worden, 1991, p. 15). Part of the insidious nature of surviving multiple AIDS-related loss are the multilayered losses present in each loss.

It often helps survivors to create a timeline of their losses. Include all losses, not just death events, but also points of realization that a global or collective loss had occurred. The deaths of famous people can come to embody more than the death of that person and should be included if they are significant to the survivor. The timeline can be a useful tool for the kind of methodical grief work necessitated by accumulated grief. Also, it provides survivors with a comprehensive perspective of their experience. Inevitably, no matter how aware survivors are of the impact of multiple loss on their lives, actually seeing their scope of loss is enlightening. Again, this helps the survivors to normalize the abnormality of their experience.

An approach developed by Volkan (1975) called "re-grief" therapy may be particularly useful because it is "designed to help the patient bring into consciousness some time after the death his memories of the one he has lost" and to work on issues characteristic of "*established* pathological grief" (p. 334). Re-grief therapy was designed as short-term therapy, with four sessions per week recommended. This therapeutic approach was laid out before the AIDS epoch and addresses a single-event loss, but many of the principles seem relevant to survivors of multiple AIDS-related loss. More clinical experience and study are needed.

Re-grief therapy begins by conducting a history-taking where survivors are asked to recount the circumstances of the death, their reactions, and memories about the memorial service. A photograph of the deceased is brought in and survivors are asked to describe the appearance of the deceased. The point of this work is to put the survivor "in a state of contact with the dead individual" (Volkan, 1975, p. 337) while also building boundaries between the survivor and the deceased. Next, the survivor is asked to examine dreams and fantasies, with attention paid to any signs of ambivalence or guilt. This approach may be beneficial to treatment of survivors of cumulative, unresolved loss because of its direct approach, which could be applied successively to many losses, including losses that are not strictly death events. It keeps the focus of therapy on grief by methodically forcing the issues left unresolved in the survivor's experience. Each loss requires the reminiscing, story-telling, memory sharing, and acknowledgment of lost dreams required in any grieving.

Ongoing Loss

Grief work normally proceeds on the assumption that loss has occurred in the past. Recovery efforts can focus on an event that is no longer causing additional loss. Grieving, for the survivor of multiple AIDS-related loss, however, inevitably includes the reality that additional loss will likely occur. Grief work will be interrupted by fresh experiences of loss. How should these fresh grief incidents be incorporated into the task of working through accumulated grief?

It is pointless to establish a rigid approach to recovery from this disaster. The reality of fresh grief events must be accommodated. New losses, which are grieved contemporaneously, prevent an accumulation of further unresolved grief. Therefore, many survivors learn to "do it right this time." This typically means that the survivor dedicates him- or herself to fully grieving: pulling out photos and letters and allowing emotions to be expressed, attending the memorial service, and seeking and using the support available when the death is recent.

AIDS provides the paradoxical benefit of allowing grief to begin early. Although grieving is prolonged, it can also be planned. The opportunity to finish unfinished business, say proper good-byes, and plan for the event of death can be useful and comforting for survivors. A common point of advice offered by survivors in Shrader's (1992) study was to leave nothing unsaid between the survivor and the person with AIDS. "Subjects felt it was important to discuss the 'uncomfortable' topics, such as death and loss with the person with the disease" (p. 141). The task of talking about these normally avoided topics is inevitably uncomfortable at first, but survivors get used to it and find immeasurable comfort in leaving nothing unsaid.

Grieving Global Losses

Global losses are the all-encompassing, collective, and community-wide losses that result from multiple AIDS-related loss. Global losses include aggregate individual losses that comprise the survivor's experience; their recognition ac-knowledges a distinctive feature of this disaster, namely its broad-based impact on the environment of survivors, especially those in the gay community. Indi-vidual griefs add up and accumulate so that survivors feel "the total sum of AIDS-related losses as one big loss" (Shrader, 1992, p. 114). Almost nothing has been written about coping with global loss. Traditional grief theory provides no foundation for this work, so survivors of multiple AIDS-related loss are pioneering new territory.

Grieving global losses is a task that must be included in recovery efforts for survivors of this disaster. Aspects of global loss inevitably come up, so it helps survivors to name them; this is part of normalizing the abnormal. It helps when a counselor can address the issues directly. Survivors should engage in grieving global loss directly. Making a timeline of loss helps present the per-spective of total environmental disruption faced by many survivors. Talking about the specific issues of global loss is essential.

- Losses to the overall community. How has the gay community changed in the absence of 200,000 members?
- Losses of a sexual lifestyle.
- Losses of a sense of safety, predictability, and expectations about the future.
- Losses brought about by constantly living under a death imprint, includ-ing a lack of spontaneity, fun, and ability to be carefree.

Jewish response to the Holocaust is an example of a community's ability to recognize that the sum of its individual losses resulted in a broader global loss to the community. An example of the Jewish capacity to recognize loss in a global and community-wide context is the kaddish prayer, which "moves the private trauma of death into a sanctified place within the community" and has been "said for the destruction of Jewish sacred objects, for fallen leaders, for martyrs, and for victims of Nazi murder. The prayer binds one's particular loss to the losses of the people" (Jay, 1994, pp. 31–32).

Memorials that commemorate aggregate losses arising from a particular disaster are not new, and their creation, existence, and maintenance is a source of solace for survivors of the Holocaust and of the Vietnam War. AIDS has inspired a superb commemorative ritual to honor aggregate and individual losses: the Names Quilt.

The Names Project AIDS Memorial Quilt is composed of 3×6 foot quilt panels. Each panel is unique, individually made to commemorate someone who has died from AIDS. When the Quilt was first displayed in Washington, DC, it was about a city block long. In October 1996, when the Quilt was displayed again on the Mall in Washington, DC, it stretched for a mile from the Washing-ton Monument to the Capitol ("Mile-long AIDS quilt," 1996). Even that space was insufficient. Blocks of panels were displayed under the trees that surround the Mall and over 4,000 new Quilt panels were added during the display. Most panels are made by those who loved someone who died of AIDS and provide an excellent ritual for grieving. Viewing the Quilt is both overwhelming and healing. One survivor of multiple loss described his experience in October 1996:

> At first I walked all the way from one end of the display to the other. A mile of names stretching further than I could see. Later, I started walking the aisles, paying attention to individual panels. Every now and then one of the panels would grab my attention. I would think about how much potential was lost in that one person. Then, my eyes would look up, and I would see all the thousands and thousands of panels around me.

Over 40,000 people are represented in the AIDS Quilt, only a fraction of the total number who have died of AIDS in the United States.

The author visited the 1996 Quilt display on the Mall and was impressed by the support available to the families, friends, and observers. A continual cadence of names was read over loudspeakers that surrounded the Mall. The coordinators gave the readers a list to read, and at the end the reader inevitably added the names of their own loved ones. All over the Mall, one could observe clutches of people hugging each other, sharing each other's grief, and healing.

Beyond the Quilt, other efforts to commemorate AIDS losses are arising. In San Francisco, for example, the AIDS Memorial Grove is a special place designed to mark the community's losses to AIDS. The 15-acre site in Golden Gate Park received designation as a national landmark in late 1996. Kerry Enright, executive director of the AIDS Memorial Grove, observed that "this is not just a place for mourning; it is a living and breathing space where people can experience the pathos of AIDS" ("Legislation approved," 1996, p. 7). He noted that the Grove allows survivors "to grieve openly without being stigmatized and to experience the feelings of renewal and hope inspired by nature" (p. 7).

Traumatic Grief

Many survivors of multiple AIDS-related loss will suffer the effects of trauma interconnected with their experience of grief (see chapter 7). Approaches "incorporating both bereavement models and traumatology are needed to serve populations affected by HIV/AIDS" (Bidgood, 1992, p. 242). Although not all survivors have been traumatized, many have, and their recovery depends on addressing issues of trauma. The treatment of traumatic grief "requires introspection and increased levels of self-awareness for survivor-victims after the traumatic death of a loved one" (Sprang & McNeil, 1995, p. 118). Unfortunately, almost no attention has been devoted to the traumatic effect of multiple AIDS-related loss and none to treating it.

Many survivors of multiple AIDS-related loss are caregivers to people with AIDS and others who have worked in the front lines of AIDS services. These survivors often suffer from secondary stress disorder (see chapter 5). Unfortunately, models of treatment for secondary stress "have yet to be widely developed" (Dutton & Rubinstein, 1995, p. 97). The next chapter addresses prevention strategies for caregivers whose work places them at high risk for secondary stress reactions.

It is assumed that many approaches developed to treat trauma will be useful to this experience; many good sources exist for information about treatment. However, this event combines grief as a normal component of the survivor's experience and usually includes ongoing traumatization—two factors that complicate traditional treatment approaches.

Trauma and grief work must occur concurrently because it is impossible to divide the effects from each other, and it is futile to try. As mentioned above, an overshadowing death that remains unresolved will stymie recovery efforts, so grief must be addressed up front. The effects of trauma can, however, hinder grief resolution work, so they need to be addressed early on as well. Trauma work with survivors of multiple loss usually includes the following tasks.

Assessment and Evaluation   Assessment and evaluation of the survivor's traumatic response should be a two-way process. It is not optimal for a professional to take full responsibility for assessing, evaluating, and planning treatment. A professional obviously needs to monitor for risks to the survivor's personal safety. Yet, a vital component of recovery must include the survivor in the process of assessing the traumatic impact of multiple loss on his or her life and planning the recovery effort.

An excellent resource for this process is the *DSM–IV* (American Psychiatric Association, 1994). Chris Tollfree (personal communication, March 10, 1996) lays the *DSM–IV* in front of his clients and has them look at each symptom of trauma under the diagnosis of posttraumatic stress disorder, then decide whether it applies. This approach helps clients feel empowered in their assessment and treatment while providing a context for the symptoms they may be experiencing. It is remarkable how much relief survivors of multiple AIDS-related loss will express when they understand their problems in terms of being traumatized for the first time. Ochberg (1993), who regularly uses this approach in posttraumatic therapy, noted that "responses vary, from satisfaction that the symptoms are officially recognized, to surprise that anybody else has a similar syndrome. Some patients take pride in making their own diagnosis, pointing out exactly which symptoms apply" (p. 775).

Assurance and Stability   Treatment of trauma normally involves first removing the victim of trauma from the source of traumatization. That option is unavailable to survivors of multiple AIDS-related loss. Acknowledging this regrettable reality bolsters the approach of normalizing the abnormal.

Professional psychotherapy is indicated for survivors who suffer trauma. Survivors live in a world of uncertainty and vulnerability. Survivors "may confuse the abnormality of the trauma with abnormality of themselves" (Ochberg, 1993, p. 773). The counseling environment needs to be stable, predictable, safe, and competent and should provide guidance. To the extent possible, the therapist should outline the course of treatment. Educating survivors about the normal effects of trauma and the traumatic stress recovery process is important. "For example, it is not unusual for trauma survivors to be preoccupied with fear of loss of control over powerful emotions" (Scurfield, 1993, p. 881). Survivors need to be forewarned that the process of recovery is not linear, that cycles of feeling better and feeling worse are inevitable.

Therapy needs to have a well-planned end point without surprise and shock. With multiple, ongoing loss, this is particularly important because of the risk of recreating the traumatic event within therapy.

Expression of Recollections and Emotions   Survivors need "to verbally and emotionally process the traumatic event, though emotional responses are generally constricted initially" (Sprang & McNeil, 1995, p. 127). This task is necessary for recovery from trauma and grief; the same venting assists both. Friends and family of survivors may have grown tired of hearing about the same old issues, so the empathetic ear of a counselor is often important. "Sometimes it is therapeutic merely to verbally share one's thoughts, feelings, and memories of a trauma experience" (Scurfield, 1993, p. 881).

A modulated and dosed recollection of distressing memories is important. The most successful therapists maintain "a steady expectant, but nondemanding, presence which facilitate(s) gradual release of affect-laden material, as well as permission *not* to reveal that which the patient [is] not ready to convey" (Lindy et al., 1983, p. 607) Survivors need to move back and forth between intense recollection of emotion-laden memories and more benign "chat." For example, the survivor of multiple AIDS-related loss may talk about the horrors of his partner's final days and the terrible pain the partner suffered *and* talk about plans for dinner that night.

Provide Support   Throughout this difficult process, survivors need to feel supported. For the survivor who is intensely isolated and withdrawn, a psychotherapist may be the primary source of support. Ochberg (1993) gave advice to counselors of trauma survivors that explains the importance of their supportive role. "The client should feel your presence at that moment [of sharing their traumatic story]. The purpose is more than catharsis. It is partnership in survival" (p. 780).

Referrals to peer support groups or other sources of support is appropriate. Peer support is especially useful for victims of multiple AIDS-related loss, who frequently complain that no one understands. Among Vietnam War veterans, for example, "peers offer a special role in terms of identification, self-worth, familiarity with the trauma context, and reality-based feedback" (Scurfield, 1993, p. 880). The same is true for survivors of this event.

Being listened to can provide survivors with a sense of empowerment.

> Usually, the victims of disaster need to change passivity into activity through talk-ing and working-through the stressful and overwhelming aspects of the trauma they have undergone, and their specific role in the event. This represents the kind of emotional support that is most beneficial to restoring the normal stress recovery process. (Eranen & Liebkind, 1993, p. 962)

Changing passivity into activity involves more than a change in attitude. Survi-vors, especially those who suffer problems related to learned helplessness, may require directive therapy. This is another reason that framing recovery as work is so important. It provides a sense of control and renews belief in personal efficacy.

Restore a Sense of Control and Mastery   Wherever possible, survivors must be encouraged to regain a sense of control and mastery to counter feelings of helplessness inherent in this disaster. Empowering survivors restores a sense of control that is usually severely shaken by traumatic stress. Clients seek coun-seling in a vulnerable position with relatively little power. Their lack of power is the reason they are seeking help (Cowger, 1994).

Ochberg (1993) asserted that the empowering principle of traumatic recov-ery includes the implication that the "therapeutic relationship must be collabora-tive, leading to empowerment of one who has been diminished in dignity and security" (p. 774). Cowger (1994) provided valuable information about empow-ering clients. In this approach,

> clients give direction to the helping process, take charge and control of their per-sonal lives, get their "heads straight," learn new ways to think about their situa-tions, and adopt new behaviors that give them more satisfying and rewarding out-comes. Personal empowerment recognizes the uniqueness of each client. (Cowger, p. 263)

Survivors of multiple, ongoing loss need to have a perspective of personal em-powerment because of the powerlessness generated by their experience.

"According to the theory of reciprocity, a feeling of independence requires reciprocal give and take" (Eranen & Liebkind, 1993, p. 962). That is why it is so important to include survivors collaboratively in therapy from the very be-ginning. To have a perception of "mastery of one's life, one just needs to have an internal locus of control" (Flannery, 1989, p. 223).

The reason the term *survivor* rather than *victim* is used throughout this book has precisely to do with the necessity for empowerment. Every survivor must realize that he or she is indeed a survivor. Many have committed intentional or subintentional suicide or succumbed to lives of mere existence or chronic abuse of mood-altering chemicals. Survivors of multiple AIDS-related loss who are working at recovery are always a strong and brave group; they need to hear that fact and be encouraged to adopt this perspective about themselves.

One technique that is particularly helpful with survivors of multiple AIDS-related loss is focusing on the future. When the survivor is ready, questions directed toward future goals and planning are healing and foster personal empowerment. If the client is not yet able to think about the future, questions such as "If you were not overwhelmed with your losses now, what would you be doing/feeling/thinking?" can help to change the survivor's perspective.

Survivors of multiple AIDS-related loss will need to remake their assumptive world, challenging almost all expectations that were shattered by this disaster. This is why encouraging a purposeful search for meaning is so important. It provides survivors a renewed sense of personal empowerment in terms of their values, their spirituality, and their expectations about the future. In the later stages of recovery, it is important to facilitate the discovery and appreciation of positive aspects of the traumatic experience (Scurfield, 1993).

Survivors who suffer debilitating grief, symptoms of traumatization that include withdrawal and numbing, or traits of learned helplessness usually need behavior-based changes in patterns that established themselves in response to multiple AIDS-related loss. Seligman (1975) asserted the importance of "forced exposure to the fact that responding produces reinforcement" (p. 99). This is another reason volunteer work, social involvement, and psychotherapy are effective; they all provide survivors with direct positive reinforcement contingent on their effort.

CONCLUSION

Grief is a primary response to surviving multiple AIDS-related loss. The preceding section focused on the characteristics of surviving this disaster that require a unique response. The accumulation of grief so characteristic of the survivor's experience must be addressed head on. Realization that ongoing loss will affect recovery must be acknowledged. The reality of both individual and global losses must be grieved. The fact of concurrent traumatization has implications and must be treated. Grief response and grief recovery require a flexible approach based on the unique characteristics of surviving multiple AIDS-related loss.

This chapter stressed the importance of helping survivors realize that their struggle with multiple, ongoing loss is profoundly difficult. Survivors who can take a proactive stance to responding to this crisis are better off than survivors who respond from the stance of a victim. In the next chapter, constructive suggestions are offered to help survivors thrive in the face of this disaster.

Chapter 11

Tools and Techniques
for Surviving and Thriving

The question of desirable grief and pain or the necessity for it must also be faced. Is growth and self-fulfillment possible at all without pain and grief and sorrow and turmoil?—Abraham Maslow (1968, p. 8)

Survivors who fare better share certain similarities in attitude and outlook. These are discussed at the beginning of this chapter. Support groups help to fulfill this need and many others. Specific suggestions for forming and facilitating support groups specifically for survivors of multiple AIDS-related loss are offered in this chapter. Although there is tremendous variety in the specific techniques used by survivors to commemorate or ritualize their losses, most survivors develop personally meaningful ways to mark them. The chapter concludes by enumerating a number of rituals used by survivors.

OUTLOOK AND ATTITUDE

Survivors who report faring best in response to multiple AIDS-related loss seem to share certain outlooks and attitudes. They recognize that they are living through an abnormal set of life circumstances. Instead of exclusively focusing on themselves as victims, they are able to form responses that are self-affirming and proactive. Although they may regularly assist people with AIDS and have extensive contact with other survivors, they are able to balance their engagement with, and detachment from, AIDS. Bearing witness to their experience is seen as vitally important.

NORMALIZING THE ABNORMAL

Surviving multiple AIDS-related loss is an abnormal experience. Survivors who fare better realize that they are living through a historically unique disaster. It is perfectly understandable that their responses to it are, at times, intense, unsteady, emotional, and "crazy." As one survivor said, "We are not living through normal times; how can I be expected to be normal?" After some period of time, survivors give up the strained effort necessary to always maintain equilibrium. There is tremendous relief in the realization that it is normal to react "abnormally" to an abnormal experience.

Throughout this book, normalizing the abnormal has been encouraged because of the solid theoretical rationale underlying it. In the field of bereavement, the benefits of educating the bereaved about the grief process as a way of normalizing their experiences are well accepted. Martocchio (1985) concluded that grieving persons are helped by "recognizing the 'normal' nature of their feelings and experiences" (p. 328). Ochberg (1993) observed that survivors of trauma "may confuse the abnormality of the trauma with abnormality of themselves" (p. 773). In a normal grief or trauma experience, the bereaved will at times feel like they are going crazy. Most probably, they are not, and anyone working with these survivors should constantly normalize the experience.

Recovering survivors of multiple AIDS-related loss are able to internalize this advice and have come to truly understand that they are living through an abnormal experience. Their responses may seem crazy, but they themselves are not crazy. This vital attitudinal shift is crucial for survivors. For survivors struggling with survivor's guilt, healing is handicapped as long as they feel guilty about feeling guilty. For survivors who are self-medicating anxiety, healing is handicapped as long as they feel anxious about feeling anxious. Once free of the paralyzing fear that they are abnormal because their responses to multiple AIDS-related loss are sometimes extreme, survivors are free to be more creative and spontaneous in their healing journey.

SHIFT FROM VICTIM TO SURVIVOR

Instead of viewing their response to AIDS as pathological, survivors' outlook shifts to view their responses from an attitude of empowerment. The realization that they have lived through something truly dreadful and have somehow survived is met with a sense of justifiable pride and accomplishment. Mancoske and Lindhorst (1995) compared the ongoing traumatic experience of battered women to gay men living in the age of AIDS. "The paradigm shift from pathology to empowerment of the oppressed is challenged to expand yet again to models of empowerment of the oppressed who are living with ongoing trauma" (p. 31).

Survivors who move to this place of empowerment are able to make decisions that support themselves in the AIDS epoch. A more balanced perspective develops. Instead of focusing solely on those dying of AIDS and viewing themselves as suffering victims of this disaster, survivors can develop an attitude that finds possibilities and opportunities for themselves. A self-focused healing and growth cycle is encouraged. Krystal (1981) observed that Holocaust survivors who showed successful completion of mourning and integration of the survivor's life were able to bring themselves "to the position of being able to own up to all of his or her living as his or her own" (p. 184). Social support, community involvement, and fostering a sense of purpose are useful to this goal.

These survivors are able to tolerate and express their feelings. The act of expressing feelings, with the intent of receiving support, is self-empowering. It says that one's feelings are important and deserve to be heard. Sharing feelings has a number of benefits that have a synergistically positive effect. Sharing counteracts feelings of alienation and isolation by permitting support, inevitably lessening survivor's guilt, helping in the search for meaning, fulfilling a need for catharsis, and fostering a sense of choice and control.

BALANCING ENGAGEMENT AND DETACHMENT

For many survivors, the early years of the AIDS epoch were marked by utter denial and avoidance of anything related to AIDS or near-total immersion and obsession with AIDS. Either of these options became untenable as the years went by.

Carmack (1992) studied the management skills of gay men living in an urban setting who had suffered multiple losses. "Balancing engagement and detachment was identified as the basic social-psychosocial process that described how gay individuals struggled to reach an optimal balance in their involvement in the needs of individuals and the community" (Carmack, p. 9). Conflicting needs are recognized. Individuals need to take care of themselves. Many people are suffering and need care. Survivors who develop a healthy balance are able to balance these conflicting needs "to detach and protect themselves while still mattering and making a difference to others" (Carmack, p. 9). It is very difficult to say no when there is a need. "The individual who repeatedly watches his friends die after prolonged illness may develop a 'compassionate detachment' that allows him to continue to be involved" (Klein, 1994, p. 16). This balance is achieved by the phenomenon of ongoing self monitoring.

"Having a life outside of AIDS" is frequently mentioned by survivors who have achieved this balance. Survivors are sometimes quite structured in scheduling time that is time away from AIDS. Meditation, prayer, or pleasurable reading time fits this need for many. Garfield (1995) provided advice to care-givers who suffer burnout, saying "caregivers *must* have a life outside of AIDS caregiving" (p. 278). He recommended the establishment of a regular and en-joyable exercise routine, adoption of stress reduction techniques, and weaving "revitalizing activities into your life" (pp. 271–272). Some survivors make a point of taking vacations away from AIDS. When they are socially surrounded by friends with AIDS, this often means a vacation out of town.

Fostering a sense of humor has been important for many. Survivors in Shrader's (1992) study "believed that humor was a very important piece in their healing, and advised that survivors should not be afraid to laugh" (p. 144). George Bernard Shaw said, "Life does not cease to be funny when people die any more than it ceases to be serious when people laugh" (as cited in Klein, 1994, p. 23). Many survivors intentionally seek out comedy in order to laugh for a while.

BEARING WITNESS

The need to bear witness is a common theme voiced by survivors of multiple AIDS-related loss. "No one must ever forget." Bearing witness has two impor-tant components. First, there is the necessity of never forgetting, of remember-ing those who have died and the lives that have been forever disrupted. Second, there is a longing to have the survivor experience acknowledged. "Bearing wit-ness is not only an acknowledgment of the event, it is an acknowledgment and understanding of the *experience* of those who have lived it" (Odets, 1995, p. 267).

Keeping alive memories of the deceased is not prioritized in cultures of most Western nations. There are exceptions, but traditional psychotherapeutic approaches, along with the medical model of healing, encourage the idea of getting past, getting over, and moving on. Successful healing implies forget-ting more than remembering. Memory need not, however, be a wedge between pathology and health; it can be a bridge between experience and integrity.

At the beginning of the High Holidays, during the Jewish Selichot service, the following prayer is offered: "In these days and in the days to come, O Lord our God, You have set for us a terrible and difficult task: to remember." For Jewish people, "in the post-Holocaust world, the concept of 'healing' is an affront to the rupture, but trying to hold on to the memory of those who were cut away is a necessity and a responsibility" (Jay, 1994, p. 34). Krystal (1981) wrote powerfully about the Jewish need to incorporate memory: "The process of making peace with oneself becomes impossible when it brings back the help-lessness and shame of the past. Many survivors would experience this self-healing as 'granting Hitler a posthumous victory,' and they therefore angrily reject it" (p. 178). Even before any realistic hope for the end of AIDS, one finds the same stubborn insistence that those who died not be forgotten.

Latino cultures are likely to maintain "attachment beyond the grave" (Shapiro,

1995, p. 165). Detachment and forgetting are antithetical. The Mexican Day of the Dead is a perfect example of explicit, socially sanctioned remembrances of the dead. There has been some effort to establish a similar tradition in San Francisco. Remembering is seen as a community responsibility.

Part of the urgency expressed by survivors includes not only the desire to persuade society to remember but the desire to get people to notice in the first place. There is a fear that if a cure for AIDS were discovered, the survivor's experience would disappear and become meaningless. Those who have died and the pain of survivors will become insignificant, relegated to the history of a disenfranchised minority.

Affirmation from those outside the zone of impact recognizes the legitimacy of the survivor's pain, struggles, and triumphs. Survivors want to know that society respects this experience as something significant and meaningful. Odets (1995) explained his personal perspective on this need, and it is one shared by many survivors.

> Although Dan and I might have borne witness to each other's experience, the shared witness of only two is usually not enough for big, enduring social events. It is broad social recognition—particularly of painful, isolating, and seemingly meaningless experience—that transforms the subjective experience from a personal delusion or *folie a deux* into a witnessed, real, meaningful, and therefore bearable one. (p. 267)

Denial about the impact of AIDS is an affront to the idea of bearing witness but is still prevalent in society as a whole and even within the gay community. The need to bear witness manifests itself in many indirect ways. For example, some gay survivors find it extremely important to get their family of origin to acknowledge the terrible suffering they are enduring through the deaths of so many friends. If they could get their parents' recognition, their experience would be meaningful.

The desire to bear witness addresses the need to recognize the global, community-wide losses that occur with multiple AIDS-related loss. Bearing witness is an attitude on the part of survivors, but it is also a task for individuals and community. There are a number of ways to bear witness. Many authors have already accomplished this task, including Paul Monette, David Feinberg, Andrew Holleran, Walter Odets, Larry Kramer, Randy Shilts, and others. This book is an explicit effort to bear witness. Support groups for survivors of multiple AIDS-related loss are another means to bear witness.

SUPPORT GROUPS

Peer-based support groups with trained facilitators are an optimal setting for fostering recovery from multiple AIDS-related loss. Support groups are valuable because they are a source of emotional reassurance, provide information, promote social contact, and serve the valuable function of witnessing a survivor's experience. Well-trained facilitators bring in a therapeutic component that promotes healing.

Value of Support Groups

Interaction with other survivors of multiple AIDS-related loss is beneficial for many reasons. Peer-based support offers assurance that the survivor's experience is understood. Shrader (1992) determined that support groups were the most helpful therapeutic resource for survivors of multiple AIDS-related loss because of interaction and reciprocal sharing opportunities (pp. 119–120). Peer-based support groups are used with success with a number of populations, including persons with cancer or alcoholism, widows, and the bereaved. At this point, little empirical research exists to support the efficacy of self-help support groups (Lieberman, 1993) and studies "have netted mixed results" (Rando, 1993, p. 341), but anecdotal evidence of their effectiveness for certain survivors abounds.

Groups encourage both mutual aid and self-help. Reciprocity, inherent in group contact, is extraordinarily helpful. The support group is an excellent resource for information and education. Often, confusion surrounds the world of AIDS; new medications, alternative support resources, and rumors create anxiety. Emotional reassurance may be the most important benefit survivors derive. It is common for members to voice concern that they are crazy only to be reassured that others have felt the same way. Providing a sense of universality is one of the chief functions of groups; survivors "express great relief at discovering that they are not alone" (Yalom, 1985, p. 9). This is especially important for survivors of multiple AIDS-related loss.

Grief, especially disenfranchised grief, is best dealt with in a social setting. Groups counteract feelings of isolation and alienation. "Groups can be instrumental in helping people feel less isolated as they move at their own pace in their own way in working through their grief" (Corey & Corey, 1992, p. 424). Survivors can express their grief, putting it out in the open and knowing that their experience is witnessed. One survivor described the value of her weekly support group.

> It helps to come to group each week and dump my stuff. It is the only time all week when I feel understood. I think it helps all week long too because I know that come Wednesday night, I'll have my group and I'll be understood.

The group provides a place to validate losses, allowing the survivor's experience to be appreciated. The benefits of support are readily available through the group, especially when relationships between members deepen. Groups, especially closed groups, build community. Groups provide a structured setting for survivors to consistently lean into the pain of grief work.

Structure of Support Groups

The optimal support group for survivors of multiple AIDS-related loss is closed, is facilitated by two trained peers, has 6 to 10 regular participants, and has membership that is self-selected through the process of a previously open group choosing to close. The group focuses on multiple AIDS-related loss, not a vague and diluted topic like AIDS or hemophilia, although it defines losses from AIDS broadly and liberally. Ongoing loss necessitates ongoing groups. Existing models for bereavement groups usually emphasize the need for time-limited groups. However, ongoing groups replicate the real-life experience of group members and provide a preventative function by allowing group members to support each other in preparing for additional deaths. When these deaths occur, the quality of support is enhanced.

Providing a structured and safe environment is crucial when forming a group for survivors of multiple AIDS-related loss. Emotional support groups that are "unstructured seem to provoke anxiety," therefore "groups are more effective when planned and structured" (Dworkin & Pincu, 1993, p. 277). Survivors of multiple loss face enough uncertainty without their support group fostering more. It is important that the group facilitators be reliable and consistent; the group needs to begin and end on time (an hour and a half works well); the group needs to agree on rules that foster safety and trust. These rules usually include agreements to maintain confidentiality and to respect each other's feelings. "In *any* well-run group, safety can mean only one thing: any honest expression of feelings or thoughts will be received and tolerated by the group, and an attempt will be made to honestly respond to it" (Odets, 1995, p. 274).

Developing groups composed of the subpopulations of people affected by multiple loss may have value. Recall Debra's story in chapter 1, in which she speaks of the discomfort some members in the hemophiliac community have associating with gay men. Hemophiliacs may wish to form their own support groups for multiple loss. Klein and Fletcher (1987) suggested that the number of issues unique to gay men's grief suggest the need for specifically gay groups. A group composed of lesbians and gay men could focus on "other problems related to oppressive life circumstances" such as "the host of intrapersonal implications from living in a hostile social environment" (Mancoske & Lindhorst, 1995, p. 37). Similarly, inner-city heterosexuals may prefer their own group. In Seattle, no attempt to divide survivors of multiple AIDS-related loss was made, and these groups, although diverse, are well integrated.

A closed group of committed members is ideal. A closed group permits safety and community to develop in a way that is impossible for an open group where different people attend each week and where members come and go. It is usually not possible, however, to start a group with a collection of precommitted individuals. Ideally, the group self-selects members through a process of attrition that may occur naturally over several months.

In Seattle, one multiple-loss group began as an open group. Because it was well advertised and the need for such a group was established, the first meeting had 14 participants, too many for regular meetings. After a few months, the decision was made to close one group and open another. The closed group initially agreed to stay open to anyone who had previously attended, but after a few months decided to close, only including the 8–10 consistently attending members. The other group remains open with the option to someday close. Closing the group has fostered an experience of community among members that is complemented by a sense of responsibility among group members for regular attendance and mutual, reciprocal support.

Cofacilitators

Two facilitators are preferable to one. Using cofacilitators provides each facilitator peer support, offers an opportunity to explore different perspectives, and lessens the stress that would be placed on only one (Klein & Fletcher, 1987). Cofacilitation helps to balance and stabilize the group, augment any deficiencies in one of the facilitators, provide for continuity when one facilitator is absent, and improve understanding among the facilitators. How much emotional distance facilitators should keep between themselves and group members is controversial. There are some who maintain that strict boundaries are important. The more therapeutic the group's focus, the more the distinction between members and facilitator is important. However, there is value in peer-based facilitation that includes the facilitators as participants. Although this approach involves some risk, group members (and certainly facilitators) benefit from involvement of the facilitators in the group process.

"The single most critical issue with any group is the quality of the facilitation, regardless of the credential of the facilitator" (Odets, 1995, p. 272). Facilitators must be prepared to handle conflict and work to provide a safe container for strong emotions that may include intense anger. Facilitators will set the tone of the group early in its existence by modeling supportive behavior and by explicitly stating the group's values and objectives. In a multiple-loss group, it is important in early sessions to repeatedly define multiple loss in the broadest terms. Members will wonder whether their issues really qualify. They almost always do because losses from AIDS permeate all parts of the survivor's life.

The nature of the issues inevitably raised in group can lead to an exclusively negative focus marked more by doom than hope. Yalom (1985) asserted the need for group leaders to instill and maintain hope. It is useless to contrive hope in the face of the reality of AIDS; one way, however, that the facilitator can imbue hope is to call "attention to the improvements that members have made" (p. 7). These are often more substantial than the individual survivor recognizes.

A certain amount of education about the grief process and theoretical understanding related to multiple AIDS-related loss is ideal. Ideal times to present this information arise naturally at the beginning and end of the group and can be directly connected to the group process as it is unfolding. For example, it helps to inform participants that grief work is painful but that unresolved grief is usually more troublesome. Mainly, "the educational process is implicit" (Yalom, 1985, p. 10). Ideally, when facilitators participate in the group they inevitably share material or process that is helpful.

Support groups whose only goal is providing emotional support are less helpful to survivors than groups that include a therapeutic component, although this part should remain nondirective, unobtrusive, and subtle. Members of the group may not even realize that a therapeutic element is regularly introduced; this requires the skillful intervention of facilitators. A group whose sole purpose is to provide support will inevitably encourage "the development or strengthening of existing psychological defenses against conflict, rather than clarification and resolution of the conflict" (Odets, 1995, p. 272). A weekly gathering to make members feel better is not the optimal goal; the group should "help people attain the insight that allows them to make themselves feel better" (Odets, 1995, p. 275).

Facilitators need to receive support for their work. Multiple-loss groups tend to be intense experiences with a wide variety of issues presented each week. Facilitators should prepare for each week's session and, most important, take time after the meeting to debrief. This is an opportunity to express emotions that arose during the group so they are not carried away, becoming a burden on the facilitator. It is also a time to plan any interventions that may be necessary.

RITUALS FOR HEALING

Rituals are extremely useful to commemorate loss, provide a point of separation, and mark memories. Although greatly varied, rituals of one kind or another provide survivors of multiple AIDS-related loss with a valuable tool for healing. Rituals are rites, formal procedures, solemn observances, customs that are practiced to commemorate something. They symbolize transition, healing, and continuity (van der Hart, 1983). They derive their power from the participant; possessing no innate magic, the survivor invests the ritual with meaning. Rituals are a form of holistic healing, as evidenced by "the way they affect our minds, will, and heart. Rituals stir passions" (Kollar, 1989, p. 272).

"Rituals can be particularly helpful in assisting an individual or family to successfully resolve grief" (Rando, 1984, p. 105). Rituals are an excellent way to actualize the loss, symbolizing its irrevocable nature. Rituals that persist over time, on a schedule, provide a structured time for remembering and bearing witness. Shared rituals counteract isolation and strengthen communities. For survivors of multiple AIDS-related loss, rituals are particularly important in providing a means of communicating suffering, especially given the fact that survivors experience stigmatization in regard to their grief (Hodge, 1993). The disenfranchised griever is alienated, so community rituals are even more important (Kollar, 1989). Shrader (1992) discovered that some survivors found certain rituals to be helpful and includes an example from one survivor.

> What I ended up doing was I took the address book, I've gone through three of them now, you fill in the names of those who have died and scratch them off. I just took the pages out, of the scratched off names, and . . . said a little prayer for them, and then burned it up, and that really, that was helpful. You know, it's gone, this physical act of getting rid of it and watching as it goes up in smoke. (p. 122)

Leave-Taking Ceremonies

Leave-taking ceremonies such as memorial services, funerals, and wakes are the most common form of ritual for most deaths, including AIDS. These are extremely important to the survivor's healing. These ceremonies fulfill a number of valuable functions (Fulton, 1995). They interrupt the routine of daily life, make the loss real, permit expression of authentic emotion, provide public recognition of the loss, offer opportunities for support, and provide a point of transition in the connection between the survivor and the deceased.

> They allow us to assemble, to experience feelings about the losses, to see that others experience apparently similar feelings, and (perhaps) to understand our own. In such shared events, the losses become real and important, instead of simply remaining disturbing figments of subjective experience. It is in this sense that bearing witness is most powerful and important: that we recognize and share each other's internal experience of the public event, and thus supply the event with public meaning that can be reinternalized by the grieving individual. Thus shared and formed by social recognition, the subjective grief somehow becomes more bearable. (Odets, 1995, p. 268)

Ideally, a leave-taking ceremony demonstrates "the community's understanding of the relationship of the living to those who have died" (Kollar, 1989, p. 274), which serves to counteract the negative effect of stigmatization and disenfranchised grief. "Sorrows tend to be diminished by the knowledge that another sorrows with us" (Fulton, 1995, p. 269).

In the gay community, memorial services have become routine, and survivors have developed various ways of incorporating them into their lives. Shrader (1992) explained,

> Memorial service, funerals, and "celebrations of life" have become part of the mainstay of urban Gay existence. While the sheer numbers of memorial service were seen as overwhelming, many of the subjects found that, for the people the survivors were close to, the services have become a way to honor and truly celebrate the deceased. . . . Another way of taking care of themselves, for many of the men, however, was giving themselves permission to stop going to memorial services, except for people to whom they were close. (p. 122)

Opinion is divided regarding the necessity for survivors to attend memorial services. Of course, some survivors could not attend every service for every person they knew who died of AIDS. However, to miss the services of those who are close to the survivor (see the Circles of Relationship, Figure 1 in chapter 3) is inviting complications. First, the decision to avoid memorial services may indicate a tendency to avoid the work of grief and may fit a pattern of accumulating unresolved grief. Second, to miss the memorial service is to miss an ideal opportunity to grieve and receive support. Third, there is only one opportunity to participate in a deceased person's memorial service, and many survivors report feeling regret, and sometimes guilt, after missing the service. Unless attendance at the memorial service is replaced by another ritual that fulfills most of the same functions, survivors set themselves up for accumulated, unresolved grief. In most cases, decisions to give oneself permission to miss a service are actually denial-based avoidance decisions that are self-defeating.

A Variety of Rituals

The variety of rituals used by survivors of multiple AIDS-related loss is impressive and offers so many possibilities that anyone can find some that are personally meaningful. Rituals that have been helpful to survivors are discussed below. This list is by no means exhaustive, but it is provided to present the variety of options available.

The Names Project Quilt   Although the Quilt has grown too large to display in one place except in very special circumstances, sections of the Quilt are regularly displayed. Witnessing the Quilt can be done individually or collectively. Solitary survivors walk the aisles between the panels and personally commemorate and remember their losses. Small groups view the panels together, hugging and providing each other support.

Keeping Lists and Boxes   Some survivors have endeavored to keep lists of all their losses to AIDS. Most, however, gave up trying to keep track long ago. Others have kept letters, photos, memorial service programs, and other objects of remembrance in a box they can return to whenever it seems appropriate. Mitch, a survivor of multiple loss, described himself as "a curator without a museum." One survivor described her method.

> I started out with one box several years ago. But, you know, over the years it turned into two boxes and now it's three. I don't know what I am ever going to do with all this stuff but it helps to know it's there. The boxes also keep it contained. At first, these things were spread all over my home.

Collecting Photographs   Photos take on a special importance in the age of AIDS. Survivors often make a special point of having photos of all their loved ones. Survivors without photos are often distressed when they cannot recall the face of a certain friend. These provide tangible ways to remember.

A number of survivors keep scrapbooks that include photos but may also include other things such as programs from memorial services. Lately, videos have been used to allow the people with AIDS to say what they want to those who will survive their deaths. The video offers a more satisfying way to remember those who have died than a photograph. For children who are orphaned by AIDS

> a "life book" which is composed of photographs or pictures and the child's own life story, including the parents and other family members, can be created and read to the child. This book can accompany him or her in future placements, and added to as appropriate. (Dubik-Unruh, 1989, p. 10)

One survivor carefully selects a frame whenever a close friend dies and displays the photo, along with many others, above his living room fireplace mantel. "I combine photos of my grandparents who have died along with my friends who have died. When I am sitting on the couch and look up at the wall, I remember. It's a way for me to always remember."

Marking Anniversary Dates Birthdays, deathdays, holidays, and other special days are sometimes commemorated each year in memory of a special loved one's death. This is an excellent way to acknowledge an anniversary and counter the negative effects that may arise on anniversary dates. One survivor buys a gift for his dead partner each year, even wrapping it in special paper.

Mementos People who are dying of AIDS sometimes make special efforts to leave mementos to their friends and family. These are especially treasured because they give the survivor something physical to hold that was meaningful to the deceased. These mementos are sometimes distributed at the memorial service and include shells, Christmas ornaments, and, in at least one case, the ashes of the deceased divided into small envelopes.

Spreading Ashes Most people who die from AIDS are cremated, leaving the ashes to their family or an especially close friend. The journey to a special place, and the act of spreading the ashes, is a wonderful—if painful—opportunity for families of choice and origin to come together for healing. In some cities, where a large number of gay men have died from AIDS, a special location becomes known for having been the "final resting spot" for many people who died of AIDS. Morgan, who had survived many AIDS losses before his death from AIDS, talked about "going to the Arboretum and looking at the plants and flowers and knowing that many of my friends were there."

Installing a Permanent Marker The traditional marker for a death is a gravestone, but the prevalence of cremation and scattering of ashes has left many survivors without a physical place to visit. Some survivors have placed a bench in a park or planted a tree to commemorate their loved one.

Writing the Obituary   When a person dies, writing the obituary may be a collective effort. It provides an excellent opportunity to reminisce. Many who die from AIDS have life histories that are divided between family of choice and the early years and their friends and adult lives. The writing of the obituary provides a time to bring these parts of the deceased's life together.

Building a Shrine or Special Place   Some survivors have built a special place where certain mementos and personally significant symbols help them commemorate losses. Many light a special candle or several small ones. The ritual place may include photos of special loved ones, shells, souvenirs, or jewelry. It is entirely individual and derives its meaning from its evolving character.

Visiting a Special Site   Survivors may select a special site where they go to remember. It might be a place they previously visited with a certain loved one or it may be a location with a view or by water. It is a place where some survivors report being able to talk with their deceased loved one. They can go there and feel reconnected.

Releasing Balloons   Memorial services sometimes include helium balloons tied to the chairs in which the mourners sit. After the service, survivors are invited to take a balloon outside where they can release it. This ritual allows each survivor to individually invest the balloon and its release with meaning. Because it is done in a group, and is witnessed, it helps validate the final "letting-go" act of releasing the balloon.

Weekly Support Groups   Weekly support groups can take on an element of ritual for many survivors. Those who have HIV and attended a group with others who have now died see their weekly attendance at group as important to commemorating the losses and remembering former group members.

CONCLUSION

Survivors of multiple AIDS-related loss face a disaster with unique characteristics for which new treatment and recovery approaches are being developed. The next two chapters are most certainly not the final word on the issue. Rather, they are meant as a starting point for survivors, clinicians, professionals, and scholars. Toward the end of this second decade of the AIDS epoch, attention is shifting away from explaining the problems arising from surviving multiple AIDS-related loss toward finding helpful ways for survivors to promote their own recovery. Clinical interventions are being developed for treating survivors This is a process in its very early stages. Those who are working in this field need to do so collaboratively so that insights and approaches are shared to benefit survivors.

Chapter 12

Professional Issues in the Treatment of Survivors

If I am not for myself, who will be for me?
But if I am only for myself, what am I?
And if not now, when?
—Hillel, a Jewish teacher from the 1st century B.C.

This chapter is addressed to the professional who works with survivors of multiple AIDS-related loss. Although counselors are referred to throughout this chapter, it is directed at psychotherapists and social workers and could also be useful to volunteer caregivers such as persons who offer emotional support. Many survivors seek professional help for coping with the significant issues that arise from living in the AIDS epoch. This chapter covers the characteristics that make a therapist most effective. The counselor needs to be aware of the unique issues that this disaster presents. Functions of therapy include education, the need to mitigate social support breakdowns, empowerment of the client, and bearing witness to the client's experience. Assessment should include an evaluation of the client's strengths, coping skills, previous losses, concurrent stressors, and extent of impact from multiple loss. Professionals, and others, are often perplexed by the continuation or resumption of behaviors that place

noninfected persons at high risk for contracting HIV. An analysis of the psychodynamic reasons for this behavior is offered. Countertransference issues may be
a concern, especially for lesbian and gay therapists. The chapter concludes by
discussing ways to prevent the effects of secondary traumatization from working with these clients and discusses the importance of self-care.

Survivors of multiple AIDS-related loss are motivated to seek professional
counseling or therapy for a number of reasons. Although clients may come to
therapy seeking relief from problems and pain, the therapist should maintain a
perspective of opportunity. The survivor can be challenged to undertake much
personal growth and integration of values through this experience.

Research has supported the self-evident reasons that survivors will seek
professional help. Martin (1988) found a correlation between psychological distress and the number of deaths a survivor faced and concluded that bereaved
men were "significantly more likely to seek psychological help" than nonbereaved
men (p. 861). Martin and Dean (1993a) found that "nearly four times as many
bereaved men increased or initiated visits to psychologists or psychiatrists in an
effort to cope with fears about AIDS" (p. 327). Sometimes "the only available
support for dealing with their grief issues is that provided by a mental health
professional" (Klein, 1994, p. 19).

CHARACTERISTICS AND ATTRIBUTES OF THE COUNSELOR

The most helpful counselor is one who has the fundamental skills necessary for
psychotherapeutic work and is aware of the special issues confronted in multiple
AIDS-related loss. The personal qualities of the caregiver significantly affect
quality of care; "some persons are better suited to offer bereavement care than
others" (Martocchio, 1985, p. 337). Lindy et al. (1983) studied the characteristics of successful therapeutic engagement for survivors of the Beverly Hills
Supper Club Fire. They determined that trust between client and counselor was
required. The client needs to feel comfortable. Second, the more successful
"therapist was genuinely moved by the survivor and his experience" (Lindy et
al., p. 606). The best counselors will possess the following characteristics:

- good communication skills
- empathy, sensitivity, and compassion
- personal presence, the ability to be with people
- awareness of personal limitations (Lattanzi, 1982).

Features of this disaster and characteristics of survivors also suggest the importance of other characteristics in the counselor. Those with a solid grounding in
treating complicated bereavement and traumatization bring a foundation of skills
necessary to this work. It is useful to have a background in existential psychotherapy given the inevitability of these issues being raised by survivors of
multiple loss (see chapter 9).

Counselors must assess whether they are comfortable working with the population most likely to be affected by multiple AIDS-related loss, especially homosexuals and IVDUs. A variety of researchers have observed that minority groups often receive ineffective or harmful mental health treatment (Acosta, Yamamoto, & Evans, 1982). A history of homophobia in mental health professionals has been well documented (DeCrescenzo, 1985; Riley & Greene, 1993).

Counselors must have an attitude that is not simply tolerant of or accepting of differences but, ideally, closer to an attitude that cherishes diversity and appreciates the unique concerns of these populations. Klein (1994) asserted that the counselor is required to have "a great deal of self-awareness regarding attitudes, thoughts, and responses" to alternative lifestyles. "There is no place for therapists who question the validity of the client's sexual orientation" (p. 20). "If the therapist's awareness and information about these communities and lifestyles is limited, the client should be referred to a practitioner knowledgeable of the client's community patterns" (Siegal & Hoefer, 1981, pp. 523–524). Multiple AIDS-related loss in the gay community "can only be dealt with in the context of the gay and lesbian life experience" (Dworkin & Kaufer, 1995, p. 56).

The counselor must also possess a competent level of knowledge about AIDS. Clients prefer therapists with special training or experience working with people with AIDS (Neimeyer & Stewart, in press). Nothing alienates a survivor faster than questions that demonstrate ignorance about AIDS; clients should not have to stop their therapeutic process to educate the counselor. The fact that so much of society ignores or minimizes losses from AIDS makes survivors particularly sensitive to any perception that the counselor is similarly ignorant. Knowledge about AIDS should include information about community resources, especially support group options.

FUNCTIONS OF THERAPY

Counselors are in an ideal position to bear witness to survivors of multiple AIDS-related loss. Simply the act of being present and listening to the survivor's story is healing. Odets (1995) noted that

> Psychotherapists bear witness to the feelings and insights of patients, and this is one reason that so much good psychotherapy is conducted with the therapist's silence, or with his or her spare reflections or clarifications, which the patient can reinternalize. . . . I am always surprised by how much psychotherapy is accomplished by simply allowing patients to exist *as themselves* in front of me. (p. 268)

A simple, sincerely empathetic presence will go a long way toward facilitating the client's recovery because it directly counteracts the impact of disenfranchised grief, stigmatization, and isolation while mitigating survivor's guilt and anxiety. The "therapist and client both benefit from remembering that the goal of psychotherapy is to provide comfort and support rather than a 'cure' for death anxiety, depression or the AIDS virus itself" (Neimeyer & Stewart, in press).

The traumatic effects of multiple, ongoing loss have a dehumanizing effect. Titchener and Kapp (1976) observed that "every disaster places man at the mercy of forces beyond his control. The feelings of being a pawn of fate is dehumanizing—people feel without appeal, beyond empathy, and cannot be persuaded or assuaged" (p. 299). They concluded, however, that "dehumanization may be mitigated by corrective experiences with empathic people in the helping professions" (p. 299). This is a useful perspective for the counselor to maintain. At times, work with survivors may seem perpetually ineffective because of the overwhelming and continual nature of this disaster, but healing does occur when the survivor is encountered at a human level.

Psychoeducational efforts are a primary intervention that should be used when counseling survivors of multiple loss. First, all survivors need to hear and hear again that they are living through an abnormal phenomenon. Whenever a client judgmentally questions his or her responses to this disaster, the therapist must return again to normalizing the abnormal. Statements such as these are appropriate:

"Of course you feel overwhelmed and anxious. Who wouldn't after going through what you are going through?

"It's perfectly natural that you break down and cry unpredictably."

"It's understandable that you are very, very angry."

"Your children are dying of AIDS, all of your nephews have died, many friends are dead or dying. Who wouldn't feel like their life was crumbling?"

As mentioned earlier in this book, the client must be persuaded to understand that recovery from multiple AIDS-related loss is hard work. It will absolutely require a diligent, committed, consistent effort, and it will, at times, be painful. There is no way through the work without pain. This reality implies that the survivor who undertakes the work is a strong person, motivated and interested in self-improvement. The attributes that allow the survivor to pursue this work should regularly be explicitly stated during therapy because of the tendency of survivors to feel out of control and, therefore, weak and powerless.

This type of encouragement serves to empower the client. It is important that the counselor not focus exclusively on the problems presented by the client. "Deficit, disease, and dysfunction metaphors are deeply rooted in clinical social work" (Cowger, 1994, p. 262), and the emphasis has, according to Cowger, been on diagnosing abnormality and pathology.

> Promoting empowerment means believing that people are capable of making their own choices and decisions. It means not only that human beings possess the strengths and potential to resolve their own difficult life situations, but also that they increase their strength and contribute to society by doing so. (p. 264)

A better summarization of the counselor's role with survivors of multiple AIDS-related loss could not be written. The counselor should help clients assess their own situation, identify what they want, explore alternative ways to achieve those goals, and encourage them in their efforts to meet them.

ASSESSMENT ISSUES

Assessment is a collaborative effort, guided by an informed professional who is well aware of the many complications suffered by survivors of multiple AIDS-related loss. The trained professional must always assess a client's risk to him- or herself or others, especially because suicidal risk may be implicit and indirect. Clients will present with a variety of problems, including anxiety, debilitating anhedonia, other symptoms of depression, mood-altering chemical abuse, relationship problems, developmental crises, existential angst, somatic complaints, and others. The counselor who is informed about issues of multiple AIDS-related loss will be alert to the possibility that survivor's issues may be an underlying contributing factor, especially when a client comes from a high-risk group for being a survivor (e.g., hemophiliac, homosexual, IVDU, inner-city minority).

If the clinician suspects that multiple AIDS-related loss may be a factor, certain inquiries should be made. Clients may be oblivious to any link between multiple loss and their complaints. In normal grief situations, "many times people come for medical or psychiatric care unaware of the dynamics of grief, and this requires that the clinician help make the diagnosis" (Worden, 1991, p. 75). Uroda (1977) believed that "intake interviews should always get information on the significant losses in a client's life" (p. 191). These can begin generally and become more specific when warranted. For example,

> **Counselor:** *What is your history with loss?*
> **Client:** *I don't know. I've had a few but so has everybody.*
> **Counselor:** *What loss is most important to you?*
> **Client:** *Oh, that's easy. John. He died of AIDS several years ago and I just don't seem to be able to get him off my mind. It still hurts terribly.*
> **Counselor:** *How many other losses have you had to AIDS?*
> **Client:** *Oh! I don't know. I've never kept track. Twenty, 30? If you count everyone I know, I guess it may be 50 or more. (Angrily) Why are you asking me about that? I came in here to get help with my depression. Is that so hard for you to understand?*

In this hypothetical exchange, the counselor has already received four pieces of important information: The client has suffered multiple loss, has an overshadowing death, does not yet possess insight about the affect of multiple loss on his life, and appears to become easily angry. Later, after a period of building trust as a foundation of the therapeutic relationship, the counselor should return to the issues of multiple loss as a possible cause of the depression with which the client presented. Assessment may take several sessions, and the counselor should not rush the process, trying to finish assessing in the first meeting with the client. For clients without the insight to connect their experience of multiple loss with their presenting symptom, a rushed approach will likely result in the client's deciding that the counselor does not understand. This eventuality is particularly dangerous because it may color the client's perspective on counseling as a helpful way to cope with multiple loss.

The manner in which the survivor of multiple loss has coped with not only AIDS-related loss but other losses is information that should be obtained in the assessment process. Positive adjustment to prior losses and stresses can be therapeutic by teaching the mourner what is necessary to cope and what strategies have been helpful and unhelpful (Rando, 1993). Asking outright "How have you coped with those losses?" can yield valuable information because it inevitably says much about healthy and unhealthy coping skills. For lesbian and gay clients, assessment of previous loss must include direct questions about their coming-out process, family of origin, and early history in coming to terms with their own sexuality. Answers to this and follow-up questions will be useful in planning future interventions.

Questions that elicit information about preexisting problems and concurrent stressors that may be affecting the client's response to AIDS are valuable. Many survivors of multiple AIDS-related loss have preexisting psychiatric concerns such as depression, personality disorder, or substance abuse. Those with preexisting Axis II diagnosis will have a much more difficult time because of the impact this condition has on establishing and maintaining necessary social support. However, clients who bring strong skills and sound mental health to their experience with AIDS will fare better.

> To the extent that the mourner brings sound mental health, achievement of appropriate object relationship, good ego strength, hardiness, healthy self-esteem, effective communication skills, emotional resilience, appropriate coping resources, capacity to express emotion, a mature personality, optimism, and a transcendent belief system to bear on mourning, it appears clear that the individual will have an advantage. (Rando, 1993, p. 461)

When inquiry turns to the effect of AIDS on the client's life, one of the first lines of questions might include determining what attributions the survivor makes about AIDS. Again, begin generally and become more specific. Answers to these questions may inform the counselor about the impact of stigmatization and disenfranchisement on the client's grief process. How others in the client's life have been supportive, or not, may elicit information about the client's families of origin and choice. The counselor may learn that he or she is the only source of social support available to the client at this time.

Assessments with this population must include evaluating the impact of traumatization. In survivors of non-AIDS-related trauma, presentation of trauma as the issue necessitating the need for counseling is rare.

> Few people who have been traumatized feel enough outside confirmation to present trauma as their problem; instead, they present issues such as difficulty in relationships, depression, or substance abuse, even though trauma may be the core of the suffering. (Jay, 1994, p. 32)

As mentioned in the previous chapter, collaborative use of the *Diagnostic and Statistical Manual of Mental Disorders* (American Psychiatric Association, 1994) is a valuable resource for assisting clients to recognize their experiences as traumatic.

Gradually, clients who are suffering the effects of multiple AIDS-related loss will connect their history of loss with symptoms they are experiencing. This process is helped by a counselor who educates the survivor on the characteristics of unresolved grief, complicated bereavement, and traumatization.

CONTINUED HIV INFECTION RISK BEHAVIORS

Great perplexity is expressed about why people continue to engage in high-risk behaviors for contracting HIV. Questions such as the following are expressed and thought: "Why does she continue to make love with him without a condom?" "Why don't they use clean needles?" "Why do gay men continue to engage in unprotected anal intercourse?" All of these questions come from a perspective outside the world of multiple AIDS-related loss and show a lack of understanding of the psychological dimension of life in the center of the AIDS epoch. The psychological implications embedded in the destruction of the survivor's assumptive world have everything to do with the reason why some people continue to engage in risky behaviors and why public education campaigns to discourage risky behaviors have been only marginally effective. HIV infection continues to happen at rates that alarm many. Between 40,000 and 80,000 people become infected with HIV each year in the United States (Neergaard, 1996).

Because little information is available about continued risky behaviors involving male-to-female sex or sharing of needles, the following discussion focuses on the behavior most heavily studied in connection with HIV prevention: gay male sex. There is, however, no reason to suppose that the psychological issues faced by gay male survivors of multiple loss are altogether different than those faced by other survivors. The same psychodynamics are applicable to a variety of people who behave in ways that are patently dangerous for contracting HIV.

Focus groups sponsored by the Department of Public Health to identify issues that might be causing gay and bisexual men to continue practicing unsafe sex found remarkable similarity among participants, according to Van Gorder (1994).

These issues included powerful feelings of depression, numbness and denial about the epidemic, overwhelming grief and loss, low self-esteem and the effects of rampant homophobia and racism, ageism and a fear of growing older, the need for greater intimacy, a desire to live fuller sexual lives, the need to feel that others care about them, the need for a greater sense of community, and a poorly defined sense of future. (p. 2)

Most of these issues have precisely to do with violations to the survivor's assumptive world, especially concerns for greater community and a predictable future. Surely, these men did not grow up expecting, or preparing, to deal with overwhelming grief and loss, forced isolation, or the threat of psychological disintegration. How could these survivors be anything but ill equipped to cope with multiple AIDS-related loss?

Odets (1995) offered a psychological interpretation of high-risk gay sex that is both insightful and chilling.

From a psychological perspective, when educated gay men engage in unprotected anal intercourse with serodiscordant or sero-unknown partners, we must assume that the behavior has meaning that should be understood. When protected sex would be appropriate, ambivalence about it or the failure to practice it suggests in part that a man is experiencing ambivalence about surviving the epidemic and his identity as HIV-negative. The knowing exposure of oneself to HIV suggests in part the desire, usually ambivalent and unconscious, not to survive. (p. 188)

Unprotected sex and sharing needles are ways to avoid being a survivor of multiple AIDS-related loss. The risk involved in such behavior is the motive for engaging in it.

The assumptive world of the gay survivor of multiple AIDS-related loss is turned upside down. Instead of assuming that one will live to an average old age, the assumption becomes an early death from AIDS. Many gay men have a sense of inevitability about contracting HIV (Odets, 1994, p. 11). Why not get it over with and escape the anxiety of uncertainty? One survivor of multiple AIDS-related loss was seen by the author in psychotherapy. Brian chose to regularly expose himself to HIV by visiting adult video stores and public parks where he would have sex with strangers, usually as the receptive partner of unprotected anal intercourse. At the same time, Brian reported extreme anxiety about his HIV status and regularly (every month or two) got tested for HIV. Each time the test was negative, he was troubled by his contradictory reaction of relief and disappointment. Brian felt out of control and was terribly upset over his inability to stop putting himself at high risk for HIV. Yet, underneath his words was a longing for the inevitable day when the uncertainty would end with a positive HIV test. When therapy began to focus on his feelings and thoughts about surviving when so many had not, Brian abruptly terminated therapy. Looking at issues around surviving contradicted his assumption that he could not survive, which evoked an anxiety worse that the threat of HIV infection.

Deciding to quit worrying about gradations of risk calms the survivor. In this light, other self-destructive behaviors become understandable. Sex had been readily combined with alcohol and drug abuse before AIDS. If survivors shut down their worry about contracting HIV by adopting a carefree attitude toward sex, there is little reason to prohibit themselves from using drugs and enjoying themselves to the fullest. Many survivors derive great comfort and relief by giving in to an assumptive world that presupposes an early death from AIDS.

This sense of inevitability easily translates into a sense of hopelessness and helplessness. Assumptions that include a future of continuing loss and personal vulnerability easily transform into depression, anhedonia, suicidal ideation, sleep disturbances, anxiety, diffuse rage, and personality changes.

HIV prevention campaigns have almost exclusively focused on biological survival as the entire motive for HIV risk reduction. This approach ignores the fundamental dilemma posed by existence amid an incredible amount of suffering and threat. Lives must be worth living. It should surprise no one when a survivor of multiple AIDS-related loss is unwilling to exert effort to merely exist in a world that assumes a continuation of overwhelming pain and loss. Unfortunately, professional caregivers, social workers, and psychotherapists often collude with this cycle. Those who continue to test negative for HIV are discouraged from contemplating the reasonableness of choosing not to survive. How, then, can they be expected to authentically contemplate what it means to choose to survive?

COUNTERTRANSFERENCE AND OVERIDENTIFICATION

Multiple AIDS-related loss provokes a number of topics that may overlap with the counselor's own issues and concerns. Countertransference can be understood as the therapist's responses to a given client and what that client represents to the therapist (Pearlman & Saakvitne, 1995). It is an unconscious process involving the therapist's unresolved conflicts, both positive and negative (Dunkel & Hatfield, 1986). "Countertransference feelings, if not recognized, can raise havoc in treatment" (Cerney, 1995, p. 135).

A number of issues related to surviving multiple AIDS-related loss, or being a member of one of the high-risk populations, can provoke countertransference. These can include fear of the unknown, fear of contagion, fear of dying and death, fear of helplessness, fear of homosexuality, overidentification, anger, and the need for professional omnipotence (Dunkel & Hatfield, 1986). The counselor might share the experience of stigmatization with a devalued population and, perhaps, unresolved concerns about his or her own sexual identity. Strong experiences and emotions in the client may be taken on by the counselor. This can make counselors "feel inept and inadequate when they become aware of their own countertransference feelings and behavior" (Cerney, 1995, p. 133).

Survivors of multiple, ongoing loss are likely to feel fearful of abandonment and may transfer these fears onto the counselor. If counselors take on this potential role as an abandoner, they might either carry it out or so strongly seek to avoid carrying it out that they avoid taking vacations and sick days. Psychotherapists, as a group, are more "prone to experiencing survivor's guilt" (Odets, 1995, p. 43). Issues of survivor's guilt can get very complicated and convoluted; therefore, counselors who experience it will need to be particularly aware and cautious that their guilt does not collude with or promote the survivors'.

Counselors can experience particular difficulty in hearing clients talk about some of the physical symptoms that frequently accompany AIDS. They may feel revulsion and disgust. They may think to themselves that the client is exaggerating. "I can't believe anyone has seen this much suffering or experienced that many deaths." Detachment can look like objectivity and replace empathy.

Counselors working with gay men and lesbians face unique issues of countertransference. Work with persons affected by AIDS may challenge the counselor's level of comfort in working with gay men and lesbians (Mancoske & Lindhorst, 1995, p. 35). If a counselor feels disgust or judgment when a gay man discusses his gay lifestyle, therapy will be negatively affected. After listening to a gay man discuss a sexual history that is far from the counselor's experience, the counselor may develop an attitude that "those gays are getting what they deserve."

Widespread stigmatization presupposes that some counselors will feel either sympathetic or critical of the stigmatized. Countertransference issues, based on the perceived culpability of survivors, is an issue that demands attention. Sprang and McNeil (1995) wrote that

> The attitude of the clinician then becomes a primary therapeutic issue. To deal effectively with the surviving family and friends after a stigmatized death, the clinician must assume an attitude that communicates, unequivocally, a nonjudgmental acceptance of the bereaved and must allow for open catharsis within the safety of the therapeutic relationship. (p. 170)

Sprang and McNeil went on to acknowledge the counselor who is struggling with these issues but is willing to attempt a sincere effort at working effectively with survivors of stigmatizing grief. First, they recommended education appropriate to the concerns at hand. Second, resolution of the counselor's personal issues "is an essential component in a healthy therapeutic relationship" (p. 171). Counselors who are well educated about issues relevant to gays and lesbians and counselors who have had exposure to gays and lesbians are best able to work with this population.

Counselors who are themselves survivors of multiple AIDS-related loss are prone to feelings of overidentification. Many of the same counselors who now work with survivors were brought to this work through their early and prolonged work connected to AIDS. Those therapists who have worked with clients of multiple loss or been active in caregiving for people with AIDS are particularly susceptible to countertransference.

> Vicarious traumatization increases the therapist's susceptibility to certain counter-transference responses. If one is suffering from vicarious traumatization, one's countertransference responses may be less readily recognizable and can become problematic in the therapy with adult survivors. (Pearlman & Saakvitne, 1995, p. 156)

With overidentification, the ability to return to an objective stance is compromised. "This can result in the worker's investing unrealistic amounts of time and energy in the client, fusing personal needs and professional responsibilities, and, in extreme cases, generating symptom formation" (Dunkel & Hatfield, 1986, p. 116).

Gay therapists are in an ideal position to understand the concerns and feelings of their clients who are gay survivors. Although they have "an awareness of pertinent issues from personal and social experience," they "may not have analyzed or conceptualized their observations" (Dworkin & Kaufer, 1995, p. 54). For a gay therapist who identifies strongly with many of the issues presented by a gay client suffering multiple loss, overidentification is almost certainly a concern. Overidentification can be a problem for a therapist when a patient comes from a similar background in terms of culture, social values, and experience (Cerney, 1995). Alternatively, counselors may tend to minimize, negate, or invalidate aspects of the client's experience if the patient comes from a different background (Fischman, 1991). Thus, a gay therapist may minimize the experience of a hemophiliac mother or an inner-city Hispanic person.

"Methods for dealing with countertransference reactions include recognition of the value of these reactions in guiding the therapeutic process and willingness to monitor these feelings on a continuous basis" (Dunkel & Hatfield, 1986, p. 116). Many good sources exist to further the clinician's understanding of countertransference. Countertransference is not only a problem to be solved. It offers an opportunity for the counselor to understand the client's experience.

PREVENTING SECONDARY STRESS COMPLICATIONS

The professional counselor, and other caregivers, are well positioned to develop symptoms of secondary stress disorder, as discussed in chapter 7, on traumatization. Prevention is far and away the best approach to dealing with secondary stress. Yassen (1995) provided a useful resource for counselors interested in prevention of secondary traumatic stress. He offered a useful analysis on the concept of prevention, offered a number of specific components that comprise a dedicated prevention program, and discussed implementation of a prevention plan.

Staff training programs should incorporate "information on stress and its management, as well as on the physical and psychological impact of trauma, into emergency worker training programs" (McCammon & Allison, 1995, p. 117). Although the focus of secondary stress prevention is on individuals, "it is important to stress that it is not the individual's sole responsibility to prevent individual STSD [secondary traumatic stress disorder]" (Yassen, 1995, p. 206). Fortunately, many AIDS service organizations recognize the unique brand of stress arising from work in this crisis. Many, in fact, have strict rules about the number of client contact hours permitted and require a period of rejuvenation after a client's death. Regular support meetings, with opportunities to debrief, are useful. Caregivers who are given the regular opportunity to ventilate feelings are less likely to develop complications due to secondary stress. "Much secondary trauma can be avoided or its effects ameliorated if therapists seek regular supervision or consultation" (Cerney, 1995, p. 139).

Preventing secondary trauma involves strengthening social networks. Many AIDS service organizations have a strong sense of community. According to Munroe et al. (1995), the ideal context in which to prevent and treat secondary traumatization is through community.

> A community absorbs the traumatic experience of an individual by diffusing its effects among many people and demonstrating that the survivor's feelings are understood. . . . The community that validates the survivor and continues to include him or her as a valued member provides roles and relationship patterns that are not repetitions of the trauma. A team that validates the therapist's responses to secondary trauma . . . provides valued roles for its members. (p. 215)

Team members, in the community, can provide to survivors the conviction that there is meaning in the work they are doing and enable the counselor to maintain the valued role as healer.

In addition, despite the value of community, many preventative tasks—such as meditation, exercise, adequate sleep, proper nutrition, creative expression, contact with nature, humor, social support, and fostering a sense of balance—require the intent of the individual caregiver. AIDS work regularly draws people who have been deeply personally affected by the pandemic. If AIDS becomes the overriding focus of the professional and private life, secondary stress reactions are inevitable. This risk is heightened in the counselor who has come to this work as a result of personal losses and the need to make a difference. Often, the line between personal and professional lives becomes blurred. Counselors must work to foster balance in their lives. Pearlman and Saakvitne (1995) emphasized the need to maintain a personal life: "To combat the effects of vicarious traumatization, it is essential to have a fulfilling personal life . . . balancing work, play, and rest is essential to healthy functioning" (p. 166).

Needless to say, no one can treat or care for all survivors of multiple loss who are in need. A counselor must develop the skill of saying no. The difficulty in this goal should not be minimized. The needs are great; it is hard to see people suffer, and the counselor may know that he or she could make a helpful difference. A sense of heroism can develop among AIDS caregivers that fosters the belief that one can do a little more and one's work is indispensable. Despite this warning, which is repeated in nearly every psychotherapy class and article on self-care, "studies continue to find that many therapists hold the irrational belief that they must operate at peak efficiency and competence at all times with all patients" (Cerney, 1995, p. 139).

Self-care is absolutely critical for caregivers in the AIDS epoch. It is important not only for the counselor's health but also for effective work with clients. Garfield (1995) referred to the importance of self-acceptance in the wounded healer.

> Self-acceptance allows caregivers to face the challenge of AIDS work with a minimum of self-blame and severe self-doubt. Self-acceptance lets us say "yes" to life. It means I am a friend to myself, I care for myself—I am the same kind of compassionate caregiver to myself that I try to be for a client. (p. 255)

When prevention of secondary stress disorder has not proven adequate and the counselor requires therapeutic help, it is imperative that professional help be sought. This is not always easy, given the reluctance of some counselors to admit the need for help and the fear that this admission will indicate incompetence in their clinical abilities. "Because therapists who suffer secondary trauma exhibit many of the same symptoms as their patients, some of the same treatment methods can be effective" (Cerney, 1995, p. 141). Harris (1995) suggested a number of specific intervention suggestions. McCammon and Allison (1995) suggested eye movement desensitization and reprocessing as a treatment of choice for emergency workers to reduce the emotional impact of traumatic situations.

Garfield (1995) strongly advised, "If someone you know, or you yourself are experiencing burnout, or incipient traumatic stress syndrome, then serious intervention strategies are necessary, such as complete withdrawal from frontline caregiving, or even from AIDS work entirely, and/or professional help" (p. 265). This is a difficult situation for the professional and one likely to provoke feelings of shame and failure. Yet, personal health and professional effectiveness require that it be addressed periodically.

CONCLUSION

The professional who decides to work with survivors of multiple AIDS-related loss must only do so after carefully questioning his or her aptitude, attitudes, and motivation. Survivors are ill served by a therapist who is well meaning but who lacks the necessary knowledge to work effectively with clients who may come from different cultural backgrounds and may be dealing with specific issues about which the client will assume a level of expertise. Survivors have good reason to be impatient with professionals who continually break the flow of work to ask for explanations about AIDS treatments, opportunistic infections, sexual practices, or slang. Working with survivors of multiple loss also requires proficiency in grief and loss counseling and may require skill in working with traumatization. Professionals should take seriously their role in bearing witness to the survivor's story. The intervention of normalizing the abnormal will be repeatedly relevant.

It will be easy for the professional to miss the fact that the client's primary issue is surviving multiple AIDS-related loss. The client may complain of secondary concerns, and the professional may easily be distracted by a number of concurrent complaints. Although adequate assessment must include explication of problems, it should also emphasize determination of client strengths. These will be useful tools for the client's recovery process.

Supervision and regular case consultation is recommended not only because of the complexity of issues raised but also because of the propensity for professionals to have personal issues provoked by this work. Countertransference can be an asset in working with these clients, but it can also become a serious liability. The professional must be willing to hear honest feedback about the content of her or his work and any signs of secondary stress complications. Working with survivors of multiple loss is challenging work that will require the professional to pioneer new treatment approaches. Although work with survivors can be frustrating, difficult, and confusing, it can also be tremendously rewarding by providing opportunities for professional education and personal growth.

Chapter 13

Conclusions

Whoever does not, some time or other, . . . give his full consent, his full and joyous consent to the dreadfulness of life, can never take possession of the unutterable abundance and power of our existence; can only walk on its edge, and one day, when the judgment is given, will have been neither alive or dead—Rainer Maria Rilke (as cited in Garfield, 1995)

Surviving multiple AIDS-related loss is a historically unique disaster. This is not true because of the number of people affected. History has many examples of widespread disaster, although this one comes at a unique time in social history. Advances in science and medicine were supposed by many to have relegated such disasters to the past. AIDS proves that humans are still exposed to the whims of natural powers that sometimes dwarf human powers. What mainly makes multiple AIDS-related loss unique is the interconnection of so many social, psychological, political, and cultural factors that exacerbate its impact on survivors. Now, at the conclusion of this book, the reader is challenged to not view the various characteristics and factors of this phenomenon as separate influences on survivors' experiences. They all interrelate. The politics of AIDS, stigmatization, characteristics of the disease, lack of public support, cumulative and ongoing nature of this disaster, preponderance of unresolved grief and complicated bereavement symptoms, traumatization, etiology of HIV, multiplicity of losses, primary impact on minorities, and collective nature of loss all occur together, at the same time, to primarily the same people.

Other disasters imprint the public consciousness with much more impact, effect, and response than multiple AIDS-related loss. This is partly explained by the longevity of the AIDS epoch. Events that succinctly produce anguish are more efficient at provoking the public's short attention span and, therefore, better meet the commercial needs of profit-making news sources. Survivors of multiple loss notice the lack of attention their predicament receives. They are affronted, galled, exasperated, and furious about it. Survivors justifiably want their pain acknowledged, and they deserve compassion for their ongoing distress.

Multiple AIDS-related loss is minimized and belittled in comparison to other disasters. Survivors of multiple loss care about the pain that survivors of other disasters experience. In fact, their experience seems to strengthen their empathy for other victims. Nevertheless, the outpouring of attention that other disasters receive, even when they are comparatively minor in terms of the quantity of people affected, usually evokes a degree of bitterness. The Oklahoma City bombing, Tylenol contamination scare, toxic shock syndrome, O. J. Simpson trial, or Legionnaires Disease physically and tangibly affected very few people. Survivors of multiple AIDS-related loss rightly believe they deserve widespread public support for what they have endured.

Each of the events mentioned above stands out as a distinct event in public perception in a way that multiple AIDS-related loss still does not. The stark contrast between public perception and support for survivors is explainable by a number of factors. The fact that AIDS has focused its attention on disenfranchised, prestigmatized, and shunned groups is significant. The fact that the phenomenon of multiple AIDS-related loss has been evolving over nearly two decades makes it less attention provoking.

To comprehend this phenomenon requires a look at existential issues of meaning, responsibility, nonbeing, and essential isolation. It nearly always provokes challenges to spiritual beliefs. These are not issues in which modern society shows much interest. They always evoke an angst that is, at minimum, uncomfortable and, at most, shakes the very foundation of a person's existence. These are issues that most prefer to avoid.

Elie Wiesel, Victor Frankl, Bruno Bettelheim, and others have proven that a person did not need have survived the horrors of the death camps to learn from the experience of those who did. Similarly, one does not have to survive the impact of multiple AIDS-related loss to learn from, and benefit from, this experience.

This disaster challenges society on a number of fronts. From its impact on families of choice, the value of these families and the inadequacy of existing vocabulary to describe nontraditional relationships are exposed. Language must catch up with the social realities it now minimizes and belittles. Burkett (1995) asserted that AIDS demands not just an acknowledgment of a massive new medical crisis, but an admission that the nation's deepest problems—from racism to a crumbling health care system, from the corrupt relationship between corporations and researchers to teen alcoholism—still have not been solved. AIDS unmasks all of America's illusions about itself as modern, sophisticated, tolerant, even competent. The challenge of AIDS exceeds the national attention span and overloads the national capacity for self-reflection. (p. 304)

The long-range perspective that AIDS demands is needed but unlikely. AIDS has lost its crisis appeal and now must be addressed as the long-standing social disaster it is. Although this must happen, it probably will not. For example, the horrific medical mistreatment and shocking rejection of people with AIDS that were common in the early years of the AIDS epoch have mainly been replaced by better care and increased compassion. But what about the underlying issues that allowed these shameful acts to occur in the first place? Why has so much attention been paid to AIDS in Western postindustrial nations while so little has been paid to its staggering impact in parts of Africa? What social forces contribute to the reality of young homosexual men living lives that involve so much overt and subintentional suicide? AIDS has cast a bright light on some of society's greatest shortcomings.

Multiple AIDS-related loss has been instructive about issues that apply to social concerns other than AIDS. The impact of multiple loss had rarely been acknowledged or analyzed before this phenomenon. As a result of AIDS, much more is known about the impact of multiple, ongoing loss. Recovery and treatment issues are being developed because the need for them outstrips current theories and interventions. These new approaches may help other survivors of similar disasters. Many of the implications that this book presents are likely to apply to other forms of multiple, ongoing loss such as abuse and living in dangerous environments. Theories about grief and trauma are stretched by the circumstances of this event. Even a single death is a multiple loss, a fact borne out in the extreme realities of multiple deaths. The importance of incorporating existential and spiritual inquiry into the work of persons who have experienced major life disruption is illuminated. From the experience of survivors who are faring best, the value of helping others as a way to help one's self is proven.

THE FUTURE AND ITS CHALLENGES

The limitations of existing psychological diagnostic criteria are plainly seen in light of the multiple-loss survivor's experience. The lack of options available to professionals means that consideration must be given to developing diagnostic criteria that encompass the experience of people. Writing about the lack of a diagnosis for complicated bereavement, Rando (1993) concluded that "caregivers are forced to assign other diagnoses that have clinical implications unacceptable to many bereaved individuals" (p. 13). A number of authorities have argued for the need for diagnostic criteria that encompass the range of grieving responses, especially one that results in symptoms characteristic of complicated bereavement.

Although multiple AIDS-related loss is not strictly a bereavement issue, its affect on survivors, and the symptoms that result, demand a diagnostic category that adequately encompasses it. As mentioned in the conclusion of chapter 7 on trauma, the unique consequences of this disaster warrant the naming of a new syndrome: *multiple AIDS-related loss syndrome.*

What about the survivors of multiple AIDS-related loss after AIDS? There is little reason yet to assume a time after AIDS, but recent advances are making it increasingly likely that AIDS will become a chronic, if inevitably fatal condition. Life expectancy for persons with HIV continues to increase. Prophylactic treatments that prevent many opportunistic infections already make the horrors of the disease process less severe. A shift in the infected person's prognosis would result in profound changes in the survivor's experience. The roller coaster experience of survivors would become a great deal smoother, leveled out by increasing gaps of time between deaths. Survivors would have increased time to work through their grief between deaths. A sense of equilibrium would be easier to maintain with a slower pace of sickness and death.

Even with the potential for improvement in the characteristics of AIDS, which make unresolved grief and traumatization so likely, survivors will be left with scars for the rest of their lives. Some of the impact and pain of loss will endure. Historic precedent bears out this conclusion. "Even after the Holocaust, the feeling of loss did not subside" (Kaminer & Lavie, 1993, p. 331). After the plague had run its course, in Camus's book, survivors went on living by its standards (Camus, 1948). Those standards vary by survivor and are not all bad.

Many survivors report personal growth and a deepening of interpersonal relationships that they gratefully credit to their experience with AIDS. These survivors will cling to the advantages AIDS has fostered. The experience of surviving this disaster may "inoculate" survivors to the adverse effects of future life traumas. This outcome is true for those who have "successful experiences in coping with trauma" (Sprang & McNeil, 1995, p. 113). After a flood in southeastern Kentucky, Norris and Murrell (1988) found support for an inoculation hypothesis. Comparing the victims of a southeastern Kentucky flood with previous flood experience to flood-naive victims, they found an advantage for the "inoculated" survivors. They developed less postdisaster psychiatric disturbance. Those who have been relatively successful in coping with multiple AIDS-related loss may be better able to cope with future life stresses.

However, survivors whose basic ability to trust has been compromised, whose interpersonal relationships have become marked by distance, and who have developed self-destructive coping responses may find these negative consequences enduring for the rest of their life. At the very least, difficult and long-term psychotherapeutic help may be necessary.

Experience with prior disasters has provided evidence that the negative impact on survivors' lives continues. Among Holocaust survivors, Krystal (1981) observed that these "survivors continue to experience problems of chronic depression, masochistic life patterns, chronic anxiety, psychosomatic disease" (p. 167), anhedonia, and survivor's guilt. Among these survivors, aging imposed "the inescapable necessity of facing one's past" (Krystal, p. 177). Survivors of multiple AIDS-related loss either accept the past, integrating the experience into their lives, or reject it angrily and live in disgust and despair. As years passed, the gap between those who developed positive and negative coping styles widened in Holocaust survivors. Symptoms in those who fared poorly increased (Kaminer & Lavie, 1993). This outcome can be predicted for survivors of multiple AIDS-related loss as well.

Despite this dire outlook for some survivors, it is also evident that many have benefited from their experience. One survivor summed up his paradoxical evaluation of watching most of his friends die.

> I know it may sound sick and I have trouble admitting it, but in a lot of ways I am grateful for AIDS. Don't get me wrong, I would turn back history in a second and get my friend back, but . . . there have also been benefits. I'm a lot more mature and spiritual than I was. I have worked through a lot of issues that were holding me back. I am more loving of others and myself. I am less selfish. I never want to go back to being the person I was before AIDS.

Surviving multiple loss has been a devastating experience, but many survivors note that what has been devastated most is their naivete, their immaturity, their alienation from spirituality. Those survivors who have taken up the challenge of personal growth have benefited and recognize it. Without exception, however, survivors want their losses from AIDS to end. Another survivor said: "I know that AIDS has taught me a lot but enough already. I have learned enough!"

A serious dearth of research currently exists about the effects of this phenomenon or the treatment of its consequences. More study is essential, and those who take up the challenge of developing treatment interventions or conducting research about the effects of multiple, ongoing loss will provide important ground-breaking knowledge.

This book is a beginning. Almost nothing has been previously written about the experience of multiple AIDS-related loss or the generic experience of multiple, ongoing loss. How well this analysis stands up to the test of time remains to be seen. At the very least, this book bears witness to the survivor's experience. It places in the archives of history the horrors and hopes of those who have survived multiple AIDS-related loss.

This book has combined the poignant experience of survivors with an analysis of the psychological, sociological, and cultural implications of this historic experience. It is hoped that this book has contributed both to comprehension of, and emotional appreciation for, the survivor's experience. Those who gain a better understanding from this book are in an excellent position to help.

The Author's Experience
with Multiple AIDS-Related Loss

Forget your personal tragedy. We are all bitched from the start and you especially have to be hurt like hell before you can write seriously. But when you get the damned hurt use it—don't cheat with it. Be as faithful to it as a scientist.—Ernest Hemingway in a letter to F. Scott Fitzgerald, Baker (1981, p. 408)

I am tired of people dying. I would feel fortunate to have written this book as a neutral observer, as merely a witness to the pain of a generation. How soothing it would be to read this book as the history of someone else's pain; but fate had a different plan. I write this book as a survivor of multiple AIDS-related loss. I am living through this experience. I sink into sadness, despair in helplessness, and labor toward recovery. I have two conflicting minds about my journey with multiple, ongoing loss. Certainly, it is a heartbreaking disaster for which my expectations, or even my worst fears, never prepared me. However, it is also a rich opportunity to grow stronger, to deepen my spirituality, and to foster greater intimacies with those I love. This book is written from a fusion of my experiences as a survivor, a gay man, a witness, a psychotherapist, and an author; there is no way to separate these.

I was at Whitman College in the early 1980s when the distant rumblings of some homosexual disease eked their way into the local newspaper of Walla Walla, Washington. I faintly recall a twinge of anxiety, nothing more. In the mid-1980s, posters appeared in bars showing men at risk for AIDS; they did not look like me. I comforted myself with the belief that this danger was striking the "bad" elements of our community, the ones who were older and did the things I did not do. In late 1985, on a trip to southern California, I drank too much, did some drugs, and took a chance. Later, alone in bed, I realized that my life had changed forever, something irrevocable had shifted. Early in 1986, I was sick with the classic symptoms of early HIV infection. I tested positive and have lived with that overshadowing reality ever since.

The world was different in 1986. Only the bravest of the brave admitted their infection, and I was not brave. Desperate for some kind of support, I turned to my father and his wife. I was scared and hoped only for comfort and the sense of security that would come from hearing them say that they would stand by me. Instead, I was told that I had done this to myself and not to come begging for support and sympathy. I shut down and went into a hard, protective shell, reliving my early years hiding my sexuality. Instead of hiding magazines and sneaking into bars, I hid AZT and snuck into doctor's offices.

I lived alone with my fears until I decided to volunteer for Shanti, a volunteer organization that provides emotional support for persons affected by AIDS. Their training is intense, both emotionally challenging and utterly safe. For the first time in my life, I learned to feel my feelings and risk sharing them. Shanti requires participation in weekly support groups. Through my group, I was able to open up and met two friends who have been my buttress against the worst of life and my cocelebrants through its best. From my work with Shanti, and later volunteer work, I learned the importance of friends and created my family of choice.

My first Shanti client and my first contact with AIDS was through John, a Black man who gave me more and taught me more than I ever offered him. We met for a few hours every week as I tried to fulfill my role of providing him emotional support. I was sometimes severely challenged. Besides the complications of AIDS, which were severe, he was troubled by paranoid fears and condemning voices. There were times when we were close friends, and there were times when he accused me of being in league with the devil to kill him. There were times when we would walk down Broadway together like two friends, and there were times when he couldn't dress himself. Later, the simplest goals took on profound significance for John because the effort they required prevented him from achieving them without help. Simply to go to a convenience store was so satisfying, even the center of his week. Yet this simple task required so much: It meant dressing him, hurting him as I put on his pants and socks, twisting his body into the wheelchair, inching him into my truck as his now-worthless legs became an awkward hindrance, lifting his tall body into my truck, trying to get a seatbelt around him, folding up the wheelchair and placing it in the back, driving to the store, worrying about what people would think, unpacking the wheelchair, getting John out and into it without hurting him too much more, assisting him at the store while people stared, and then having to set time limits on his only outing from his dark apartment for the week. Then, the whole process was repeated in reverse.

In the final days of his life, he was moved to a nursing home that had never before admitted a person with AIDS. On his first day there I went to visit. The place reeked of stale urine. Once I found his room, I tried to smile and carry on a casual banter but my insides churned as I averted my eyes from the dried vomit that was encrusted throughout his unshaven beard and caked onto his flimsy hospital gown. After a short time, I excused myself to find a nurse to help clean him up. I went to the nursing station and explained John's situation. "He has dried vomit on him. Can someone clean it off?" The nurse hushed me up and motioned me to one side.

"Don't you know?"

"Know what?" I asked.

"He has AIDS!"

"Yes, of course I know," I said, "What does that have to do with cleaning up the vomit?"

"I'll see what we can do," the nurse replied.

"No, I'll clean it up," I said. "Will you please give me a towel or wash-cloth?"

The nurse looked around and told me she couldn't find any.

"What about paper towels?" I asked with a patience I did not know I possessed.

She couldn't locate any of those either. I told her I was going back to his room and expected some supplies right away. A few minutes later I looked up when I heard knocking on the open door. The nurse was standing in the hallway with her toes on the line between the room and hall. "I found some tissues," she said, with her arm stretched out as far as it would go. She wouldn't enter his room, so I walked over to get the box of flimsy tissues. It is not easy to clean up dried vomit with wet tissues.

John's mother was furious about the quality of care her son received. Many of my visits were punctuated by her screams and threats to the nursing home staff. By this time, John was nearly constantly in pain. He liked to get out of bed and move to a window, but every move caused him excruciating pain in his legs and feet. It is a hard thing to both help and hurt a friend. There were times I wished he would die so his suffering would end. That too is a hard thing. Between his pain, his mother's out-of-control anger, and my frustration with his quality of care, I felt harried and over my head. I was enraged, frustrated, and powerless. Sometimes, in my self-centered moments, I feared that I was looking at my future in John's present. There was one particularly bad day. John's mother was yelling in the background, John was suffering, and everything seemed out of control. I asked him, "John, how do you handle all this?" He was looking out into the distance with a rare composure and serenity.

"David," he said, struggling to lift his twitching right arm and show me his clenched hand, "These troubles don't do me no good so I just take them in my hand here and throw them to the wind."

I was speechless and humbled, like I would be so many times in the coming years. Here was a dying man, in pain, surrounded by disorder, and still he was able to transcend it and find a way to comfort me.

A few days later I had been visiting him and went home to rest. I was napping when I felt a tug at one of my feet. It woke me, and I knew with an absolute certainty that John was calling me to him. I drove to the nursing home and found him breathing hard but slow. It was the death rattle that I would later grow accustomed to. Gradually, his gasping breaths came at longer and longer intervals. Then they stopped. John had gone.

I kissed his forehead and closed his eyes. I sat with him for a while, and then I found the one nurse who cared for John and asked him to come with me. He was a big Black man who let out a deep, deep sob and then started singing a spiritual. It was a sacred moment, one that is forever imprinted on my soul.

A few weeks later, John's mother and I took a small boat out onto Puget Sound where we spread his ashes. It was the first time I felt the weight of a friend's cremated ashes in my fingers. It was the first time I heard the beautiful tinkling sound they make as they are spread over the water. It was the first time I watched the fragments of a friend settle down and spread out in the water. Neither of us saw the sea gull arrive, but he appeared just beyond the area where we cast John's remains. When we were finished the sea gull was gone, but neither of us saw him leave.

John was the first. There have been others, many others.

I would like to give some estimate as to how many friends and acquaintances I have lost, but I do not think I can. Certainly more than 50, probably more than 100. There are so many who simply disappeared. Those are especially hard to deal with because I find it hard to grieve for a person who has vanished. Maybe it's more than 200. I feel pathetic for not knowing. Some stand out in my mind. Steve was a handsome man and former fling who withered in weeks from PML, a disease that turned his brain to mush. Charles was a brilliant, if eccentric, spirit who lived a lot longer than I expected. Larry could make anyone laugh and always had a positive attitude, but a few days before his death he confided in me that he "wouldn't wish this on anyone." Keith watched his brother die from AIDS and worried about the pain his death would cause his mother; he kept trying to live until the end. Morgan was a role model of strength and grace who died sitting up in his living room chair. Gary was an inventive, creative, and generous soul who loved art, but years of potential were cut off his life. Victor was an ex-lover who worked hard to wake up an apathetic public; however, his vigorous fury was not enough. Brett and I had tremendous fun together—I remember dancing together at a Prince concert—but he moved home to Idaho to live with his Christian parents, and I never heard from him again. Robin was a mentor of mine at Shanti; he taught me to be competent at compassion, but gradually he withered. Terry was a friend from the time I was a boy, the son of family friends with whom we went camping and fishing. I marveled at his lively, funny spirit, but he died too. Bryan and I went to college together, forming a bond although neither of us knew the other was gay; I found out he died from a notice in the alumni news. I will not take up the space to write about Joe, Richard, Lou, Billy, David, and so many others who took a piece of my life with them when they left here. There are a slew of acquaintances and casual friends. Sometimes I see an obituary and gasp. More often, they simply disappear. I wonder what happened to them, then I forget. Sooner or later someone will tell me of their death.

I associate myself with other persons with AIDS. Somehow I feel bonded to them all, even when we never meet. Each time a man dies of AIDS, I feel that a brother has died. When I look at the *Bay Area Reporter* and see the 10 or 20 faces in the obituaries every week, I feel like they are related to me and I feel sad for them. Some of the celebrities who have died strike me particularly hard. Paul Monette was a star to me, and I mourn the loss of his literary genius. Randy Shilts was an honest reporter, but he is no longer. John Boswell wrote ground-breaking histories about gays in history, but he will educate no more. Pedro Zamora was a young role model. And this list is never complete, and I am frustrated by the fact that I know I am failing to remember many.

It is not fair! A man in his 30s should not be spreading ashes, reading obituaries, cleaning up vomit, changing diapers, carrying rubber gloves, becoming a critic of memorial services, or knowing the layout of so many hospitals. Not infrequently I want to be the pretender in Jackson Browne's song who "packs his lunch in the morning and goes to work each day." How did I get stuck in the middle of all this?

Over the years, my experience surviving multiple AIDS-related loss has evolved. I was bitter for many years, and sometimes still am. I dread the day Ronald Reagan dies and is transformed into a "hero" like Nixon. I don't know how I will handle it; my hate for him is so strong. He could have done so much to prevent so much suffering.

My anger boils over the top at times. A few months ago, I was sitting in a coffee shop proofreading one of the chapters of this book. A handsome young man was sitting at a table next to mine. We struck up a conversation, and I was thinking about what a nice guy he seemed to be. He reached for something across his table. His cane, which I had not previously noticed, fell to the ground. I started shaking with rage, saying to myself, "I am sick of seeing young, handsome men with canes!" I was so furious I couldn't speak. I gathered my things and flew out of the coffee shop. Fortunately I found a phone and was able to reach a friend who patiently listened to me rant. It infuriates me that I will never know a time, for the rest of my life, when I won't be surrounded by young men with canes, dying friends, and anxiety about existence.

At the end of the movie *Longtime Companion* (Wlodkowsky & Rene, 1990), the only remaining friends from a large group of friends wonder aloud what it will be like the day after they find a cure.

"It seems inconceivable, doesn't it, when we didn't wake up every day wondering who's sick now? Who else is gone?"

One friend says, "I just want to be there, if they ever do find a cure."

"Can you imagine what it would be like?"

"Like the end of World War II."

Then the scene changes and a long line of those who have died stream down the boardwalk onto the beach. They are all there amid hugs, laughter, and tears of joy. They are not really gone. It was all a bad dream.

But the fantasy is short lived. Once again, it is only three friends, and the movie ends with one saying, "I just want to be there." So do I.

I still cannot watch that scene without sobbing. Something about it rips at my gut: the impossible chance to see my friends one more time, the hopeless longing I have for the relief of a day when no one is dying of AIDS, the stupid wish that I could rewind my life to a time before AIDS, the futile hope that a cure will ever be found.

How I long to hear the words "It's over now. They've quit dying. You can rest." It would comfort me to know, at least, that it will end at my death; but it won't. I will die knowing that there are people I love dearly who will outlive me and still die young. The pain will carry on after me. So, for me, it is a perpetual fall that death won't surcease.

I have learned to look despair in the eyes. I do not shrink from its threat. My lifetime partner has been baffled by the existential titles I read and the thoughts I express. At times, he finds me morbid and depressing. But he is beginning to learn what I learned. One has to go through despair to reach the other side. Like grief, there is no way around it, only through it. Once we face despair, we can make honest choices, and life becomes richer, more complete than it ever was in a protected existence of mediocrity.

I have learned to live in the paradox of continual despair and investment in life. My journey back to life has required work. I was not willing to shut down and die emotionally and spiritually like I have seen so many others do. I have told myself, over and over, "AIDS is a full-time job." Part of that job is grieving. When I grieve, I grieve hard. I let the emotions flow and I don't inhibit them. There was a period of time when I chose to skip some memorial services, but the regret from those decisions lingers and those sores still fester. Now, I go to memorial services of friends because it helps to hurt.

I have been greatly helped by the various forms of volunteer work I have done and continue to do. Whether it is organized or not, helping others cope with AIDS always makes me feel better because it provides me a sense of meaningfulness. At times, I have gone overboard, doing too much. Then, I feel the burnout, resentment, and rage that tells me I have let my life get out of balance. Though I have learned the lesson over and over, I still need to be reminded. My friends help me a lot with this. Life is not all AIDS. Always, a trip to the ocean or into the woods will revive me and remind me of the larger spiritual truths that remain true in spite of the pain that seems to overwhelm every truth.

It helps me to remain active in voicing the concerns of survivors while honoring the concerns of those with AIDS. I understand both. I regularly train volunteers and professionals on grief and the variety of losses encompassed by the AIDS epoch. I began the first group for survivors of multiple loss in Seattle. The group members have taught me so very much, and they have constantly let me know that I am not alone. They lovingly refuse to let me be the facilitator and demand that I take my place as a member.

More still needs to be done. Very few survivors face their survival head on. I want to be part of a movement that educates survivors about the need to grieve, the need to feel despair, the need to find meaning in a seemingly mean-ingless world. Community-wide validation of our experience is necessary and should be demanded. We deserve recognition commensurate with our suffering. We must work together in community to commemorate ourselves, to bear wit-ness to our experience, especially if others will not do it. The Names Project is a superb starting point, but more is needed. Communities heal as communities, not as fractured individuals. We need to establish shrines and rituals that allow the community of survivors to share in each other's pain and share in each other's recovery.

Writing this book has certainly been cathartic and helped me to find mean-ing in my experience. Many, many times I would be writing something and suddenly begin crying. I learned to let myself cry. Then, I would go back to writing. This book has extracted a lot of my pain by giving me an outlet, but it has also been a consistent meditation on AIDS. One day I was writing and a friend, Mark, called to say, "Joe died last night. I thought you'd want to know." I had known Joe was sick but had not heard anything in months. So typical of AIDS, here I was confronted with another death. Then, I went back to writing.

References

Acevedo, J. R. (1986). Impact of risk reduction on mental health. In L. McKusick (Ed.), *What to do about AIDS* (pp. 95–102). Berkeley: University of California Press.

Acosta, F., Yamamoto, J., & Evans, L. (1982*). Effective psychotherapy for low-income and minority patients.* New York: Plenum.

AIDS agency says epidemic leveled off in Western Europe. (1995, November 26). *Seattle Times,* p. A13.

AIDS Caregivers Support Network. (1996). AIDS facts. *AIDS Caregivers Quarterly, 6*(1), 6.

Allport, G. (1959). Preface. In V. E. Frankl, *Man's search for meaning* (pp. 9–13). New York: Washington Square Press.

American Psychiatric Association. (1994*). Diagnostic and statistical manual of mental disorders* (4th ed.). Washington, DC: Author.

Anderson, G. R., Gurdin, P., & Thomas, A. (1989). Dual disenfranchisement: Foster parenting children with AIDS. In K. J. Doka (Ed.), *Disenfranchised grief: Recognizing hidden sorrow* (pp. 43–53). Lexington, MA: Lexington Books.

Appelby, G. A. (1995). AIDS and homophobia/heterosexism. *Journal of Gay and Lesbian Social Services, 2,* 1–23.

Atwood, J. D. (1993). AIDS in African American and Hispanic adolescents: A multisystemic approach. *The American Journal of Family Therapy, 21*(4), 333–349.

Attenborough, R., & Eastman, B. (1993). *Shadowlands.* Savoy Pictures.

Baker, C. (Ed.). (1981). *Ernest Hemingway: Selected letters 1917–1961.* New York: Charles Scribner's Sons.

Bardach, A. L. (1995, June 5). The white cloud: Latino America's stealth virus. *The New Republic,* 27–31.

Barrett, W. (1962). *Irrational man: A study in existential philosophy.* New York: Anchor Books. (Original published 1958)

Bartlett, J. (1968). *Familiar quotations* (14th ed.), E. M. Beck (Ed.). Boston: Little, Brown, and Company.

Beaton, R. D., & Murphy, S. A. (1995). Working with people in crisis: Research implications. In C. R. Figley (Ed.), *Compassion fatigue: Coping with secondary stress disorder in those who treat the traumatized* (pp. 51–81). New York: Brunner/Mazel.

Beck, A. T., Rush, A. J., Shaw, B. F., & Emery, G. (1979). *Cognitive therapy of depression.* New York: Guilford Press.

Bell, J. P. (1988). AIDS and the hidden epidemic of grief: A personal experience. *American Journal of Hospice Care,* 25–31.

Bess, J. (1969). Grief is. In A. H. Kutscher (Ed.), *Death and bereavement* (pp. 202–203). Springfield, IL: Charles C. Thomas.

Bettelheim, B. (1980a). The Holocaust—One generation later. In *Surviving and other essays* (pp. 84–104). New York: Vintage Books. (Original published 1952)

Bettelheim, B. (1980b). The ultimate limit. In *Surviving and other essays* (pp. 3–18). New York: Vintage Books. (Original published 1952)

Bibring, E. (1953). The mechanism of depression. In P. Greenacre (Ed.), *Affective disorders* (pp. 13–48). New York: International Universities Press.

Bickelhaupt, E. E. (1995). Alcoholism and drug abuse in gay and lesbian persons: A review of incidence studies. *Journal of Gay and Lesbian Social Services, 2,* 5–14.

Bidgood, R. (1992). Coping with the trauma of AIDS losses. In H. Land (Ed.), *AIDS: Complete guide to psychosocial intervention* (pp. 239–252). Milwaukee, WI: Family Service America.

Biller, R., & Rice, S. (1990). Experiencing multiple loss of persons with AIDS: Grief and bereavement issues. *Health & Social Work, 15,* 283–290.

Bivens, A. J., Neimeyer, R. A., Kirchberg, T. M., & Moore, M. K. (1994). Death concern and religious beliefs among gays and bisexuals of variable proximity to AIDS. *Omega, 30*(2), 105–120.

Blankfield, A. (1989). Grief, alcohol dependence and women. *Drug and Alcohol Dependence, 24*(1), 45–49.

Booth, L. (1995). Spirituality and the gay community. *Journal of Gay & Lesbian Social Services, 2*(1), 57–65.

Bor, R., Elford, J., Hart, G., & Sherr, L. (1993). The family and HIV disease. *AIDS Care, 5*(1), 3–6.

Bor, R., Miller, R., & Goldman, E. (1992). *Theory and practice of HIV counseling: A systemic approach.* London: Cassell.

Bowlby, J. (1980). *Attachment and loss: Loss, sadness, and depression* (Vol. 3). New York: Basic Books.

Bowman, T. (1994). *Loss of dreams: A special kind of grief.* St. Paul, MN: Ted Bowman.

Boykin, F. F. (1991). The AIDS crisis and gay male survivor guilt. *Smith College Studies in Social Work, 6*(3), 247–259.

Bozett, F. W., & Sussman, M. B. (1990). Homosexuality and family relations: View and research issues. In F. W. Bozett & M. B. Sussman (Eds.), *Homosexuality and family relations.* New York: Haworth Press.

Bradshaw, J. (1988). *Bradshaw on: Healing the shame that binds you.* Deerfield Beach, FL: Health Communications.

Bridgewater, D. (1992). A gay male survivor of antigay violence. In S. H. Dworkin & F. J. Gutierrez (Eds.), *Counseling gay men & lesbians: Journey to the end of the rainbow* (pp. 219–230). Alexandria, VA: American Association for Counseling and Development.

Britton, P. J., Zarski, J. J., & Hobfoll, S. E. (1993). Psychological distress and the role of significant others in a population of gay/bisexual men in the era of HIV. *AIDS Care, 5*(1), 43–54.

Bronski, M. (1988). Death and the erotic imagination. In J. Preston (Ed.), *Personal dispatches: Writers confront AIDS*. New York: St. Martin's Press.

Brookmeyer, R. (1991, August). Reconstruction and future trends of the AIDS epidemic in the United States. *Science, 253*, 37–42.

Brown, L. K., & DeMaio, D. M. (1992). The impact of secrets in hemophilia and HIV disorders. *Journal of Psychosocial Oncology, 10*(3), 91–101.

Buber, M. (1970). *I and thou* (W. Kaufman, Trans.). New York: Scribner's.

Bugen, L. (1979). Human grief: A model for prediction and intervention. In L. Bugen (Ed.), *Death and dying: Theory, research, practice*. Dubuque, IA: William C. Brown.

Burgess, A. W., & Holmstrom, L. (1974). Rape trauma syndrome. *American Journal of Psychiatry, 131*, 981–986.

Burkett, E. (1995). *The gravest show on Earth: America in the Age of AIDS*. New York: Houghton Mifflin.

Callen, M. (1988, May 3). I will survive. *Village Voice*, pp. 34–35.

Campbell, J. (1988). *Historical atlas of the world mythology. Volume I: The way of the animal powers*. New York: Harper & Row.

Camus, A. (1946). *The stranger*. New York: Alfred A. Knopf.

Camus, A. (1948). *The plague*. New York: Random House.

Carl, D. (1990). *Counseling same-sex couples*. New York: W. W. Norton.

Carmack, B. J. (1992). Balancing engagement/detachment in AIDS-related multiple loss. *Image: Journal of Nursing Scholarship, 24*(1), 9–14.

Cass, V. C. (1979). Homosexual identity formation: A theoretical model. *Journal of Homosexuality, 4*(3), 219–235.

Cass, V. C. (1984). Homosexual identity: A concept in need of definition. *Journal of Homosexuality, 9*, 105–126.

Catania, J. A., Binson, D., Dolcini, M. M., Stall, R., Choi, K.-H., Pollack, L. M., Hudes, E. S., Canchola, J., Phillips, K., Moskowitz, J. T., & Coates, T. J. (1995). Risk facts for HIV and other sexually transmitted diseases and prevention practices among U.S. heterosexual adults: Changes from 1990 to 1992. *American Journal of Public Health, 85*(11), 1492–1499.

Centers for Disease Control. (1987). *Morbidity & Mortality Weekly Report, 36*, 801–804.

Centers for Disease Control. (1995, 3rd quarter). Demographic characteristics of cumulative AIDS cases—King County, other WA counties, all WA State. *U.S. HIV/AIDS Quarterly Epidemiology Report, 3*.

Cerney, M. S. (1995). Treating the "heroic treaters." In C. R. Figley (Ed.), *Compassion fatigue: Coping with secondary stress disorder in those who treat the traumatized* (pp. 131–149). New York: Brunner/Mazel.

Chachkes, E., & Jennings, R. (1992). Latino communities: Coping with death. In B. O. Dane & C. Levine (Eds.), *AIDS and the new orphans: Coping with death* (pp. 77–100). Westport, CT: Auburn House.

Christ, G. H., & Weiner, L. S. (1985). Psychosocial issues in AIDS. In V. T. De Vita Jr., S. Hellmman, & S. A. Rosenbers (Eds.), *AIDS, etiology, diagnosis, treatment and prevention*. Philadelphia: Lippincott.

Chu, S. Y., Peterman, T. S., Doll, L. S., Buehler, J. W., & Curran, J. W. (1992). AIDS in bisexual men in the United States: Epidemiology and transmission to women. *American Journal of Public Health, 82*, 1757–1759.

Church, J. A., Kocsis, A. E., & Green, J. (1988). Effects on lovers of caring for HIV infected individuals related to perceptions of cognitive, behavioral, and personality changes in the sufferer (Abstract No. 8592). *Fourth International Conference on AIDS*.

Clark, J. M., Brown, J. C., & Hochstein, L. M. (1989). Institutional religion and gay/lesbian oppression. *Marriage and Family Review, 14*, 89–115.

Cohen, B. B. (1991). Holocaust survivors and the crises of aging. *Families in Society, 72*, 226–231.

Cohen, M. A., & Weisman, H. W. (1986). A biopsychological approach to AIDS. *Psychosomatics, 245–249.*

Colburn, K. A., & Malena, D. (1988). Bereavement issues for survivors of persons with AIDS: Coping with society's pressure. *The American Journal of Hospice Care, 5,* 20–25.

Coleman, S. (1980). Incomplete mourning and addict family transactions: A theory for understanding heroin abuse. In D. Lettieri (Ed.), *Theories on drug abuse.* Washington, DC: U.S. Government Printing Office.

Corey, M. S., & Corey, G. (1992). *Groups: Process and practice* (4th ed.). Belmont, CA: Brooks/Cole.

Cowger, C. D. (1994). Assessing client strengths: Clinical assessment for client empowerment. *Social Work, 39*(3), 262–268.

Crawford, R. (1994). The boundaries of the self and the unhealthy other: Reflections on health, culture and AIDS. *Social Science Medicine, 38*(10), 1347–1365.

Crow, H. E. (1991). How to help patients understand and conquer grief: Avoiding depression in the midst of sadness. *Postgraduate Medicine, 89,* 117–123.

Dalton, H. L. (1989). AIDS in blackface. *Daedalus, 118,* 205–227.

Dane, B. O. (1992). Death and bereavement. In B. O. Dane & C. Levine (Eds.), *AIDS and the new orphans: Coping with death* (pp. 13–32). Westport, CT: Auburn House

Danieli, Y. (1985). The treatment and prevention of long-term effects and intergenerational transmission of victimization: A lesson from Holocaust survivors and their children. In C. R. Figley (Ed.), *Trauma and its wake: The study and treatment of post-traumatic stress disorder* (pp. 298–301). New York: Brunner/Mazel.

Davis, M., & Wallbridge, D. (1990). *Boundary and space: An introduction to the work of D. W. Winicott.* New York: Bruner-Mazel.

Dean, L., Hall, W. E., & Martin, J. L. (1988). Chronic and intermittent AIDS-related bereavement in a panel of homosexual men in New York City. *Journal of Palliative Care, 4,* 54–57.

Deck, E. S., & Folta, J. R. (1989). The friend-griever. In K. J. Doka (Ed.), *Disenfranchised grief: Recognizing hidden sorrow* (pp. 77–89). Lexington, MA: Lexington Books.

DeCrescenzo, T. A. (1985). Homophobia: A study of attitudes of mental health professionals toward homosexuality. In R. Schoenberg, R. S. Goldberg, & D. A. Shod (Eds.), *With compassion toward some: Homosexuality and social work in America* (pp. 115–136). New York: Harrington Park Press.

Defoe, D. (1969). *A Journal of the plague year.* New York: Signet Classics. (Original published 1721)

Delaney, M. (1996, July 17). *Strategies for survival and update from the XI International Conference on AIDS.* Presentation at the close of the National Lesbian and Gay Health Association conference, Seattle, WA.

Deutsch, H. (1937). Absence of grief. *Psychoanalytic Quarterly, 6,* 12–22.

de Wit, J. B. F., van den Hoek, J. A. R., Sandfort, T. G. M., & van Griensven, G. J. P. (1993). Increase in unprotected anogenital intercourse among homosexual men. *American Journal of Public Health, 83,* 1451–1453.

Dillard, J. M. (1983). *Multicultural counseling: Toward ethnic and cultural relevance in human encounters.* Chicago: Nelson-Hall.

Doka, K. J. (1987). Silent sorrow: Grief and the loss of significant others. *Death Studies, 11,* 455–469.

Doka, K. J. (1992). Suffer the little children: The child and spirituality in the AIDS crisis. In B. O. Dane & C. Levine (Eds.), *AIDS and the new orphans: Coping with death* (pp. 33–42). Westport, CT: Auburn House.

Dubik-Unruh, S. (1989). Children of chaos: Planning for the emotional survival of dying children of dying families. *Journal of Palliative Care, 5*(2), 10–15.

Dunkel, S., & Hatfield, S. (1986). Countertransference & AIDS. *Social Work, 31,* 114–117.

Dutton, M. A., & Rubinstein, F. L. (1995). Working with people with PTSD: Research implications. In C. R. Figley (Ed.), *Compassion fatigue: Coping with secondary stress disorder in those who treat the traumatized* (pp. 82–100). New York: Brunner/Mazel.

Dworkin, S. H., & Pincu, L. (1993). Counseling in the era of AIDS. *Journal of Counseling and Development 71,* 275–281.

Dworkin, S. H., & Kaufer, D. (1995). Social services and bereavement in the lesbian and gay community. *Journal of Gay and Lesbian Social Services, 2*(3/4), 41–60.

Ellen, J. M., Kohn, R. P., Bolan, G. A., Shiboski, S., & Krieger, N. (1995, November). Socio-economic differences in sexually transmitted disease rates among Black and White adolescents, San Francisco, 1990 to 1992. *American Journal of Public Health, 85,* 1546–1548.

Eranen, L., & Liebkind, K. (1993). Coping with disaster: The helping behavior of communities and individuals. In J. P. Wilson & B. Raphael (Eds.*), International handbook of traumatic stress syndrome* (pp. 957–963). New York: Plenum Press.

Erikson, E. H. (1950). *Childhood and society.* New York: W. W. Norton.

Erikson, E. H. (1980). *Identity and the life cycle.* New York: W. W. Norton. (Original published 1959)

Erikson, K. T. (1976). Loss of communality at Buffalo Creek. *American Journal of Psychiatry, 133,* 302–305.

Eth, S., & Pynoos, R. S. (1985). Developmental perspective on psychic trauma in childhood. In C. R. Figley (Ed.), *Trauma and its wake: The study and treatment of post-traumatic stress disorder* (pp. 36–52). New York: Brunner/Mazel.

Faulstich, M. E. (1987). Psychiatric aspects of AIDS. *American Journal of Psychiatry, 142,* 82–85.

Figley, C. R. (1985a). Introduction. In C. R. Figley (Ed.*), Trauma and its wake: The study and treatment of post-traumatic stress disorder* (pp. xviii–xix). New York: Brunner/Mazel.

Figley, C. R. (1985b). From victim to survivor: Social responsibility in the wake of catastrophe. In C. R. Figley (Ed.), *Trauma and its wake: The study and treatment of post-traumatic stress disorder* (pp. 398–415). New York: Brunner/Mazel.

Figley, C. R. (1995). Compassion fatigue as secondary traumatic stress disorder: An overview. In C. R. Figley (Ed.), *Compassion fatigue: Coping with secondary stress disorder in those who treat the traumatized* (pp. 1–20). New York: Brunner/Mazel.

Fischman, Y. (1991). Interacting with trauma: Clinicians' responses to treating psychological aftereffects of political repression. *American Journal of Orthopsychiatry, 61,* 179–185.

Flannery, R. B. (1989). From victim to survivor: A stress management approach in the treatment of learned helplessness. In B. A. van der Kolk (Ed.), *Psychological trauma* (pp. 217–231). Washington, DC: American Psychiatric Press.

Frankl, V. (1984). *Man's search for meaning.* New York: Washington Square Press. (Original published 1959)

Franks, K., Templer, D. I., Cappelletty, G. G., & Kauffman, I. (1990). Exploration of death anxiety as a function of religious variables in gay men with and without AIDS. *Omega, 22*(1), 43–50.

Freeman, E. M. (1984). Multiple losses in the elderly: An ecological approach. *Social Caseworker, 65,* 287–296.

Freud, S. (1957). Mourning and melancholia. In J. Rickman (Ed.), *A general selection from the works of Sigmund Freud* (pp. 124–140). Garden City, NY: Doubleday Anchor Books. (Original published 1917)

Friedman, M. (1985). Toward a reconceptualization of guilt. *Contemporary Psychoanalysis, 21*(4), 501–547.

Fudin, C. E., & Devore, W. (1981). The unidentified bereaved. In O. S. Margolis, H. C. Raether, A. H. Kutscher, J. B. Powers, I. B. Seeland, R. De Bellis, & D. J. Cherico (Eds.), *Acute grief: Counseling the bereaved* (pp. 133–139). New York: Columbia University Press.

Fuller, R. L., Geis, S. B., & Rush, J. (1989). Loves and significant others. In K. J. Doka (Ed.), *Disenfranchised grief: Recognizing hidden sorrow* (pp. 33–41). Lexington, MA: Lexington Books.

Fulton, R. (1995). The contemporary funeral: Functional or dysfunctional? In H. Wass & R. A. Neimeyer (Eds.), *Dying: Facing the facts* (pp. 185–206). Washington, DC: Taylor & Francis.

Gallagher, D., & Thompson, L. W. (1989). Bereavement and adjustment disorders. In E. W. Busse & D. G. Blazer (Eds.), *Geriatric psychiatry* (pp. 459–473). Washington, DC: American Psychiatric Press.

Garfield, C. (1995). *Sometimes my heart goes numb: Love and caregiving in a time of AIDS.* San Francisco: Jossey-Bass.

Gay City Health Project. (1995). *Welcome to gay city.* Seattle, WA: Gay City.

Goering, L. (1995, March 6). Brazil sexual culture makes fighting AIDS an uphill battle. *The Seattle Times,* p. A12.

Goffman, E. (1963). *Stigma: Notes on the management of spoiled identity.* New York: Simon & Schuster.

Goldman, E., Miller, R., & Lee, C. A. (1993). A family with HIV and haemophilia. *AIDS Care, 5*(1), 79–89.

Gordon, J. H., Ulrich, C., Feeley, M., & Pollack, S. (1993). Staff distress among haemophilia nurses. *AIDS Care, 5*(3), 359–367.

Goss, P. (1994, November). 10,000 will die. *National Hemophiliac Foundation Congressional Update, 1*(4).

Gottfried, H., & Boggart, P. (1988). *Torch Song Trilogy.* New Line Cinema.

Gough, J. (1996). Help wanted: Caregivers needed, no experience necessary. *Caregivers Quarterly, 6*(1). Seattle, WA: AIDS Caregivers Support Network.

Green, B. L. (1993). Identifying survivors at risk: Trauma and stressors across events. In J. P. Wilson & B. Raphael (Eds.), *International handbook of traumatic stress syndrome* (pp. 135–143). New York: Plenum Press.

Green, S. K., & Bobele, M. (1994). Family therapists' response to AIDS: An examination of attitudes, knowledge, and contact. *Journal of Marital and Family Therapy, 20*(4), 349–367.

Haney, D. Q. (1996, February 11). HIV spreading among young men despite warnings, study shows. *The Seattle Times,* p. A11.

Harel, Z., Kahana, B., & Kahana, E. (1993). Social resources and the mental health of aging Nazi Holocaust survivors and immigrants. In J. P. Wilson & B. Raphael (Eds.), *International handbook of traumatic stress syndrome* (pp. 241–251). New York: Plenum Press.

Harris, C. J. (1995). Sensory-based therapy for crisis counselors. In C. R. Figley (Ed.), *Compassion fatigue: Coping with secondary stress disorder in those who treat the traumatized* (pp. 101–114). New York: Brunner/Mazel.

Haskell, M. (1994). *Northwest AIDS Foundation annual report.* Seattle, WA: NWAF.

Hay, L. L. (1988). *The AIDS book: Creating a positive approach.* Santa Monica, CA: Hay House.

Hays, R. B., Chauncey, S., & Tobey, L. A. (1990). The social support networks of gay men with AIDS. *Journal of Community Psychology, 18,* 374–385.

Heidegger, M. (1962). *Being and time* (J. Macquarrie & E. Robinson, Trans.). San Francisco: Harper & Row. (Original published 1926)

Hemingway, E. (1929). *A farewell to arms.* New York: Charles Scribner's Sons.

Herek, G. M., & Glunt, E. K. (1988). An epidemic of stigma: Public reactions to AIDS. *American Psychologist, 43,* 886–891.

Herek, G. M., & Capitanio, J. P. (1993). Public reactions to AIDS in the United States: A second decade of stigma. *American Journal of Public Health, 83*(4), 574–577.

Hesse, H. (1956). *The journey to the East.* New York: Noonday Press.

Hill, K. (1996, April 19). AIDS rises among blacks, women: Cumulative cases in U.S. pass half-million mark. *Seattle Times,* p. A5.

Hintze, J., Templer, D. I., Cappelletty, G. G., & Frederick, W. (1994). Death depression and death anxiety in HIV-infected males. In R. A. Neimeyer (Ed.), *Death anxiety handbook: Research, instrumentation, & application* (193–200). Washington, DC: Taylor & Francis.

Hodge, B. (1993). *Supporting gay men in grieving an AIDS death: With an emphasis on the use of ritual.* Unpublished manuscript.

Horowitz, M. J. (1976a). Diagnosis and treatment of stress response syndromes. In H. J. Parad, H. L. P. Resnik, & L. G. Parad (Eds.), *Emergency and disaster management* (pp. 259–269). Bowie, MD: Charles Press.

Horowitz, M. J. (1976b). *Stress response syndromes.* New York: Jason Aronson.

Horowitz, M. J. (1985). Disasters and psychological responses to stress. *Psychiatric Annals, 15*(3), 161–167.

Horowitz, M. J., Wilner, N., Marmar, C., & Krupnick, J. (1980). Pathological grief and the activation of latent self images. *American Journal of Psychiatry, 137,* 1157–1162.

Houseman, C., & Pheifer, W. G. (1988). Potential for unresolved grief in survivors of persons with AIDS. *Archives of Psychiatric Nursing, 2,* 296–301.

Hudson, R., & Davidson, S. (1986). *Rock Hudson: His story.* New York: William Morrow.

Ingram, R. E. (1986). *Information processing approaches to clinical psychology.* New York: Academic Press.

Interview with Randy Shilts. (1995, December 31). In *60 Minutes.* CBS

James, J. S. (1996). Fewer AIDS deaths: San Francisco information. *AIDS Treatment News, 260,* 3.

Janoff-Bulman, R. (1985). The aftermath of victimization: Rebuilding shattered assumption. In C. R. Figley (Ed.), *Trauma and its wake: The study and treatment of post-traumatic stress disorder* (pp. 15–33). New York: Brunner/Mazel.

Janoff-Bulman, R. (1992). *Shattered assumption: Towards a new psychology of trauma.* New York: Free Press.

Jason, J. M., Stehr-Green, J., Holman, R. C., Evatt, B. L., & Hemophilia-AIDS Collaborative Study Group. (1988). Human immunodeficiency virus infection in hemophiliac children. *Pediatrics, 82,* 565–570.

Jay, J. (1994, May/June). Walls for wailing. *Common Boundary,* 30–35.

Johnson-Moore, P. & Phillips, L. J. (1994). Black American communities: Coping with death. In B. O. Dane & C. Levine (Eds.), *AIDS and the new orphans: Coping with death.* Westport, CT: Auburn House.

Jones, E. E., Farina, A., Hastorf, A. H., Markus, H., Miller, D. T., & Scott, R. A. (1984). *Social stigma: The psychology of marked relationships.* New York: W. H. Freeman.

Jue, S. (1994, June). Psychosocial issues of AIDS long-term survivors. Families in society: *The Journal of Contemporary Human Services, 6,* 324–332.

Kaminer, H., & Lavie, P. (1993). Sleep and dreams in well-adjusted and less adjusted Holocaust survivors. In M. S. Stroebe, W. Stroebe, & R. O. Hansson (Eds.), *Handbook of bereavement: Theory, research, & intervention* (pp. 331–345). New York: Cambridge University Press.

Kastenbaum, R. J. (1969). Death and bereavement in later life. In A. H. Kutscher (Ed.), *Death and bereavement* (pp. 28–54). Springfield, IL: Charles C. Thomas.

Kastenbaum, R. J. (1977). *Death, society, & human experience.* St. Louis, MO: C. V. Mosby.

Kauffman, J. (1989). Intrapsychic dimensions of disenfranchised grief. In K. J. Doka (Ed.), *Disenfranchised grief: Recognizing hidden sorrow* (pp. 25–29). Lexington, MA: Lexington Books.

Kayal, P. M. (1994). Communalization and homophile organization membership: Gay volunteerism before and during AIDS. *Journal of Gay & Lesbian Social Services, 1*(1), 33–57.

Kerr, M. E., & Bowen, M. (1988). *Family evaluation: An approach based on Bowen theory.* New York: W. W. Norton.

Kierkegaard, S. (1989). *The sickness unto death* (A. Hannay, Trans.). London: Penguin. (Original published 1849)

Kimmelman, M. (1989, March 19). Bitter Harvest: AIDS & the arts. *New York Times,* p. 2.

King, W. (1996, July 8). Anger dominates start of AIDS conference. *Seattle Times,* p. A1.

Klein, S. J. (1994). AIDS-related multiple loss syndrome. *Illness, Crises and Loss, 4*(1), 13–25.

Klein, S. J., & Fletcher, W. (1987). Gay grief: An examination of its uniqueness brought to light by the AIDS crisis. *Journal of Psychosocial Oncology, 4,* 15–25.

Kliman, A. S. (1981). Facilitation of mourning after a natural disaster. In O. S. Margolis, H. C. Raether, A. H. Kutscher, J. B. Powers, I. B. Seeland, R. De Bellis, & D. J. Cherico (Eds.), *Acute grief: Counseling the bereaved* (pp. 71–76). New York: Columbia University Press.

Kohn, R., & Levav, I. (1990). Bereavement in disaster: An overview of the research. *International Journal of Mental Health, 19*(2), 61–76.

Kollar, N. R. (1989). Rituals and the disenfranchised griever. In K. J. Doka (Ed.), *Disenfranchised grief: Recognizing hidden sorrow* (pp. 271–285). Lexington, MA: Lexington Books.

Kominars, S. B. (1995). Homophobia: The heart of the darkness. *Journal of Gay & Lesbian Social Services, 2*(1), 29–40.

Kramer, L. (1983, March 14–27). 1,112 and counting. *New York Native, 59.*

Kramer, L. (1994). *Reports from the Holocaust: The story of an AIDS activist.* New York: St. Martin's Press.

Krupp, G. (1972). Maladaptive reactions to the death of a family member. *Social Caseworker, 53,* 425–434.

Krystal, H. (1975). Affect tolerance. *The Annual of Psychoanalysis, 3,* 179–219.

Krystal, H. (1979). Alexithymia and psychotherapy. *American Journal of Psychotherapy, 33*(1), 17–31.

Krystal, H. (1981). The aging survivor of the Holocaust: Integration and self-healing in post-traumatic states. *Journal of Geriatric Psychiatry, 14*(2), 165–189.

Kubler-Ross, E. (1969). *On death and dying.* New York: Macmillan.

Kubler-Ross, E. (1987). *AIDS: The ultimate challenge.* New York: Macmillan.

Kurath, B. (1996, April). Blood math. *POZ, 17.*

Kurdek, L. A., & Siesky, G. (1990). The nature and correlates of psychological adjustment in gay men with AIDS-related conditions. *Journal of Applied Social Psychology, 20,* 846–860.

Kushner, T. (1994). *Angels in America. Part Two: Perestroika.* New York: Theater Communications Group.

Lattanzi, M. E. (1982). Hospice bereavement services: Creating networks of support. *Death Education, 8,* 54–63.

Lazare, A. (1979). Unresolved grief. In A. Lazare (Ed.), *Outpatient psychiatry: Diagnosis and treatment* (pp. 498–512). Baltimore: Williams & Wilkins.

Legislation approved for S. F. AIDS memorial grove. (1996, October 18), *Seattle Gay News,* p. 7.

Lennon, M. C., Martin, J. L., & Dean, L. (1990). The influence of social support on AIDS-related grief reaction among gay men. *Social Science Medicine, 31,* 477–483.

Levine, C. (1992) The new orphans and grieving in the time of AIDS. In B. O. Dane & C. Levine (Eds.), *AIDS and the new orphans: Coping with death* (pp. 1–13). Westport, CT: Auburn House.

Lewis, C. S. (1961). *A grief observed.* New York: Bantam.

Lieberman, M. A. (1993). Bereavement self-help groups: A review of conceptual and methodological issues. In M. S. Stroebe, W. Stroebe, & R. O. Hansson (Eds.), *Handbook of bereavement: Theory, research, & intervention* (pp. 411–426). New York: Cambridge University Press.

Lifton, R. J. (1979). *The broken connection: On death and the continuity of life.* New York: Simon & Schuster.

Lifton, R. J. (1993). From Hiroshima to the Nazi doctors: The evolution of psychoformative approaches to understanding traumatic stress syndromes. In J. P. Wilson & B. Raphael (Eds.), *International handbook of traumatic stress syndrome* (pp. 11–23.) New York: Plenum Press

Lifton, R. J., & Olson, E. (1976). Death imprint in Buffalo Creek. In H. J. Parad, H. L. P. Resnik, & L. G. Parad (Eds.), *Emergency and disaster management* (pp. 295–308). Bowie, MD: Charles Press.

Lima, G., Lo Presto, C. T., Sherman, M. F., & Sobelman, S. A. (1993). The relationship between homophobia and self-esteem in gay males with AIDS. *Journal of Homosexuality, 25,* 69–75.

Lindemann, E. (1944). Symptomatology and management of acute grief. *The American Journal of Psychiatry, 101,* 141–148.

Lindstrom, B. (1983). Operating a hospice bereavement program. In C. A. Corr & D. M. Corr (Eds.), *Hospice care: Principles and practice* (pp. 266–278). New York: Springer.

Lindy, J. D. (1985). The trauma membrane and other clinical concepts derived from psychotherapeutic work with survivors of natural disasters. *Psychiatric Annals, 15*(3), 153–160.

Lindy, J. D., Green, B. L., Grace, J., & Titchener, J. (1983). Psychotherapy with survivors of the Beverly Hills Supper Club fire. *American Journal of Psychotherapy, 37,* 593–610.

Lippmann, S. B., James, W. A., & Frierson, R. L. (1993). AIDS and the family: Implications for counselling. *AIDS Care, 5*(1), 71–78.

Lloyd, G. A. (1992). Contextual and clinical issues in providing services to gay men. In H. Land (Ed.), *AIDS: Complete guide to psychosocial intervention* (pp. 91–106). Milwaukee, WI: Family Service America.

Lovejoy, N. C. (1990). AIDS: Impact on the gay man's homosexual and heterosexual families. *Marriage and Family Review, 14,* 285–317.

Macklin, E. (1988). AIDS: Implications for families. *Family Relations, 37,* 141–149.

Maddison, D., & Walker, W. (1967). Factors affecting the outcome of conjugal bereavement. *British Journal of Psychiatry, 113,* 1057–1067.

Mancoske, R. J., & Lindhorst, T. (1995). The ecological context of HIV/AIDS counseling: Issues for lesbians and gays and their significant others. *Journal of Gay & Lesbian Social Services, 2*(3/4), 25–40.

Marino, T. W. (1996). Grief counseling broadens its definition. *Counseling Today, 38*(11) 11–14.

Martin, J. L. (1987). The impact of AIDS on gay male sexual behavior patterns in New York City. *American Journal of Public Health, 77*(5), 578–581.

Martin, J. L. (1988). Psychological consequences of AIDS-related bereavement among gay men. *Journal of Counseling and Clinical Psychology, 61,* 856–862.

Martin, J. L., & Dean, L. (1993a). Bereavement following death from AIDS: Unique problems, reactions, and special needs. In M. S. Stroebe, W. Stroebe, & R. O. Hansson (Eds.), *Handbook of bereavement: Theory, research, & intervention* (pp. 316–330). New York: Cambridge University Press.

Martin, J. L., & Dean, L. (1993b). Effects of AIDS-related bereavement and HIV-related illness on psychological distress among gay men: A 7-year longitudinal study, 1985-1991. *Journal of Consulting and Clinical Psychology, 61,* 94–103.

Martocchio, B. C. (1982). *Living while dying.* Bowie, MD: Robert J. Brady.

Martocchio, B. C. (1985). Grief and bereavement: Healing through the hurt. *Nursing Clinics of North America, 20*(2), 327–341.

Maslow, A. H. (1968). *Toward a psychology of being* (2nd ed.) New York: Van Nostrand.

Mason, P. J., Olson, R. A., Myers, J. G., Huszti, H. C., & Kenning, M. (1989). AIDS and hemophilia: Implications for interventions with families. *Journal of Pediatric Psychology, 14*(3), 341–355.

May, R. (1981). *Freedom and destiny.* New York: Dell.

May, R. (1983). *The discovery of being: Writings in existential psychology.* New York: W. W. Norton.

McCammon, S. L., & Allison, E. J. (1995). Debriefing and treating emergency workers. In C. R. Figley (Ed.), *Compassion fatigue: Coping with secondary stress disorder in those who treat the traumatized* (pp. 115–130). New York: Brunner/Mazel.

McCann, I. L., & Pearlman, L. A. (1990). A framework for understanding the psychological effects of working with victims. *Journal of Traumatic Stress, 3*(1), 3–4.

Mendola, M. (1980). *The Mendola report: A new look at gay couples.* New York: Crown.

Messiah, A., Mouret-Fourme, E., & the French National Survey on Sexual Behavior Group. (1995). Sociodemographic characteristics and sexual behavior of bisexual men in France: Implications for HIV prevention. *American Journal of Public Health, 85*(11), 1543–1546.

Middleton, W., Raphael, B., Martinek, N., & Misso, V. (1993). Pathological grief reactions. In

M. S. Stroebe, W. Stroebe, & R. O. Hansson (Eds.*), Handbook of bereavement: Theory, research, & intervention.* New York: Cambridge University Press.

Mile-long AIDS Quilt is on display. (1996, October 12). *Seattle Times,* p. A1.

Milgram. (1983). War-related trauma and victimization: Principles of traumatic stress prevention in Israel. In J. P. Wilson & B. Raphael (Eds.), *International handbook of traumatic stress syndrome.* New York: Plenum Press.

Mogenson, G. (1992). *Greeting the angels: An imaginal view of the mourning process.* New York: Baywood.

Morales, J. (1995). Gay Latinos and AIDS: A framework for HIV/AIDS prevention curriculum. *Journal of Gay & Lesbian Social Services, 2,* 89–106.

Munroe, J. F., Shay, J., Fisher, L., Makary, C., Rapperport, K., & Zimering, R. (1995). Preventing compassion fatigue: A team treatment model. In C. R. Figley (Ed.), *Compassion fatigue: Coping with secondary stress disorder in those who treat the traumatized* (pp. 209–231). New York: Brunner/Mazel.

Musaph, H. (1990). Anniversary reactions as a symptom of grief in traumatized persons. *Israel Journal of Psychiatry Related Science, 27,* 175–179.

Neergaard, L. (1995, November 24). AIDS virus infects 1 in 92 young men. *Seattle Times,* pp. A1, A23.

Neergaard, L. (1996, March 5). Too many teens not protected from AIDS, says study. *Seattle Times,* pp. A4.

Neimeyer, R. A. (1988). Death anxiety. In H. Wass, F. Berardo, & R. A. Neimeyer (Eds.), *Dying: Facing the facts* (2nd ed., pp. 97–136). Washington, DC: Hemisphere.

Neimeyer, R. A., & Stewart, A. E. (in press). AIDS-related death anxiety: A review of the literature. In H. E. Gendelman, S. Lipton, L. Epstein, & S. Swindells (Eds.), *Neurological and neuropsychiatric manifestations of HIV-1 infection.* New York: Chapman & Hall.

Neimeyer, R. A., & Van Brunt, D. (1995). Death anxiety. In H. Wass & R. A. Neimeyer (Eds.), *Dying: Facing the facts* (3rd ed., pp. 49–88). Washington, DC: Taylor & Francis.

Neugebauer, R., Rabkin, J. G., Williams, J. B. W., Remien, R. H., Goetz, R., & Gorman, J. M. (1992). Bereavement reactions in homosexual men experiencing multiple losses in the AIDS epidemic. *American Journal of Psychiatry, 149,* 1374–1378.

New data raise world total of HIV infected to 18.5 million. (1995, December 16). *Seattle Times,* p. A18.

Nichols, W. C., & Everett, C A. (1986*). Systemic family therapy: An integrative approach.* New York: Guilford Press.

Niederland, W. G. (1971). Introductory notes on the concept, definition, and range of psychic trauma. In H. Krystal & W. G. Niederland (Eds.), *Psychic traumatization: Aftereffects in individuals & communities* (pp. 1–10). Boston: Little, Brown.

Nietzsche, F. (n.d.). *Thus spake Zarathustra.* New York: Modern Library.

Nord, D. (1996a). Assessing the negative effects of multiple AIDS-related loss on the gay individual and community. *Journal of Gay and Lesbian Social Services, 4*(3), 1–34.

Nord, D. (1996b). The impact of multiple AIDS-related loss on families of origin and families of choice. *American Journal of Family Therapy, 24(2),* 129–144.

Nord, D. (1996c) Issues and implications in the counseling of survivors of multiple AIDS-related loss. *Death Studies, 20*(4), 389–414.

Norris, F. H., & Murrell, S. A. (1988). Prior experience as a moderator of disaster impact on anxiety symptoms in older adults. *American Journal of Community Psychology, 16,* 664–683.

Novello, A. C. (1991). Women and HIV infection. *Journal of the American Medical Association, 265,* 1805.

Ochberg, F. M. (1993). Posttraumatic therapy. In J. P. Wilson & B. Raphael (Eds.), *International handbook of traumatic stress syndrome* (pp. 773–783). New York: Plenum Press.

Oda, S. C. (1992). *In sympathy.* Norwalk, CT: C. R. Gibson.

Odets, W. (1994). AIDS education and harm reduction for gay men: Psychological approaches for the 21st century. *AIDS & Public Policy Journal, 9*(1), 1–16.

Odets, W. (1995). *In the shadow of the epidemic: Being HIV-negative in the age of AIDS.* Durham, NC: Duke University Press.

Oerlemans-Bunn, M. (1988). On being gay, single, and bereaved. *American Journal of Nursing, 88*(4), 472–476.

O'Neil, M. (1989). Grief & bereavement in AIDS and aging. *Generations, 13,* 80–82.

Ortega y Gasset. (1961). *Meditations on Quixote* (E. Rugg, Trans.). New York: W. W. Norton.

Osterweiss, M., Solomon, F., & Green, M. (1984). *Bereavement: Reactions, consequences and care.* Washington, DC: National Academy Press.

The Oxford Universal Dictionary (1933, 3rd ed.). Oxford, England: Clarendon Press.

Parkes, C. M. (1972). *Bereavement: Studies of grief in adult life.* New York: International Universities Press.

Parkes, C. M. (1975). Determinants of outcome following bereavement. *Omega, 6,* 101–115.

Parkes, C. M. (1987). *Bereavement: Studies of grief in adult life* (2nd ed.). Madison, CT: International Universities Press.

Parson, E. R. (1993). Posttraumatic narcissism: Healing traumatic alterations in the self through curvilinear group psychotherapy. In J. P. Wilson & B. Raphael (Eds.), *International handbook of traumatic stress syndrome* (pp. 821–840). New York: Plenum Press.

Pearlman, L. A., & Saakvitne, D. W. (1995). Treating therapists with vicarious traumatization and secondary stress disorders. In C. R. Figley (Ed.), *Compassion fatigue: Coping with secondary stress disorder in those who treat the traumatized* (pp. 150–177). New York: Brunner/Mazel.

Perga, M. A. (1995, November 29). Worldwide celebration couples education with a deep sense of concern for others. *Milwaukee Journal Sentinel,* p. A18.

Peterson, C., Maier, S. F., & Seligman, M. E. P. (1993). *Learned helplessness: A theory for the age of control.* New York: Oxford University Press.

Pohl, M. I. (1995). Chemical dependency and HIV infection. *Journal of Gay & Lesbian Social Services, 2*(1), 15–28.

Ramos, D. (1995, June 5). A second wave. *The New Republic,* 29.

Rando, T. A. (1984). *Grief, dying and death: Clinical interventions for caregivers.* Champaign, IL: Research Press.

Rando, T. A. (1986a). A comprehensive analysis of anticipatory grief: Perspective, processes, promises, and problems. In T. A. Rando (Ed.), *Loss and anticipatory grief* (pp. 3–14). Lexington, MA: Lexington Books.

Rando, T. A. (1986b). Death of the adult child. In T. A. Rando (Ed.), *Parental loss of a child.* Champaign, IL: Research Press.

Rando, T. A. (1993). *Treatment of complicated mourning.* Champaign, IL: Research Press.

Rank, O. (1945). *Will therapy and truth and reality.* New York: Alfred A. Knopf.

Raphael, B. (1983). *The anatomy of bereavement.* New York: Basic Books.

Raphael, B., & Wilson, J. P. (1993). *International handbook of traumatic stress syndrome.* New York: Plenum Press.

Remien, R., Rabkin, J., Williams, J., & Katoff, L. (1992). Coping strategies and health beliefs of AIDS long-term survivors. *Psychology and Health, 6,* 335–345.

Riley, J., & Greene, R. (1993). Influence of education on self-perceived attitudes about HIV/AIDS among human services providers. *Social Work, 38*(4), 396–401.

Roberts, T. L. (1995). African American gay males with HIV/AIDS: Building upon cultural capacities to survive. *Journal of Gay & Lesbian Social Services, 2,* 75–87.

Rosenberg, P. S. (1995, November 24). Scope of the AIDS epidemic in the United States. *Science, 270,* 1372–1375.

Rosin, H. (1995, June 5). The homecoming. *The New Republic,* 21–26.

Samuelson, R. J. (1996, January 8). Great expectations. *Newsweek,* 24–33.

Sartre, J. P. (1947). *The flies.* In *No exit and three other plays.* New York: Vintage.

Schmale, A. H., Jr. (1971). Psychic trauma during bereavement. In H. Krystal & W. G.

Niederland (Eds.), *Psychic traumatization: Aftereffects in individuals & communities* (pp. 147–168). Boston: Little, Brown.

Schochet, R. (1989, August). Psychosocial issues for seronegative gay men in San Francisco. *Focus*, p. 3.

Scurfield, R. M. (1993). Treatment of posttraumatic stress disorder among Vietnam veterans. In J. P. Wilson & B. Raphael (Eds.), *International handbook of traumatic stress syndrome* (pp. 879–888). New York: Plenum Press.

Seligman, M. E. P. (1975). *Helplessness: On depression, development and death*. San Francisco: W. H. Freeman.

Seligman, M. E. P. (1994). *What you can change & what you can't: The complete guide to successful self-improvement*. New York: Alfred A. Knopf.

Shaffer, P. (1988). *Equus*. London: Penguin. (Original published 1973)

Shanfield, S., & Swain, B. (1984). Death of adult children in traffic accidents. *Journal of Nervous and Mental Disease, 172*, 533–538.

Shapiro, E. R. (1995). Grief in family and cultural context: Learning from Latino families. *Cultural Diversity & Mental Health, 1*(2), 159–176.

Shaver, K. G. (1985). *The attributions of blame: Causality, responsibility and blameworthiness*. New York: Springer-Verlag.

Shearer, P., & McKusick, L. (1986). Counseling survivors. In L. McKusick (Ed.), *What to do about AIDS: Physicians and mental health professionals discuss the issues*. Berkeley: University of California Press.

Shilts, R. (1987). *And the band played on: Politics, people, and the AIDS epidemic*. New York: Penguin.

Shore, J. H., Tatum, E. L., & Volmer, W. M. (1986). Psychiatric reactions to disaster: The Mount St. Helens experience. *American Journal of Psychiatry, 143*, 590–595.

Shrader, G. N. (1992). A descriptive study of the effects of continuous multiple AIDS-related losses among gay male survivors. *Dissertation Abstracts International, 53*(10), 5454B. (University Microfilms No.).

Siegal, R. L., & Hoefer, D. D. (1981). Bereavement counseling for gay individuals. *American Journal of Psychotherapy, 35*, 517–525.

Siegel, B. S. (1986). *Hope and a prayer: An interview with Dr. Bernie S. Siegel*. Santa Monica, CA: Hay House.

Sipprelle, R. C. (1992). A vet center experience: Multievent trauma, delayed treatment type. In D. W. Foy (Ed.) *Treating PTSD: Cognitive-behavioral strategies* (pp. 13–37). New York: Guilford Press.

Skolnick, V. (1979). The addictions as pathological mourning: An attempt at restitution of early losses. *American Journal of Psychotherapy, 33*, 281–290.

Sontag, S. (1978). *Illness as metaphor*. New York: Vintage.

Sontag, S. (1989). *AIDS and its metaphors*. New York: Farrar, Straus & Giroux.

Sprang, G., & McNeil, J. (1995). *The many faces of bereavement: The nature and treatment of natural, traumatic, and stigmatized grief*. New York: Bruner/Mazel.

Staudacher, C. (1994). *A time to grieve: Meditations for healing after the death of a loved one*. San Francisco: Harper.

Stein, T. S. (1988). Homosexuality and new family forms: Issues in psychotherapy. *Psychiatric Annals, 18*, 12–20.

Stein, T. S., & Cohen, C. J. (1984). Psychotherapy with gay men and lesbians: An examination of homophobia, coming out, and identity. In E. S. Hetrick & T. S. Stein (Eds.), *Innovations in psychotherapy with homosexuals* (pp. 60–73). Washington, DC: American Psychiatric Press.

Steinhart, B. (1990). *Living with HIV: For adolescents with hemophilia*. New York: The National Hemophilia Foundation.

Stowe, A., Ross, W., Wodak, A., Thomas, G. V., & Larson, S. A. (1993). Significant relationships and social supports of injecting drug users and their implications for HIV/AIDS services. *AIDS Care, 5*(1), 23–33.

Stroebe, W., & Stroebe, M. S. (1983). *Bereavement and health: The psychological and physical consequences of partner loss.* Cambridge, England: Cambridge University Press.

Stulberg, I., & Smith, M. (1988). Psychosocial impact of the AIDS epidemic on the lives of gay men. *Social Work, 33,* 277–281.

Stylianos, S. K., & Vachon, M. L. S. (1993). The role of social support in bereavement. In M. S. Stroebe, W. Stroebe, & R. O. Hansson (Eds.). *Handbook of bereavement: Theory, research, & intervention* (pp. 397–410). New York: Cambridge University Press.

Sullivan, A. (1990, December 17). Gay life, gay death. *New Republic,* 19–25

Switzer, D. K. (1970). *The dynamics of grief.* New York: Abingdon Press.

Tartaglia, C. R. (1989). AIDS anxiety syndromes. In Dilley, C. Pies, & M. Helquist (Eds.), *Face to face: A guide to AIDS counseling.* San Francisco: AIDS Health Project.

Tillich, P. (1980). *The courage to be.* New Haven: Yale University Press. (Original published 1952)

Titchener, J. L., & Kapp, F. T. (1976). Family and character change at Buffalo Creek. *American Journal of Psychiatry, 133,* 295–299.

Tourse, D., & Gunderson, L. (1988). Adopting and fostering children with AIDS: Policies in progress. *Children Today, 17*(3), 17–23.

Troiden, R. R. (1979). Becoming homosexual: A model of gay identity acquisition. *Psychiatry, 42*(4), 362–373.

Troiden, R. R. (1989). The formation of homosexual identities. *Journal of Homosexuality, 17*(1–2), 43–73.

Troiden, R. R., & Goode, E. (1980). Variables related to the acquisition of a gay identity. *Journal of Homosexuality, 5*(4), 383–392.

de Unamuno, M. (1954). *Tragic sense of life* (J. E. Crawford Flitch, Trans.). New York: Dover. (Original published 1921)

Uroda, S. F. (1977, April). Counseling the bereaved. *Counseling and Values,* 185–191.

Vachon, M. (1976). Grief and bereavement following the death of a spouse. *Canadian Psychiatric Association Journal, 21,* 35–44.

Vachon, M. L. S., Sheldon, A. R., Lancee, W. J., Lyall, W. A. L., Roger, J., & Freeman, S. J. J. (1982). Correlated of enduring distress patterns following bereavement: social network, life situation and personality. *Psychological Medicine, 12,* 783–788.

van der Hart, O. (1983). *Rituals in psychotherapy: Transition and continuity.* New York: Irvington.

van der Kolk, B. A. (1989). In B. A. van der Kolk (Ed.), *Psychological trauma* (pp. 1–30). Washington, DC: American Psychiatric Press.

Van Gorder, D. (1994). We know how, but do we care if we stay HIV negative? *AIDS & Public Policy Journal,* 1–12.

Viney, L. L., Henry, R. M., Walker, B. M., & Crooks, L. (1992). The psychosocial impact of multiple deaths from AIDS. *Omega, 24,* 151–163.

Volkan, V. D. (1975). "Re-grief" therapy. In B. Schoenberg, I. Gerber, A. Wiener, A. H. Kutscher, D. Peretz, & A. C. Carr (Eds.), *Bereavement: Its psychosocial aspects* (pp. 334–350). New York: Columbia University Press.

Webster's new world dictionary of the American language. (1980). New York: Simon & Schuster.

Weinback, R. W. (1989). Sudden death and secret survivors: Helping those who grieve alone. *Social Work,* 57–60.

Weinberg, G. (1972). *Society and the healthy homosexual.* New York: St. Martin's Press.

Weston, K. (1991). *Families we choose: Lesbians, gays, kinship.* New York: Columbia University Press.

Whitney, C. K. (1989). The impact of HIV infection on the hemophilia community. *Mental Retardation, 27,* 227–228.

Williams, C. C. (1983). The mental foxhole: The Vietnam veteran's search for meaning. In R. H. Moos (Ed.), *Coping with life crises: An integrated approach.* New York: Plenum.

Wlodkowsky, S., & Rene, N. (1990). *Longtime companion.* Samuel Goldwyn Company.

Worden, J. W. (1991). *Grief counseling & grief therapy: A handbook for the mental health practitioner* (2nd ed.). New York: Springer.

Yalom, I. D. (1980). *Existential psychotherapy.* New York: Basic Books.

Yalom, I. D. (1985). *The theory and practice of group psychotherapy* (3rd ed.). New York: Basic Books.

Yassen, J. (1995). Preventing secondary stress traumatic stress disorder. In C. R. Figley (Ed.), *Compassion fatigue: Coping with secondary stress disorder in those who treat the traumatized* (pp. 178–208). New York: Brunner/Mazel.

Ziegler, P. (1969). *The black death.* New York: Harper Torchbooks.

Zisook, S., & DeVaul, R. (1983). Grief, unresolved grief, and depression. *Psychosomatics, 24*(3), 247–256.

Zisook, S., DeVaul, R., & Click, M. (1982). Measuring symptoms of grief and bereavement. *American Journal of Psychiatry, 139,* 1590–1593.

A Visualization of Multiple Loss

Guided imagery is a powerful tool for better understanding the experience of loss. Shanti, an organization that provides emotional support for the HIV/AIDS community, uses a death visualization as an integral part of their training. Trainees are taken through the experience of a person with AIDS from diagnosis through death. Volunteers consistently appreciate the effectiveness of this exercise for taking them to a new, deeper level of appreciation for the experiences of their clients. This exercise is built on that model, and some ideas are borrowed from it.

This particular exercise is primarily designed for persons who are not survivors of multiple AIDS-related loss. Presumably, survivors are already familiar with the experience. This visualization focuses attention on the affective experience of survivors and sensitizes the reader to the feelings of survivors. It focuses on the specific experience of a gay man because a specific experience is more powerful than a general one, and gay men have been the hardest hit by multiple AIDS-related loss.

This exercise is best done with at least one other person. It often provokes strong emotions, so it helps to have some time after the visualization to be supported, by another person, in your feelings. One person might read the visualization while the other, or others, participate. It is appropriate to conduct this visualization in a group setting. One could record this guided visualization and listen to it. Usually, participants find it most comfortable to lay down in a darkened room. Soft instrumental music can be played as a background. The person reading the visualization needs to be aware of its pacing. Space between sections is meant to suggest that you pause.

Participants in the visualization are encouraged to make themselves as comfortable as possible so that physical distractions do not interfere. Many find it helpful to lay down with a pillow. Some remove glasses or contact lenses, loosen shoes or clothing, or use a blanket.

It is a good idea to have facial tissues available.

MULTIPLE-LOSS VISUALIZATION

Make yourself comfortable. Settle into a space where distractions are minimized. We are going on a journey of the imagination together, a journey in which I will suggest that certain things happen to you. You are invited to have your own ideas, thoughts, and feelings. There is no right way or wrong way to experience this exercise. For some it is a very emotional experience, for others it is not. Whatever way you choose to do it will be perfectly all right. Most people find it helpful to focus on their feelings, perhaps asking from time to time throughout the exercise, "How would I feel if this were happening to me?"

In this exercise, you will be asked to imagine that you are a gay man living through the late 1970s to the early 1990s. You will be asked to contemplate the deaths of several loved ones. Try to make this experience real in your mind and allow yourself to feel the feelings that arise. If you find yourself distracted during the exercise, that is all right. Simply notice the distraction and allow yourself to return to the visualization.

After the exercise, we will have a few minutes of silence. Then you will have the opportunity to share your responses to the visualization.

Now, let us begin our journey together.

As you settle in, close your eyes and become more and more comfortable. Begin to notice your breathing. Breathing in, breathing out, notice the pattern of inhaling and exhaling. Feel your breath move into and out of your lungs. Allow yourself to feel relaxed and comfortable. Sink deeper into yourself.

With each breath, feel the weight of your body sinking down to a place of comfort and safety. Feel your thoughts sinking down deeper into your heart.

Relax. Breathing in. . . . Breathing out. . . . Now, from a calm, relaxed place, imagine the following:

Take yourself back to the late 1970s. You live in the city and have several friends. It is a time when life is improving. Your life is surrounded by upbeat, affirming people who support and cherish you and your sexuality. For the first time, you and your gay friends are feeling accepted and safeguarded.

Your life is connected with the gay community. You have your hair cut by a gay stylist. You arrange vacations with a gay travel agency. You eat meals at gay restaurants. You play softball on a gay team. You go to gay bars. You shop in gay stores.

The nightlife is wild and fun. Sexual taboos have fallen, and newfound freedom abounds.

Although some discrimination against you and your friends still exists, there is steady social and political progress for gay men and lesbians. Discussion about civil rights often include the needs of homosexuals. A few years before, the American Psychiatric Association removed homosexuality from a list of mental disorders. Many are coming out to family, friends, and employers. Friends are telling their parents and trusted coworkers that they are gay. Celebrities make news with open disclosure of their sexual orientation. Recently, you talked to your family. They are not supportive, but they also are not hostile. Never before have you felt so free, so able to be yourself and express yourself. It is a time of freedom, a time of celebration, a time of possibilities.

Maybe you are happiest about Victor, a wonderful man whom you have been seeing for some time. He's handsome, intelligent, caring, and fun. Finally, you have met "Mr. Right."

How do you feel as you reflect on the affirmative trends in your life?

It is now a Sunday morning, in the summer of 1981. You are together for brunch with your partner Victor, and your very closest friends: Tom, David, Jose, and Paul. After a delicious brunch, you and your friends settle in to read the Sunday paper and talk.

Victor has the front section and asks the group, "Has anyone seen this? Something about a gay cancer that's showing up in New York and Los Angeles."

At first, only you and Paul pay attention, but soon everyone turns their attention to Victor as he reads.

A mysterious form of cancer has been observed in gay men in New York, Los Angeles, and San Francisco. It is not clear whether or not this condition is contagious. The cause is unknown but may be linked to sexual behavior or the use of amyl nitrate.

Tom and you ask Victor to read it again. He does.

A mysterious form of cancer has been observed in gay men in New York, Los Angeles, and San Francisco. It is not clear whether or not this condition is contagious. The cause is unknown but may be linked to sexual behavior or the use of amyl nitrate.

David says that "it's all BS, just another way for the uptight right wing to keep us from having sex." Then the topic is dropped and friendly small talk continues, but you feel a dread impossible to understand.

What do you experience as you hear the newspaper article read?

In the coming months of 1981 and 1982, you hear occasional stories about gay cancer, Kaposi's sarcoma; a rare type of pneumonia, Pneumocystis carinii pneumonia. They kill gay men. Soon, it is called GRID, gay-related immune disorder. Although Victor, who reads a lot, is concerned, most of your friends never mention it. How do you feel as you hear about this strange, new disease?

One day, in the spring of 1982, you and Victor are casually shopping for your apartment together. It is a sunny, warm day with a gentle breeze. You both notice a man walking toward you. He is gaunt and leans on a cane as he slowly moves along. As you approach you notice dark blotches on his face. After a moment you realize that you are staring at him. You turn away.

Victor is quiet and so are you. Later that day, you call a friend to talk about what you saw. Your friend has seen someone like that too. He assures you that it was probably the same guy.

Does the conversation leave you feeling assured?

At Christmas 1982, your closest friends, Victor, and you gather for what is becoming an annual tradition. Even the dinner menu and cooks are the same. Jose brings candied yams; Paul, the salad; David, a couple of pies; and Tom, the stuffing; and you and Victor cook the turkey. Each year some angry and painful moments are spent talking about families. Jose and Paul were rejected by their parents as teenagers and forced to live on the street. David is prohibited by his brother from seeing his nephews and nieces. Victor hasn't told his parents that he is gay although they live nearby. Tom and you moved here from small towns.

None of your families are close. Your parents make it clear that they don't want to hear about your life, so any conversations center on the weather or work. For all of you, your biological families are not nearly as important this circle of friends, your family of choice.

On New Year's day you get a frantic phone call from Tom. Jose is in the hospital. David had found him very sick, laying alone in his apartment. Tom had gone to Jose's place after several calls went, uncharacteristically, unanswered.

At the hospital, you find some of your friends are already in the waiting room. No one has any answers. There are a lot of questions.

When you finally get to see Jose, he is hooked up to a ventilator and has an IV tube in his arm. When he tries to talk, a long cough wracks his body. He perspires heavily.

You don't know what to say. Nothing seems appropriate. When you ask Jose why he didn't call you, he says that he was afraid of what people would say and do. He was sure that he would lose his apartment and probably all his friends.

Every day after work, and sometime on lunch hours, you visit Jose. Nothing ever gets better. One day you arrive and a nurse recognizes you and tells you that Jose quit breathing that morning. He is dead.

You have no idea, at the time, that he is the first.

You offer to call Jose's parents. When his father answers the phone, you tell him that you have some very bad news about his son, that he has died of AIDS. All his father will say is that "it's for the best," and he hangs up the phone.

You and your friends are left to arrange a memorial service, something none of you has ever done before. The first funeral home that is called refuses to handle the body or service. He is cremated, and you are left to deal with the ashes. Neither you or any of his friends has ever touched human ashes before. You comment on how heavy they are and what a pretty tinkling noise they make as they are cast on the water.

That night, you and Victor hold each other for a long time trying to get to sleep.

You will not make love together again for a long, long time.

What are you thinking? How do you feel?

In mid-1983, the community around you is in confusion. You regularly see young men who look old. Almost everywhere, conversations center on new diseases, possible treatments, and who is sick.

Still, no one is certain how it is spread. Some speculate that poppers are the cause and quit using them. Others are fairly sure it's sexually transmitted and try to quit having sex. A few want to close all the bathhouses, and others vehemently condemn this approach as homophobic and antisex.

You notice that Victor is searching his body. When you ask why, he tells you that he is looking for rashes, bumps, and spots. Soon you are both checking your necks for swollen lymph nodes. You are both afraid, very afraid.

For whom are you more afraid: Victor or yourself?

A few months pass, and it is December. With Jose gone, Christmas in 1983 is especially hard. Victor and you gather together with your friends, but no one is in the spirit of the holidays. Dinner conversation is full or rumors and fears. None of you say it, but you are all wondering the same thing: Who will be next?

A swirl of rumors, dashed hopes, and fears permeate your life. Some religious conservatives proclaim that AIDS is God's punishment for deviant homosexuals. Some people talk seriously about moving homosexuals into relocation camps.

Do you ever wonder if perhaps they are right?

It is no longer uncommon to see someone with AIDS. They're easily recognizable, with faces like skulls, sunken cheeks, and deep-set eyes. At the grocery store in late February 1984, you see a man with dark purple blotches over his face. He looks horrible and vaguely familiar. He catches your eye as you look away.

How do you feel as you look away?

Your good friend Paul calls you in a panic one evening. He is sure that he has Kaposi's sarcoma. You rush over to his place and try to comfort him, but you don't know what to say. He sobs and shakes, sure that he is dying. The worst part is that you're afraid to touch him. The next morning, his doctor tells him it's only a pimple.

From then on, any cough, fever, swollen gland, bruise, sweating, sore, headache, or diarrhea elicits panic. There is no way to know who has it and who doesn't, but you are sure that you probably do.

Several months later, a test is announced that will tell you whether or not you are infected. You spend a lot of time talking with friends about whether or not to get tested for HTLV-III. You all know that testing positive could mean losing your job, being denied insurance, and rejection by some friends. Hardly anyone you know is willing to get tested.

Would you get tested?

Some months later, you and Victor go together for the test. You both think it will be better to know for sure, rather than continuing to live with all the uncertainty and fear. At the test site, elaborate measures are taken to safeguard your confidentiality because of the consequences of testing positive: losing health insurance, denial of any life or disability insurance, loss of employment, and public stigma. You both are taken to separate rooms, where your blood is drawn. You are told to return next week for the results.

What do you decide to do if you test HIV positive?

The week passes torturously slow. It is hard to focus on your job. You go back and forth between believing you will test positive and believing you will test negative. During the week, you hear about a former lover who is sick.

The week drags by for you and Victor. One benefit of this crisis is that you two talk about things you never talked about before. Some of the questions are scary. What are our options? Who will we tell? Would we kill ourselves? Would we drive to Mexico for experimental medicine? Will you still love me? There are lots of questions, few answers.

Would you tell your parents?

The week finally passes. Victor and you meet in the waiting room to get your test results. You are called back first. The kindly nurse sitting across from you asks if you are sure that you want the results. For a moment you consider saying no, but you say yes.

The nurse says, "Your test came back negative."

You breath again but feel shocked and numb. After thanking the nurse over and over, you go out to the waiting room. Victor is not there yet. You are so relieved. A huge burden has been lifted.

You wonder what is happening with Victor but are sure that he will be OK too. After all, you think to yourself, "I was a lot more promiscuous than he ever was."

As soon as you see Victor, you know his test result. You think to yourself, "No, please God, don't let it be. Make it me, not him." Looking in his eyes, you know that he knows that you know, so he says nothing. In the car, you sit together for a long time without starting the engine.

When you finally speak, you tell Victor that you love him and will always be there for him. He can only mutter, "I am a dead man. I am a dead man. I am a dead man."

Do you touch him? (Pause)

What do you say?

How does it feel knowing that the man you love is going to die of AIDS?

In mid-1985, obituaries in the gay paper, which had been occasional, become weekly. You and your friends turn first to the obit page to see who died in the past week. Guys you used to see disappear; no one says what happened to them, but everyone assumes the same thing. A growing number of acquaintances and casual friends are dying.

In late 1985, Rock Hudson dies, and suddenly AIDS is a big issue in the media. Occasionally, over coming months, celebrities garner attention for AIDS. When Magic Johnson is later diagnosed with HIV, you are angry that his HIV status is more important than the thousands who preceded him.

Are you angry?

Friends just outside your closest circle of friends die. Sometimes, you think about calling somebody but remember they died. You begin crossing names out of your address book. Visits to the hospital become routine. You decide which memorial services to attend, which ones to skip.

How do you decide?

In the spring of 1986, your good friend David calls you from a phone booth. He is crying and confused. He is somewhere that he doesn't remember going. You do your best to calm him but really have no idea what to say. David has been forgetting a lot lately. Sometimes he leaves the stove on or cigarettes burning. He is admitted for neurological tests and told that he has dementia. He should no longer live alone.

Also that spring, your friend Paul tests positive for HIV. He is terrified and makes you promise not to tell anyone.

What is going to happen next?

Tom still refuses to be tested. He tells you and other friends that he would end it all if he tested positive. He says he would never go through what he has seen others go through, and you understand what he means. You hardly flinch and never even consider trying to change his mind.

The day before Thanksgiving 1986 you get a phone call from Paul, who is frantic. He says that Tom jumped off the bridge. He killed himself. He never told anyone he was being tested. His suicide note says, "I love my friends too much to put them through what we all know will come. I love you. Good-bye."

Do you blame him for killing himself? Are you angry with him?

Every time the phone rings, you begin to fear more bad news, so you answer it less and less. You quit going out with friends after work. Nothing matters anymore except your lover's and friends' health. You feel totally shut down and dead inside. It's too much for anyone to handle, but you keep trying.

Conversations center on T-cells and opportunistic infections. A new vocabulary develops: MAI, PCP, KS, CMV, CD4, AZT, HIV, ARC, and AIDS.

Everyone focuses on those who are sick or those testing positive. There doesn't seem to be anyone to talk with, especially about what it is like to test HIV negative. Most everyone you know test positive. Your concerns seem less important, and you feel very alone.

You call your mother one night. You try to tell her what you are going through, but she doesn't get it. Her advice for you is to stay away from those people so you won't keep getting hurt. "Come back home," she tells you, "we don't have AIDS here."

How does she make you feel?

Later that year, Paul and you are walking together, although it is very difficult for him to walk. His feet hurt and his legs are weak. Paul is shuffling next to you with his cane in one hand and your arm in another. You remember holding your grandpa like this.

How does it feel to see your friend so helpless and vulnerable?

In the fall of 1987, Victor develops intense night sweats. Each morning, the sheets and blankets on your bed are heavy and damp. Sometimes it is so bad that you have to get up, in the middle of the night, to change the sheets. He is both embarrassed and scared. Some nights, after he's asleep, you sneak down to the couch to sleep.

Victor grows increasingly irritable. He is constantly critical of you and everyone else. After a hard day of work you return home to a lover who is unloving. You keep reminding yourself why he is so angry, but sometimes his cynicism and rage are too much to bear. You two fight even though you know you are wasting your last days together.

Are you satisfied with life?

Christmas 1987 brings Victor, David, Paul, and you together. The absence of Tom and Jose is painful. David tries to help by making the gravy but spills it, burning himself. He lost the vision in one eye this fall and his other eye has developed floaters. He has Kaposi's sarcoma lesions on his torso and face. Something is happening to his esophagus so it hurts to eat. All the dishes are prepared as blandly as possible.

Over dinner, you talk about a new hospice that has opened for persons with AIDS. David is adamant that he will never, ever go there.

What do you think as David says that?

The first week of 1988, David is admitted to the hospice. He is too weak to clean out his apartment, so you and Victor do it for him. David sits on the couch and points out the things he wants to keep and the things he will lose. He sobs. You thought you had already hurt as bad as you would ever hurt. You were wrong. Your heart breaks as you watch your friend make these decisions. The hospice room is small, but David has refused to get rid of many possessions, so boxes are stacked to the ceiling. Victor and you agree to store some of his stuff so there is room to move around the room. No one says what you are all thinking.

Later, when you visit David at the hospice, a part of you dreads going. Whenever you look in a room you see emaciated bodies with morphine drips staring at televisions. Sometimes you encounter people you know. Patients inch down the hall grasping walkers. Family members and friends sit in the hallway and cry.

Do you look at the people who are crying?

You start making a list of everyone you know who has died of AIDS when you realize that you are forgetting some of your friends. It's hard work and you know that you are forgetting some names and faces, but it's important.

A few months later you give up on the list.

One day, driving home from work, you realize that it is only the second day in the past two weeks that you aren't going to the hospital or hospice. You certainly could, but today you choose not to go.

How does your decision make you feel?

Your New Year's resolution in 1988 is to make new friends, hopefully some friends without HIV. You volunteer as a chore worker for people with AIDS. You meet some wonderful, caring people, but you also see a lot more illness and death. Still, it helps to think you are doing something constructive about AIDS.

Paul's health continues to be stable. He is excited about the message of Louise Hay, reads her books, and listens to her tapes that promote self-love and the healing of dis-ease. He has positive messages taped on walls all around his house. "I love myself just the way I am" is his constant refrain. He is convinced that he has given up any need for his dis-ease; it was only a wake-up call to love himself more. You pray that he is right.

How much hope do you really feel?

Even though he has been in the hospice for several months, it takes David a very long time to die. Over and over his death seems imminent, but then he bounces back. He has dementia, lymphoma, and chronic pain and is mostly blind. You have been visiting him almost daily for a long time and you feel resentful but also guilty for feeling that way. He looks like bones covered in skin.

David is on a constant morphine drip for the pain. Sometimes, you are fairly certain that he knows you are there. When you and Victor visit David together, you wonder what Victor is thinking as he watches your friend die. Lately, Victor has developed a lot of skin problems.

When David finally dies, you go to his service. Even though you want to, you cannot cry. For one of your closest friends, you cannot cry.

What is it like to be so numb and cold?

In early 1989, Victor becomes too weak to work. He loses his health insurance. Social Security still hasn't been approved. He spends much of his time in the waiting rooms of government offices looking for assistance. With both of you working, there was enough money to get by. Now, there is not enough, and it hurts horribly to see him go without the medicine he needs.

How does it feel to watch your lover die?

More friends and acquaintances die. Your partner becomes sicker. You don't know how you will survive without him. You ask yourself, "What's the point in living on in this world?" The future seems to hold little more than pain and fear and loneliness. You find yourself thinking that HIV is inevitable. "Maybe I should go out and get it over with."

You have some new friends now and that does help, but new friends are different than old friends. No one really knows your history. There is no one with whom you can reminisce about anything that happened before 1980.

Who will be left in your future?

Thanksgiving day of 1989 is spent next to Victor's bed in the hospital. You hold his hand and try to communicate when he is conscious.

Your employer threatens to fire you because you have missed some work and seem distracted when at work. You tell her what is happening and your boss says, "We all lose friends, but life has to go on."

You are very angry, very bitter.
What can you do?

In early 1990, Paul develops patchy white areas in his mouth and has trouble swallowing. He also develops problems with his vision and begins daily IV treatment to slow the progression of blindness. After his veins collapse in both arms, a permanent main line catheter is installed into his chest.

You realize that once Paul and Victor are gone, there will be nobody left from that circle of friends who sat down to Sunday brunch and read that first news story about AIDS.

For the first time in a long, long time, you cry. As you do, you realize that you are not crying for your lost friends or your dying lover, you are crying for yourself.

Victor's parents, who had ignored him for years, show up at the hospital during his last days. They only let you be with him when someone else is in the room. You never again have any time alone.

Victor struggles to hold on until his 40th birthday on March 10. He does. The next day he dies.

When he dies, his parents demand, and receive, the body. They are next of kin and you don't matter. By the time you get home from the hospital, his brothers have gone into your home and stripped it of anything that might be Victor's. You cannot even find a photo of the two of you. Later, at the memorial service, you are shunned. During the eulogy you are not even mentioned.

You have run up large debts caring for Victor. When you check into his life insurance policy that he said would go to you, it is determined that he never made you the beneficiary. His family has already claimed the insurance money. When you call them to ask about it, they call you a "dirty queer who killed our son" and hang up on you.

What do you say? How do you respond?

Throughout 1991, you are like a zombie. You try to be there for Paul as he gets sicker, but you just can't do it. When he is diagnosed with lymphoma, after a series of invasive tests, you collapse. It's too much to bear.

You start drinking more and isolating yourself. Sometimes you have sex that you know is risky, but who cares? What difference does anything make, now?

Over the next few years, you try to go on. Every Christmas reminds you of Victor and your friends, so you avoid it as best as you can. Almost everyone you have known is dead. You've made some new friends, but they are only that, new friends. Some of them are dying too.

And your future holds no respite. There is still no vaccine or cure. Everyone seems to get AIDS and die.

You wonder what the future holds. Repeatedly, hopes have been raised for a vaccine or cure, but it hardly matters now.

What is the point in living?

Allow yourself some time to gently come back to this room at this time. The visualization is complete, but take some time to readjust. Realize that this has been an exercise. Take the time you need to return to your body, remember the room you are in, notice your breathing. Notice the sounds in the room. Remember that you are not alone. When you are ready, open your eyes.

Index

Recollections, expression of, in counseling, 226

Recovery
  community help in, 208
  for cumulative loss, 219, 220–222
  defined, 205–206
  global loss in, 222–224
  healing rituals in, 237–241
  improvement in, 218–219
  ongoing loss in, 222
  overshadowing death in, 219–220
  pain in, 217
  reinvestment and, 34–36
  social support and, 207–208
  from traumatic loss, 224–228
  traumatic loss in, 224–228

Reinvestment stage, of multiple loss, 34–36

Relationships
  ambivalent, 101
  avoiding, 36
  concentric circles of, 46–48
  conflicted, 220
  deepening of, 260
  distance in, 198
  extramarital, 163
  guilt of homosexual, 124–125
  improved community, 192
  loss of, 46–48
  between lovers, 163
  new, 115
  secrecy of, 96
  self-identity in, 184, 190

Religion, existential issues of, 201–203

Reminiscing, survivors loss of, 48

Responsibility, existential issues of, 196–198

Retinitis, cytomegalovirus, 58

Risk behaviors, continued, 249–251

Rituals
  commemorative, 6, 223–224
  for healing, 237–241
  leave-taking ceremonies, 238–239

Role models, loss of, 138

Roles
  family, 167–168
  loss of, 50
  in stigmatization process, 212

Safety issues, self-identity and, 191–193

Seattle AIDS Support Group (SASG), 10, 66

Secondary traumatic stress disorder (STSD)
  of caregivers, 141–143, 224–225

of counselors, 142, 253–256
diagnosis of, 156–157
of families, 142
of health care professionals, 141–143
post-traumatic stress disorder and, 142

Secrecy, 92, 96

Security, loss of, 48–49

Self-actualized person, 199–200

Self-awareness, 194, 245

Self-destructive behavior
  counseling for, 251
  guilt and, 125–126
  help for, 214–215
  in recovery process, 218

Self-esteem
  of counselors, 255
  denigration of, 122
  depression and, 108
  health and, 141
  loss of, 50
  trauma impact on, 140–141
  volunteering and, 210

Self-help support groups, 226, 233–234

Self-identity
  in community, 192–193
  connected
    to others, 187–188
    to world, 190–192
  developmental disruptions in, 185–187
  in future relationships, 190
  future self in, 185
  individual sense of, 182–184
  personality alterations and, 184–185
  positive, 187
  recapitulation in, 185–187
  reflected in others, 188–189
  sexuality and, 184
  in social system, 189–190
  trauma impact on, 144

Seligman, M., 147, 148, 149

Service organizations, community-based, 35–36

Service workers, AIDS-related (see Volunteers)

Sexual freedom, 25–26, 51

Sexual issues
  guilt and, 124
  in HIV/AIDS etiology, 59
  in nontraditional families, 164
  risk behaviors and, 249–251
  self-identity and, 184